# Maternity nursing

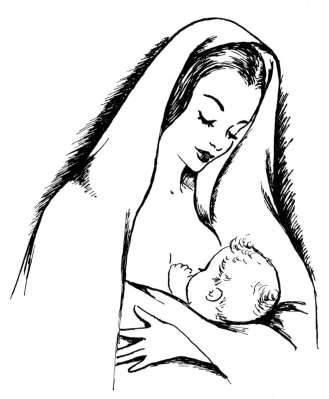

The most important person on earth is a mother. She cannot claim the honor of having built Notre Dame Cathedral. She need not. She has built something more magnificent than any cathedral—a dwelling for an immortal soul, the tiny perfection of her baby's body. . . . The angels have not been blessed with such a grace. They cannot share in God's creative miracle. . . . Only a human mother can. Mothers are closer to . . . the Creator than any other creature. . . . What on God's good earth is more glorious than this: to be a mother.

*Joseph Cardinal Mindszenty*

# Maternity nursing

## CONSTANCE LERCH
**R.N., B.S.(Ed.)**

*Runnemede, New Jersey*

*With 190 illustrations*

*Saint Louis*

## THE C. V. MOSBY COMPANY

*1970*

This book is dedicated to
students interested in the welfare of
mothers-to-be and in mothers
and their infants.

# Preface

The content of this text is planned for concurrent teaching and learning, with the subject matter divided into four units: the preparatory phase and the period of pregnancy, the period of parturition, the postpartum period, and the neonate.

With an intensive period of study, the prenatal units can be completed in one week. With completion of Chapter 10, the student is ready for a most valuable learning experience, that of counseling and teaching in the clinic.

Instructors read and hear much about comprehensive nursing care. They want to expose their students to the entire maternity cycle, but in many instances do just the opposite by restricting them to one area of maternity for a set time. The clinic experience can therefore be of value to both student and mother.

In the clinic, students are brought in contact with mothers whose pregnancies proceed normally and with those in the high-risk group. Students must be able to recognize signs and symptoms and interpret the doctor's instructions intelligently. To function adequately among these women, they need knowledge of both the normal and the abnormal. That is why I have included a chapter on high-risk pregnancy in the first unit. Preparing for co-operative childbirth is included in the first unit for the same reason; the woman prepares for this during her pregnancy, not during labor.

With concurrent teaching, students are prepared to counsel women in the prenatal clinic, give them supportive care during their labor and delivery, and continue with teaching on the postpartum unit. During the experience they are exposed to every aspect of the maternity cycle.

My hope is that this book will make many friends among instructors and their students.

I am indebted to Dr. Paul Ebner, who gave of his time to read Unit II, for his constructive criticism and suggestions, and to Dr. Ralph Warwick, who gave generously of his time to read Unit IV.

I also wish to express my appreciation to Mrs. Lida White for her interest in this textbook and her critical reading of the manuscript and to Mrs. Miriam Ward and Mrs. Helen Fletcher for preparation of the illustrations.

**Constance Lerch**

# To the student

Prior to your orientation to maternity nursing, your clinical experience has been centered chiefly around the sick individual with concern for his return to health. Your experience in maternity nursing should be quite a contrast, for now you will be in contact with healthy women who are beginning a normal physiological process—childbearing. This relationship can be a mutually profitable one in that while you are learning, teaching, and counseling you will establish foundations in preparation for your own experiences as a future parent.

Organize and plan your study time. This is just as important as it is for you to organize your work on the clinical area. If you will take time to copy subject headings from your text into your notebook, and then summarize what the author has to say about the subject and coordinate this with lecture notes, you will find your efforts will help you learn the principles of maternity nursing.

A survey of the selected readings will also prove a rewarding investment. They are specific to the subject you just completed and will enrich your knowledge.

It is your responsibility to learn the vocabulary. All new terms are defined in the glossary; learning these is the first stepping-stone to mastering the subject matter.

# Contents

UNIT IV

# The neonate

## Appendixes

UNIT I

# The preparatory phase and the period of pregnancy

## Part I The preparatory phase

## Part II The period of pregnancy— "the waiting months"

Chapter 1

# Female reproductive anatomy

Some knowledge of the anatomy of the female reproductive system is essential for understanding the physiology of the maternity cycle. The anatomical structure of the mammary glands is also discussed in this chapter as basic to the study of the physiology of lactation.

## External organs of generation

The external organs of generation are situated within the boundaries of the perineum. Collectively they are called the vulva or pudendum. (See Fig. 1-1.)

*Mons pubis, mons veneris, or mount of venus.* The area over the pubic bones is composed of adipose tissue that forms a cushionlike elevation covered by skin and hair, which is referred to as escutcheon.

*Labia majora.* Two thick pads of fat arise from either side of the mons to form the anterior commissure and are called the labia majora. They extend downward on each side of the midline, enfold into the tissues of the vulva, and form the posterior commissure. The inner surfaces are smooth, moist, and supplied with numerous blood vessels and sebaceous glands. The outer surfaces are covered with hair.

*Labia minora (nymphae).* Situated between the labia majora and ordinarily concealed are the labia minora. These two folds of tissue extend downward and merge into the labia majora. Anteriorly, they unite above and below a structure called the clitoris—above to form the prepuce and below to form a band of tissue called the frenulum. They are composed of two folds of thin, pigmented mucous membrane, are

smaller and more delicate than the labia majora, and are rich in sebaceous glands. Posteriorly, they form a transverse fold of skin, the fourchette.

*The clitoris.* The clitoris is located where the labia minora unite anteriorly. In some women the glans of the clitoris may be partially covered by the prepuce. This tiny organ is rich in nerve endings and is extremely vascular, which accounts for its erectility on sexual excitement.

*The hymen.* The fold of thin, vascularized mucous membrane that separates the vagina from the vestibule is the hymen. It varies in thickness, size, and shape and is usually torn during the first coitus. It may completely cover the vaginal orifice and is then known as an imperforate hymen.

*The vestibule.* The area between the anterior portion of the labia minora and the posterior fourchette is called the vestibule. Within the vestibule are the vaginal and urethral orifices and the ducts from Bartholin's and Skene's glands. Skene's ducts open in the posteriorlateral aspects of the urinary meatus. Bartholin's ducts open in the lateral walls of the vestibule.

*Urethral meatus.* Located in the upper part of the vestibule, somewhat posterior to the clitoris, is the urethral meatus. It is

3

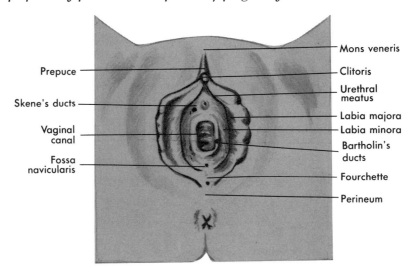

**Fig. 1-1.** Female external genitalia.

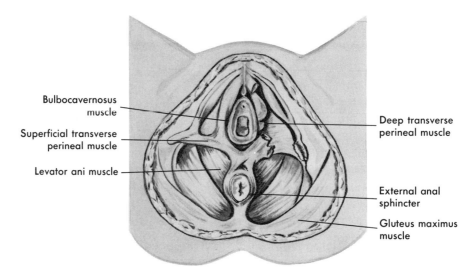

**Fig. 1-2.** Muscles of female perineum.

surrounded by many Skene's glands that are homologues of the male prostate gland. The meatus and urethral tube are often traumatized during the birth process; this is one of the reasons women have difficulty voiding after delivery.

*The fourchette.* The area formed by junction of the labia majora and the labia minora posteriorly is called the fourchette.

*Fossa navicularis.* The shallow depression located between the fourchette and the vaginal orifice is the fossa navicularis.

*The perineum.* The term perineum is used (in obstetrics) when referring to that area between the fourchette and the anus; anatomically, however, it is the area from the pubic arch to the anus. In obstetrics we also make many references to the perineal body, meaning the deep-wedged area where muscles attach, form the pelvic floor, and give support to pelvic structures. The important ones are the levator ani, transverse perinei, and sphincter ani. Study the locations of these muscles shown in Fig.

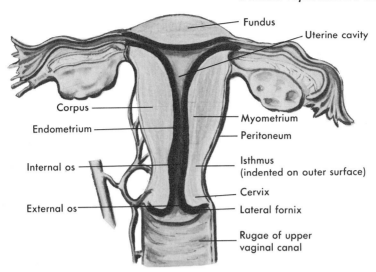

Fundus
Uterine cavity
Corpus
Myometrium
Endometrium
Peritoneum
Internal os
Isthmus (indented on outer surface)
Cervix
External os
Lateral fornix
Rugae of upper vaginal canal

**Fig. 1-3.** Section of uterus showing linings, adjacent tubes, and ovaries.

1-2. The chief source of the blood supply to the perineum is the inferior hemorrhoidal and the pudendal arteries.

### Internal organs of generation

*The vagina.* The fibromuscular tube extending from the vulva to the cervix and situated between the bladder and the rectum is called the vagina. The vagina is supported by cardinal ligaments and the levator ani muscle, extending upward and backward. Posteriorly, the vagina attaches farther up on the cervix of the uterus than it does anteriorly, thus making its anterior wall somewhat shorter than the posterior one. Where the cervix of the uterus converges with the vagina, there is a cufflike arrangement, with fornices to the right and left, anterior and posterior. The posterior fornix is in close apposition to the cul-de-sac of Douglas and separated from the peritoneal cavity by a thin wall.

The vagina is a muscular, partially collapsed, but extremely dilatable organ to facilitate copulation and the birth process. It is lined with stratified squamous epithelium that is arranged in many transverse folds called rugae (Fig. 1-3). This lining undergoes slight changes in its glycogen content under stimulation of ovarian hormones and is lubricated by mucus from the cervical glands. The vaginal fluid is normally acid, with a pH 3.8 to 4.5, due to the lactobacilli that change glycogen to lactic acid. Döderlein's bacilli flourish in these secretions and it is believed that they inhibit growth of some pathogenic bacteria because they have an acid reaction. The circular membrane (hymen) just inside the labia minora occludes the vaginal canal.

*The uterus.* The uterus is a muscular organ situated in the true pelvis between the bladder and the rectum. The uterus varies in size, but in the average adult it is approximately 3 inches in length and 2 inches in width and weighs 2 ounces. It is shaped like an inverted pear and has a narrow central canal with the anterior and posterior walls almost in direct contact. This canal has three outlets; two openings, called cornua, are on each side and near the top of the uterus where the fallopian tubes attach, and the lower opening projects into the vagina. The portion of the uterus above the tubal insertion is called the *fundus;* that portion below the insertion of the tubes is the *corpus* (body), and the lowermost portion is the *cervix.* A pouch, cul-de-sac of Douglas, separates the lower part of the uterus from the rectum. The uterus is a movable organ suspended in the pelvic cavity by ligaments and supported from below by the muscles of the pelvic floor.

The cervix is extremely muscular and is closed except for a fraction of a diameter through which the menstrual flow and cervical secretions pass. The cervix is supported by cardinal and uterosacral ligaments and is rich in mucus-secreting glands (nabothian glands).

The wall of the uterus is composed of three layers of tissue: *outer (peritoneum)*—serous membrane that covers most of the uterus, except that portion of the corpus in close contact with the bladder; *middle (myometrium)*—connective tissue and smooth muscle tissue arranged antagonistically to allow for expansion during pregnancy and to aid in the mechanism of the second and third stages of labor, and the *inner (endometrium)*—mucous membrane lining the uterus and containing many glands that protrude from underlying connective tissue. The secretions are alkaline and mucoid. This lining responds to a woman's cyclical changes under stimulation of ovarian hormones.

*Uterine ligaments.* The uterus is suspended in the pelvic cavity by transverse broad ligaments. Below these, thicker and more prominent cardinal ligaments (Mackenrodt's) offer the chief support. The round ligaments extend from the upper, lateral portion near insertion of the tubes through the inguinal canal into the labia majora. The uterosacral ligaments attach the uterus posteriorly to the sacrum.

*Blood supply.* Blood is circulated through the uterus by way of uterine and ovarian arteries and veins. The uterine arteries, branching from the hypogastric, are the major source of blood supply. The ovarian arteries (branching from the aorta) enter the uterus near the tubal insertion. (See Fig. 1-4.)

*The ovaries.* There are two ovaries that lie against the posterior surface of the broad ligaments, in close approximation to the distal end of the tube. They are suspended by folds of peritoneum called mesovarian. They are firm, grayish, oval shaped bodies, 1 to 2 inches in length, ½ to 1 inch wide, and ¼ to ½ inch in thickness (after sexual maturation). They weigh about 5 grams. Their structure consists of an outer layer called the cortex and an inner layer called the medulla. The medulla consists of many blood vessels and cell nests. The cortex is covered with germinal epithelium. The ova are contained within this layer, each housed within primordial follicles and in liquor folliculi, a clear, alkaline albuminoid fluid. During maturation process, the ova migrate to the medulla portion. At puberty the primordial follicles become graafian follicles, so called because they were discovered in 1672 by de Graaf. The

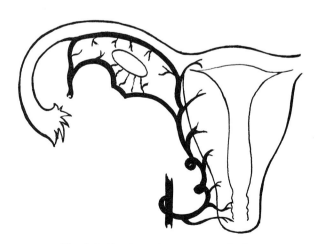

**Fig. 1-4.** Blood supply to uterus and tubes.

two main functions of the ovaries are production of the ova and secretion of the hormones estrogen and progesterone. (See Fig. 1-5.)

*Fallopian tubes (salpinges, oviducts).* These two flexible tubes, 4½ inches long and approximately ¼ inch in diameter, extend laterally from the cornu of the uterus toward the pelvic ridge; the fallopian tubes lie in close approximation to the ovaries, but are not directly attached to them (Fig. 1-5). They are suspended by folds of tissue called the mesosalpinx that continues as the outer serous coat. Anatomically, they are divided as follows: (1) *interstitial segment,* extending into the uterus proper, (2) *isthmus,* extending from the interstitial segment at the cornu of the uterus for about 1 to 1½ inches, (3) *ampulla,* more dilated, extending to the distal end, and (4) *infundibulum,* terminating in fingerlike projections termed fimbriae. The fimbriae open into the peritoneal cavity and enfold the ovary. Aided by peristaltic waves, fimbriae draw the ovum into the tube. Layers of smooth muscle form the middle coat. The lining is of columnar epithelium with secretory cells predominating at the uterine end, and cili-

ated cells distally. Ciliary and peristaltic actions combine to draw the ovum into the tube and propel it through to the uterus. The structure of the inner layer of the tube is the same as that of the uterus. These lining cells like those of the uterus undergo cyclical changes under the influence of ovarian hormones; hence the possibility of ectopic tubal pregnancies.

## Mammary glands

The mammary glands are considered accessory reproductive organs because they undergo many physiological changes during pregnancy and contribute a great deal to the physical and psychological needs of the newborn. They are located anterior to the pectoral muscle, one on each side of the chest wall. Laterally they extend from the sternum to the anterior axillary border. The contour and size vary greatly during different functional states, but in the adult they are dome shaped and weigh 100 to 200 grams. They are composed of adipose, fibrous, and glandular tissues. The gland tissue is arranged in fifteen to twenty lobes that divide into smaller lobules, radiating to the area of the nipple. The area between

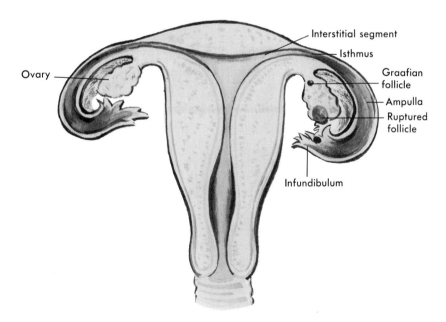

**Fig. 1-5.** Female reproductive organs showing section of uterine tubes and ovaries.

the lobes is composed of fat and connective tissue. Each lobule contains numerous acini and has its own excretory duct (lactiferous duct) (Fig. 1-6). Cooper's ligaments of fibrous tissue give support to the breasts.

In the center of the breast is a circular, pigmented area about 1.5 to 2 cm. called the areola. The pigmentation varies with functional changes from pink to brownish red. In the areola are numerous sebaceous glands, the follicles or tubercles of Montgomery (named after the man who first described them as a constellation of stars). The secretion from these glands lubricates the nipple for the process of nursing. In the center of this areola is a small, pigmented cylindrical body, the mammary papilla, or nipple. This may be flat or may project outward for a few millimeters. It contains fibromuscular tissue that becomes erectile on stimulation and contributes to the infant's ability to grasp the nipple for nursing.

Thoracic branches of the axillary, intercostal, and internal thoracic arteries furnish the main blood supply to the mammary glands. Lymphatic vessels have their origin in the walls of the lactiferous ducts. They drain into the axillary and subclavian nodes. Nerve innervation is from the fourth, fifth, and sixth thoracic nerves and the supraclavicular nerves. See p. 64 for physiology.

## STUDY QUESTIONS
### Matching

Match the terms in the first column with their apropriate definitions in the second column:

(a) Vestibule

(b) Bartholin's glands

(c) Cooper's ligaments

(d) Fundus

(e) Cardinal ligaments

(f) Skene's glands

(g) Tubercles of Montgomery

(h) Nabothian glands

(i) Cul-de-sac of Douglas

(j) Fourchette

(k) Pudendal

__Portion of the uterus above the tubal insertion

__Separates lower portion of the uterus from the rectum

__Area betwen anterior portion of the labia minora and posterior fourchette

__Ducts of these glands open in the lateral aspects of the urethral meatus

__Follicle containing immature ova

__Ducts of these glands open in the lateral walls of the vestibule

__Arranged in transverse folds called rugae

__Area formed by the junction of the labia majora and minora posteriorly

__Ligaments supporting the breasts

__Structure supported by cardinal and uterosacral ligaments

__Ligaments offering chief support to the uterus

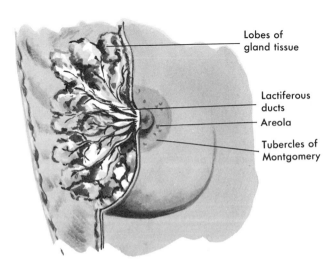

**Fig. 1-6.** Cross section of female breast.

Lobes of gland tissue

Lactiferous ducts

Areola

Tubercles of Montgomery

(1) Cervix          —Sebaceous glands in areola of the breasts
(m) Vaginal canal   —Glands of the cervix
(n) Primordial      —Artery that is chief source of blood to the perineum

## SELECTED READINGS

Boving, Bent G.: Anatomy. In Greenhill, J. P., editor: Obstetrics, ed. 13, Philadelphia, 1965, W. B. Saunders Co., chap. 1.

Eastman, Nicholson J., and Hellman, Louis M., editors: Williams' obstetrics, ed. 13, New York, 1966, Appleton-Century-Crofts, chap. 2.

Jacob, Stanley: Structure and function in man, Philadelphia, 1965, W. B. Saunders Co., chap. 17.

Oxorn, Harry, and Foote, Wm. R.: Human labor and birth, New York, 1964, Appleton-Century-Crofts, chaps. 1 to 3.

**For student's quick notes:**

# Chapter 2

# Preparation for parenthood—biological, physiological, psychological, and educational

Chapter 2 deals with the many facets involved in preparation
for parenthood—biological, physiological, psychological, and educational.
You will learn about the development of germ cells and how cyclical
changes in the ovaries and uterus, governed by hormones, prepare
a woman for the function of reproduction. The importance of
emotional and social maturity in preparation for assuming the
responsibilities of parenthood is then discussed. The chapter concludes
with a discussion of the value of educational programs in preparation
for parenthood and of the nurse's role as an educator.

## Biological preparation
### Gametogenesis

Gametogenesis, or maturation of sex cells, involves two processes of cell division—mitosis and meiosis. *Mitosis* involves division of the nucleus and results in identical nuclei. *Meiosis* involves division of the nucleus and results in the reduction of a chromosome number from the diploid number 46 to the haploid number 23. These sex cells are also referred to as germ cells, or gametes, and the organs that house them are called gonads. In the male the gonads are the testes, and in the female, the ovaries. Gametes remain in a quiescent state until sexual puberty when they become mature and active. Part of the maturation process prepares these cells for fertilization.

Within the nucleus of all body cells are minute particles called genes. They are the units of inheritance and are composed of nucleoproteins. It has been estimated that there may be many thousands in each cell. These genes are arranged within the cell nuclei in a linear order on bodies called chromosomes. In man the number of chromosomes is 46.

### Spermatogenesis

Spermatogenesis refers to development of the male germ cells (gametes) into mature spermatozoa. The *first process* of spermatogenesis is mitosis. The young cells are called *spermatogonia* and develop in the seminiferous tubules. These spermatogonia through growth and development (sexual maturity) become *primary spermatocytes*. Each primary spermatocyte divides, forming two *secondary spermatocytes*. These two secondary spermatocytes divide further into four *spermatids*, with a haploid chromosome number. This is the *second process* of spermatogenesis, *meiosis*, with chromosome reduction of the diploid number 46 to the haploid number 23. The four spermatids develop into four *spermatozoa*. Along with this specialized type of cell division a great many genetic variabilities and recombinations occur, thereby forming patterns of human inheritance.

### Oogenesis

Oogenesis refers to the development of the female germ cells into ova. In the female, before the process of maturation takes place, the germ cell is called the *oogonium*. Thousands of *oogonia* are in the cortex of the ovary at birth, lying in their primordial follicles, each with the diploid number of chromosomes.

The young oogonia develop into *oocytes* (primitive ova). Each oocyte is surrounded by a protective sac, that is, the primordial follicle that will eventually form a graafian follicle, the functional element of the ovary. Cells of the graafian follicle secrete liquor folliculi in which the oocyte floats, and they are also the source of estrogen and progesterone secretion. Some of the oocytes will continue to develop into *primary oocytes* and will undergo the first meiotic division; others will not.

When the ovum is liberated from the ovary, it has already undergone the first meiotic division. By meiotic division of the primary oocyte a functional *secondary oocyte* develops and, as in the spermatocyte, the chromosomes are reduced from the diploid to the haploid number in preparation for ovulation and fertilization. The secondary oocytes divide by *meiosis* to produce a large *ootid*, which develops into the *ovum*, and three small oocytes called *polar bodies*, which usually degenerate. This second maturation division is probably not completed until after sperm penetration.

The *phase of meiosis* is, of course, the reduction of the 46 chromosomes in each cell to 23 chromosomes in each mature ovum. When the sperm penetrates the ovum, the haploid number of chromosomes unite and the zygote starts with 46 chromosomes. The mature ovum is relatively large in comparison with the sperm, yet it is not visible to the naked eye.

## Physiological preparation
### Endocrine control of the reproductive cycle

Woman's endocrine system plays a most dramatic part in her physiology. The endocrine glands contributing toward her reproductive physiology are the pituitary, ovaries, thyroid, and adrenals. We know that our hormones are the regulators of cell activity. The hormones of the pituitary gland are called *tropins*. The tropins that stimulate these glands are called *gonadotropins*.

### Physiology of the ovarian cycle

The ovaries have three important functions: (1) they secrete the hormones responsible for the cyclic changes in the endometrium; (2) they produce the secondary oocytes; and (3) they release the oocytes. This physiology is under the rhythmic endocrine control of the adenohypophysis. This gland produces three gonadostimulating hormones: follicle-stimulating hormone (FSH), luteinizing hormone (LH), and luteotropic hormone (LTH), thought to be identical with prolactin. The action of prolactin was first thought to be limited to the breasts; hence its name. "It is now established, however, that it initiates and maintains the secretory activity of the corpus luteum, hence its new name, luteotropin."[*]

The marvelous, intricate mechanism by which these three gonadotropins govern the ovarian physiology is like the rhythm of a symphony, each contributing to the ebb and flow of the cycle. The follicle-stimulating hormone is responsible for the development and activity of the ovarian follicle and for bringing it to maturation. The luteinizing hormone stimulates ovulation and the beginning of corpus luteum formation. The luteotropic hormone stimulates luteal cells to produce progesterone; therefore, it maintains the corpus luteum, and initiates and sustains lactation.

Let us study this cycle beginning the day

---

[*]From Keele, Cyril A., and Neil, Eric, editors: Samson Wright's applied physiology, ed. 11, New York, 1965, Oxford University Press, Inc., p. 496.

following cessation of a regular period of the menses.

*Follicular phase.* (The estrogens of this phase produce the proliferative phase in the endometrium.) The secretory cells in the follicle multiply rapidly and form estrogen. The granulosa cells within the follicle thicken; the follicle becomes distended by liquor folliculi enriched with this estrogen, and in this medium the oocyte floats. It is during these 2 weeks that maturation of the oocyte is taking place (first meiotic division, p. 12) so that by the time the follicle ruptures, the ovum will be capable of being fertilized by the sperm (second meiotic division).

*Ovulatory phase.* Just what brings about the ovulatory phase? Pressure accumulates within the follicle, of course, but the consensus is that for ovulation to occur there must be a balanced activity of both the follicle-stimulating hormone and the luteinizing hormone. The estrogen level at this time (ovulation) is at its peak, which increases motility of the tubes and facilitates transportation of the sperm.

*Luteal phase.* The luteal phase after ovulation brings about the secretory phase of the endometrial cycle. Pigment cells (lutein cells) multiply in number within the follicle and form a solid mass that represents a mature corpus luteum. It is believed that this is brought about by the gonadotropic hormone LTH, which also stimulates production of progesterone.

One of two things will happen:

*If conception takes place,* secretion of corpus luteum and progesterone continues to be maintained by chorionic gonadotropin. The corpus luteum is now referred to as the "corpus luteum of pregnancy."

*If conception does not take place,* the corpus luteum reaches its maturity in about 10 to 12 days, and then regression takes place. The corpus luteum cells degenerate and leave a scar of fibrous tissue that is called corpus albicans. The estrogen and progesterone levels drop. This decrease prompts the three gonadotropic hormones to initiate the cycle once more. Active fol-

licles that do not develop completely undergo regression and are called atretic follicles.

Most women are not aware of their moment of ovulation. Some have spotting or cramplike pains in either right or left lower quadrant, depending from which ovary the graafian follicle ruptured. The spotting is attributed to the slight drop in estrogen about this time. This particular time of the cycle is referred to as mittelschmerz period, or midcycle bleeding. Ovulation does not necessarily occur with every monthly cycle, that is, there may be anovulatory menstruation.

### Physiology of the endometrial cycle

Significant forces of nature are constantly at work during the female monthly cycle. Nature, by performing a most elaborate, complex, and marvelous process, prepares the uterus each month for reception of a fertilized ovum. It is the increase and decrease in estrogen and progesterone levels of the ovulatory cycle that produce these endometrial changes, but the ultimate control stems from the hypothalamus (Fig. 2-1), the regulator of the pituitary gland. Let us study this cycle as we did the ovarian.

*Proliferative phase.* The day after the cessation of a regular period of menses the proliferative phase of the cycle begins. Under the influence of estrogen, the endometrium undergoes a change in which there is marked growth in its glands and stroma and an increased water content. This continues for about 10 days to 2 weeks.

*Secretory or progestational phase.* The secretory or progestational phase then follows and lasts about 12 days. During this time the ovum leaves the graafian follicle and the sac itself becomes a corpus luteum, which now secretes progesterone. This hormone stimulates the glands of the endometrium to secrete mucin and glycogen (uterine milk) as nourishment for the ovum. The endometrium becomes softer so that if the ovum is fertilized, it may burrow its way into this lining and receive nourishment. These changes also favor survival of the

Fig. 2-1

**HYPOTHALAMUS**
**PITUITARY** ←
**ADENOHYPOPHYSIS**
**GONADOTROPIN**

### Follicle-stimulating hormone (FSH)

Stimulates development of graafian follicle and secretion of estrogen.

### Luteinizing hormone (LH or ICSH)

Stimulates theca cells to produce estrogen. Initiates ovulation; causes FSH level to decrease with formation of corpus luteum.

### Luteotropic or lactogenic hormone (LTH)

Stimulates luteal cells to produce progesterone. Maintains corpus luteum, which reaches maturity in about 10 days. Permits corpus leteum to involute. Stimulates secretory activity of mammary glands to produce milk. Estrogen and progesterone prepare cells for milk synthesis.

**OVULATORY CYCLE**

### Follicular phase
**Days 1 to 12**
Estrogen secreted is responsible for uterine changes.

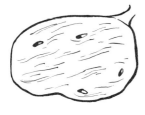

### Ovulatory phase
**Day 13 or 14**
Ovulation

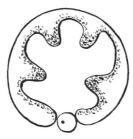

### Corpus luteum phase or postovulatory phase
**Days 14 to 24**

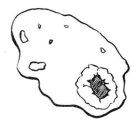

**ENDOMETRIAL CYCLE**

### Proliferative phase

Brought about mainly by estrogen from follicular phase of ovary. Endometrium thickens; water content increases along with enzymes and proteins.

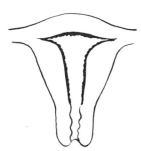

### Proliferative phase

Phase continues with no appreciable change.

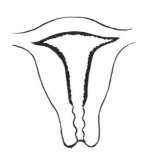

### Secretory phase

Both estrogen and progesterone contribute to further increase thickness of endometrium, with deposits of glycogen and mucin.

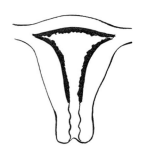

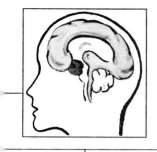

**No conception**

**Conception**
Chorionic gonadotropin stimulates corpus luteum to continue secretion of estrogen and progesterone.

trogen and progesterone levels op. Corpus luteum regresses to rpus albicans.
Days 25 to 28

Secretion of corpus luteum continues, as does estrogen and progesterone. These hormones keep myometrium in quiescent state.

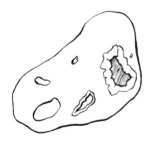 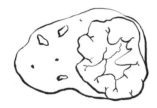

**Menstrual phase**
quamation of endometrial lining.

**Pregnant phase**
Chorionic gonadotropin secreted by cellular layer of chorion. Development of decidua and placenta. Placenta a source of estrogen, progesterone, and chorionic gonadotropin.

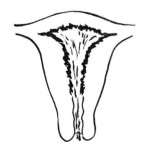 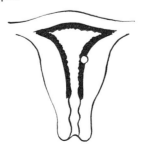

15

sperm and inhibit motility of the myometrium.

As in the ovarian cycle one of two things will occur:

*If the ovum is fertilized,* another gonadotropic hormone aids the corpus luteum—chorionic gonadotropin. It is secreted by the cellular layers of the chorion and has both luteinizing and leutotropic properties, that is, it stimulates the corpus luteum to secrete estrogen as well as progesterone. These are both essential for the maintenance of pregnancy.

*If the ovum is not fertilized,* it will be propelled down the tube and into the uterus by ciliary and peristaltic action. After about 12 days, the corpus luteum begins to regress and the progesterone decreases. Without these two hormones, the estrogen level will also decrease and the endometrium will then be in the *ischemic* stage of the cycle. The blood vessels in the endometrium are constricted, and these vascular constrictions precede the bursting of blood vessels and desquamation of the endometrial lining.

When conception fails to occur, nature then clears away the preparation; tissue is destroyed that would have been vitally important for growth and development of a new life, but worthless when conception fails to take place. The actual flow of blood is nature's lamentation because her handiwork was all in vain, but she despairs not and proceeds to rebuild again, each month, for approximately 30 years of a woman's life. In this light, then, the actual "flow" is the end result of the cyclic changes of the previous 25 days. Each woman's cycle has its own rhythm that varies in amount and length of flow. It is considered normal for the cycle to vary from 25 to 35 days.

A proteolytic enzyme formed by the endometrial glands prevents menstrual blood from normally clotting. The flow is not all blood but consists of bits of tissue and secretions from glands of the endometrium and cervix. This cycle involves not just uterine and ovarian physiology, but the "whole" woman.

## Psychological preparation
### Emotional and social

Psychologically, preparation for parenthood is an integrated process of the events from early childhood, puberty, adolescence, and marriage.

This preparation starts in the home of every little boy and girl. Their ideas and ideals of parenthood will be patterned by their home environment. The little boy is likely to pattern his thoughts concerning fatherhood from what he observes. If he can look up to his father with admiration, as a leader and master of the home, then basically the roots for psychological preparedness are being laid. If he sees strength and beauty in his mother, he looks for this in his chosen mate and is likely to have respect for women and motherhood. We need only watch the little girl at play and observe how she "mothers" her dolls and "keeps her house," and watch the little boy as he "directs her play" and observe the manner in which he commands her, and we will know something about the cultural and enviromental factors influencing the family.

If the young girl admires her mother and is prepared for the physical and psychological changes of adolescence, she will probably enjoy being a woman and look forward to marriage and parenthood. The quality and standards, then, of their parental guidance lay the foundation for psychological preparation. This should be reinforced in the school curriculum and continued in classes in preparation for marriage and parenthood.

One is physically ready for reproduction long before he or she is psychologically prepared to assume the responsibilities of parenthood. A woman is psychologically prepared for parenthood when she has attained emotional, mental, and social maturity. How and when is this attained? It is evident in her attitudes toward herself and those about her. Growth of her inner resources, such as honor, self-respect, respect for others, the ability to give and receive love, decency, loyalty, and compassion, are all nurtured by her home environment. These components become the fruits of her emotional maturity. When she recognizes that she is part of, and a contributor to, the society in which she lives, she has no doubt reached emotional and social maturity.

Psychological preparedness also means being aware of and being able to meet responsibilities. We in America seem to fall short in this aspect. It is evident that we are lax in preparation for marriage, since the divorce rates are so high. Many young couples enter into marriage without allowing time for realistic planning and, therefore, are unprepared for the responsibilities of parenthood.

Psychological preparation, then, involves a mature mind capable of mature reasoning and thinking.

## Educational preparation
*Prenatal classes—*
*the nurse as an educator*

Because of the changing nature of the family, children now leave home sooner and strive for independence at an earlier age. Years ago family ties and traditions were stable, but today this is no longer true. Young couples lean on their ideals and dreams as guides, and consequently they approach marriage and parenthood with little knowledge of what to expect. The realities they are forced to face soon outweigh their dreams.

The institution of marriage is basic to the American way of life: a home and family. However, our society sets no standards and offers very little opportunity to prepare for the important career of marriage and parenthood. True, we do have laws that forbid marriage before a set minimal age and laws regarding certain health standards, that is, serological test for syphilis, but education for marriage and parenthood is in its infancy.

Conducting such courses on marriage and the family is not within the scope of the registered nurse unless she has adequate preparation on higher levels of education, but she does plan and conduct classes in guidance and education for childbirth. Her meager 10- to 12-week experience in the clinical area of a hospital is not enough training. She needs additional education to understand the dynamics of interpersonal relationships and training in the preparation and planning of such classes.

Students should avail themselves of every opportunity to attend prenatal classes conducted by graduate nurses. One enormous problem is to locate the nurses to organize programs for expectant parents. The original objectives and plans may be good, but finding qualified, interested nurses to direct these discussions is difficult. The few nurses who are qualified usually work their 8-hour day and may not be willing to give their time to conduct these voluntary discussions. Most agencies and hospitals are reluctant to offer a paid program in education for childbirth. Fortunate is the organization that has doctors and qualified nurses willing to participate.

The prepared nurse is wise enough to know that the classes must be flexible and that it is sometimes necessary to deviate from her plans. She bases the discussions on what couples indicate they are interested in. She listens carefully so that she can determine what areas to introduce and integrate important facts pertinent to their discussion. She can detect clues to their tensions and fears. She guides them to exchange their knowledge and experiences and corrects misconceptions.

The nurse who directs the sessions usually arranges for an obstetrician, a pediatrician, and a nutritionist to participate. She arranges for the obstetrician to give several lectures on the physiology of labor, for the pediatrician to speak about the newborn infant, and for the nutritionist to discuss the importance of adequate nutrition. Many times these discussions are reinforced with films. It is through the joint effort of professional colleagues that these group discussions have been of tremendous help.

We need rapport between those giving the lectures and those who will care for the woman while she is in labor. The women are instructed in the mechanism of labor, but many times they are left alone, with no nurse to give them the encouragement they need to reinforce what was discussed during the classes. It is true that education for childbirth alleviates anxiety and fear during labor, but not if the patient is left alone in the labor room.

Attendance at these classes is voluntary; those who come are usually the mature couples who realize that they need and want knowledge concerning pregnancy, childbirth, and care of the infant. They come because they are aware that somewhere in their education this important training was neglected. These classes are beneficial to the young couple in numerous ways. They soon learn that discussion of their experiences under leadership means a better understanding of their problems.

Young married couples meet and share ideas with other couples who are in the "expectant phase" and also planning for the new member to join their family. Those awaiting their first child discuss their approaching parenthood and gain advice from the more experienced. The couples who can give each other support during all these phases are laying the foundation for a good parent-child relationship. They have the opportunity to express their negative feelings toward the pregnancy and are often relieved when they understand these feelings are normal.

They establish a good rapport (during pregnancy) with the nurses, and if they do make a visit to the maternity department, they meet hospital personnel with whom they will come in contact during the lying-in period. This strengthens the supportive relationship so desperately needed by the mother, especially upon admission to the labor room.

A "preview booklet" explaining why the admission forms must be signed and giving little hints about the mother's daily schedule may help parents to understand that hospital regulations are in the interest of both the hospital and the patient and may

eliminate the strange, cold atmosphere so many patients describe. Doctors who recognize the importance of these facets of maternity care encourage their patients to attend the classes.

One advance we have made with prenatal care is that women do seek medical advice earlier in their pregnancy. By attending classes, their mental outlook improves along with their physical condition. In these classes they soon learn that their conflicts and doubts are common to others and that sharing their experiences gives them a better perspective. The couples become enthusiastic participants in this greatest of all ventures for a woman.

The mother-to-be, important as she is and usually the center of the discussion, should not be our sole concern. The father is expecting too, and expectancy has its effect on him. Fatherhood means responsibilities; financial demands are bound to be made on him. If he is interested enough to attend with his wife, then he too wants to learn. He will then understand the meaning of "fatherhood" and together they will contemplate the wonder of it all.

If a husband is eager about his role of father, this will certainly be reflected in his wife's attitude, and together they will share in a family anticipation. If he understands something about the physiology of her pregnancy and the psychological impact it has on her, he will show more tolerance and more pride in anticipating fatherhood. He is interested in learning about the physiological changes in her body and is often puzzled and even alarmed concerning the psychological changes; one moment she needs him very much, and the next she rejects him. Her moodiness makes emotional demands on him. During the discussion he has the opportunity to learn that these changes are only temporary; and when listening to the other husbands, he realizes these changes are not as drastic as they seemed to him. He, too, needs educational preparation concerning the mechanism of labor. His concept of labor may have evolved from what he has heard others discussing; his sources of information are usually confusing. Therefore, he has unrealistic fears added to emotional conflicts about how his wife will face the ordeal. What a relief from emotional strain when he understands something about the physiology of labor, and with how much more confidence, readiness, and eagerness they both await the first warning sign that the little one is on its way.

Education does not end with the birth of their baby. A new father needs information concerning the physical and psychological changes that continue during the puerperium so that his deep concern and love will be manifested during the difficult weeks ahead. When the husband understands what his role is during the expectant phase and knows how important his reassurance is during labor and delivery, he will feel more secure in being able to meet her special needs during the puerperium.

The nurse's requisites are many; she needs to display a friendly attitude toward groups and to be tolerant of their varied differences in opinion. She encourages comments; she mixes with the group, introduces them to one another, and helps them feel at ease in expressing themselves. She must be able to recognize problems outside her scope and not ignore them, but arrange for counseling from the adequate sources. She is the one who must create an atmosphere conducive to spontaneous expression.

## STUDY QUESTIONS
### Matching

Match the terms in the first column with their appropriate definitions in the second column:

(a) Gameto-genesis    ___Layer of trophoblastic cells separating maternal from fetal blood flow

(b) Genes    ___Functional element of the ovary

(c) Spermato-genesis    ___Maturation of sex cells

(d) Langhans'    ___Development of gametes into mature sperm

(e) Mittel-schmerz    ___Prevents menstrual blood from normally clotting

(f) Oogenesis    ___Hormone responsible for development and activity of ovarian follicle

(g) Follicle-stimulating hormone    ___Midcycle bleeding

(h) Luteinizing hormone    ___Stimulates ovulation

(i) Graafian follicle    ___Stimulates luteal cells to produce progesterone and initiates and sustains lactation

(j) Luteotropic hormone    ___Development of gametes into ova

(k) Proteolytic enzyme    ___Units of inheritance, composed of nucleoproteins

## SELECTED READINGS
### Biological preparation

Corney, Gerald: Human genetics, Nurs. Times **64:** 1199, Sept. 6, 1968.

Ratcliff, J. D.: New facts about human reproduction, Reader's Digest **89:**119, Dec., 1966.

Tomasz, Alexander: Cellular factors in genetic transformation, Sci. Amer. **220:**38, Jan., 1969.

Valentine, G. H.: The chromosome disorders, Philadelphia, 1966, J. B. Lippincott Co., p. 13.

Williams, P. L., and Smith, C. P.: Basic human embryology, Philadelphia, 1966, J. B. Lippincott Co.

### Physiological preparation

Beck, A. C., and Taylor, E. Stewart: Obstetrical practice, ed. 8, Baltimore, 1966, The Williams & Wilkins Co., chaps. 1 to 3.

Bell, George H., Davidson, J. Norman, and Scarborough, Harold: Textbook of physiology and biochemistry, ed. 6, Baltimore, 1965, The Williams & Wilkins Co., chap. 51.

Brown, J. H., and Barker, S. B.: Basic endocrinology, Philadelphia, 1962, F. A. Davis Co., chap. 7.

Chiazze, Leonard, Jr., Brayer, Franklin T., Macisco, John J., Parker, Margaret P., and Duffy, Benedict J.: The length and variability of the human menstrual cycle, J.A.M.A. **203:**377, 1968.

Graber, Edward A.: Changes in endocrine system. In Barber, Hugh R. K., and Graber, Edward A., editors: Quick reference to ob-gyn procedures, Philadelphia, 1969, J. B. Lippincott Co., chap. 2.

Grollman, Arthur: Clinical endocrinology and its physiological basis, Philadelphia, 1964, J. B. Lippincott Co., chap. 21.

Guyton, Arthur: Textbook of medical physiology, Philadelphia, 1966, W. B. Saunders Co., chap. 79.

Hytten, Frank, and Leitch, Isabelle: The physiology of human pregnancy, Oxford, 1964, Blackwell Scientific Publications, Ltd., chap. 6.

Ross, Janet S., and Wilson, Kathleen J.: Foundations of anatomy and physiology, Baltimore, 1966, The Williams & Wilkins Co., chap. 16.

*Psychological preparation*

Haward, L. R.: Some psychological aspects of pregnancy, Midwives Chronicle 81:46, Feb., 1967.

Meek, Lucille: Maternal emotions and their implications in nursing, RN 32:38, April, 1969.

Meerloo, Joost: The psychological role of the father, Child Family 7:102, Spring, 1968.

Schaefer, George: The expectant father, Nurs. Outlook 14:46, Sept., 1966.

*Educational preparation*

Barren, S. L.: Social background of pregnancy, Nurs. Mirror 216:18, March 8, 1968.

Broadribb, Violet: Foundations of pediatric nursing, Philadelphia, 1967, J. B. Lippincott Co., chap. 6.

McCaffery, Margo Smith: An approach to parent education, Nurs. Forum 6:77, 1967.

Runnerstrom, Lillian: Expectant parent education, Nurs. Sci. 3:57, Feb., 1965.

**For student's quick notes:**

Chapter 3

# Diagnosis of pregnancy

Various tests are available for diagnosis of pregnancy. In this chapter you will read about these tests and also learn the clinical signs and symptoms of pregnancy. The last part of the chapter deals with the duration of pregnancy and with the calculation of the expected date of delivery.

## Pregnancy test—chorionic gonadotropic hormone

In 1928 Aschheim and Zondek discovered a substance in the urine of pregnant women that would bring about an ovulation phenomenon in the ovaries of injected mice. They also discovered that this gonadotropin was different from the three pituitary gonadotropins that we studied in Chapter 2, and they finally traced its origin to the early developing cytotrophoblasts of the chorion. This hormone is present in the urine a few days after nidation of the zygote and provides a basis for pregnancy tests as early as the tenth day after fertilization. This hormone is also present in the blood, amniotic fluid, colostrum, and milk.

After the twelfth week the titer decreases to a low level and remains so until a few weeks after delivery. This discovery did more than give a clue to the possibility of pregnancy because the hormone was also found to be present in the placenta. Therefore, the placenta also functions as an endocrine gland, since it produces hormones necessary for pregnancy.

## Clinical test—basal body temperature

You have learned about a number of changes in the female cycle attributed to hormonal influence. Another change is the variation in her basal body temperature, which varies with her cycle. This variation can be used in determining the probable date of ovulation and possible pregnancy. The hormone progesterone stimulates the thermal centers in the brain. Therefore, a woman normally has a rise in temperature at her ovulatory phase, since the progesterone level rises at this phase.

To demonstrate this fluctuation in temperature, the woman is usually instructed to keep a graphic chart at her bedside and record her temperature every morning on awakening, before any activity or mental or emotional stimulation. To facilitate reading the temperature, she may use a thermometer graded in one-tenth instead of two-tenth degree markings. After keeping this record for several months, each woman will find her cycle conforms to a fairly well-defined pattern of fluctuation or a distinct rhythm; hence the name rhythm cycle. By

**22**

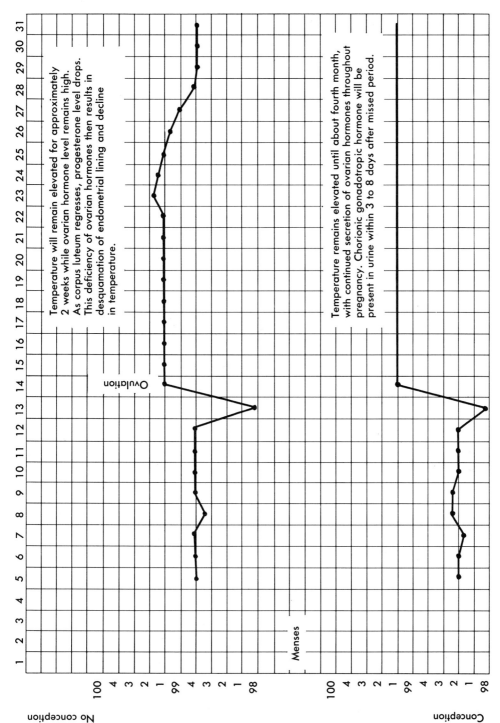

Temperature will remain elevated for approximately 2 weeks while ovarian hormone level remains high. As corpus luteum regresses, progesterone level drops. This deficiency of ovarian hormones then results in desquamation of endometrial lining and decline in temperature.

Temperature remains elevated until about fourth month, with continued secretion of ovarian hormones throughout pregnancy. Chorionic gonadotropic hormone will be present in urine within 3 to 8 days after missed period.

Ovulation

Menses

No conception

Conception

**Fig. 3-1.** Temperature table showing ovulatory curve.

starting the chart the first day after the menses cease, she will find her temperature about the same for 10 days and then one morning, the day prior to ovulation, her temperature will show a decrease of approximately 1° F. (low level of progesterone), followed by a sustained rise (ovulation) of as much as 1° F. This is her ovulatory phase.

The temperature will remain at this level for about 2 weeks; this sustained elevation is due to secretions from the corpus luteum of increased amounts of estrogen and progesterone. Persistence of this temperature for more than 2 weeks is a probable manifestation of pregnancy, since the corpus luteum and progesterone will continue to be secreted throughout pregnancy. If she does not become pregnant, the temperature will drop about 1° F. after 2 weeks of sustained elevation; this is due, of course, to the drop in progesterone. (See Fig. 3-1.)

## Duration of pregnancy and calculating estimated date of delivery

In women the average length of pregnancy is 280 days, 40 weeks, or 10 lunar (9 calendar) months, when calculated from the first day of last menses; when calculated from time of ovulation, it is 266 days. These 9 months are divided into three trimesters. Occasionally patients ask the nurse how the doctor arrives at the due date. The nurse should be familiar with Nägele's rule for estimating the date of delivery. This method of calculation is not precise, but it does give the woman and the doctor a close estimation.

**Table 3-1.** Immunodiagnostic tests*

| Name | Specimen | Test positive | Factors involved |
|---|---|---|---|
| Pregnosticon | Sheep red cells sensitized to HCG†; urine and HCG serum give characteristic doughnut-shaped sedimentation pattern | Early accuracy eighth day after missed period (95%) | 2 hours |
| Gravindex | Same as above, but latex particles used instead of red cells | Fortieth day (85% to 90%) | 5 minutes |
| *Hormone preparations* | | | |
| Primicol | Injected intradermally to produce allergic reaction in nonpregnant woman; prepared from colostrum | No bleeding within 72 hours after last injection—probably pregnant (90%) | |
| Neostigmine | 1 ml. of 1:1000, I.M., daily for 3 days | As above | |
| Delalutin | 250 mg. I.M. | No uterine bleeding within 7 days—probably pregnant | |
| Norlutin | 20 mg. orally | No uterine bleeding within 7 days—probably pregnant (95%) | |
| Enovid | 10 mg. daily for 4 days | If bleeding does not occur in 2 or 3 days—positive for pregnancy | |

*See p. 322 for other tests of pregnancy.
†Human chorionic gonadotropin.

**Nägele's rule:** To the first day of the last menstrual period, add 7 days; from this subtract 3 months.

Over one half the patients will deliver within 5 days previous to, or later than, the estimated date. It is perhaps better to speak of the period of an expected date of delivery rather than a particular day.

A woman who has regular monthly cycles over a period of years and then fails to have her menses for 1 month has as her first thought, "Am I pregnant?" This may be a young married girl, anxiously waiting for this to happen, a woman married for a number of years who has not conceived before, or a woman who may not wish to be pregnant for a variety of reasons. Regardless of what the situation may be, each woman is anxious to know as soon as possible. For a woman who is anxious for the answer before certain physiological changes in her body are discernible to the doctor, she can get her answer by having one of the pregnancy tests done (Table 3-1).

## Nursing responsibilities

It is the nurse's responsibility to be familiar with the various tests so that she can intelligently instruct the patient in order to reinforce the doctor's explanations. It is also her responsibility to understand the rhythm cycle so that she can instruct patients should the doctor request that she do so, or again to reinforce the doctor's explanation. She needs to impress on the patient the importance of daily, accurate recording and of taking the temperature before any activity, and that this is not absolutely reliable as a diagnosis of pregnancy.

If the patient is having a laboratory pregnancy test performed, the nurse needs to instruct her (1) to take no medication for 48 hours prior to collecting the specimen, (2) to restrict fluids after the evening meal, (3) to void before retiring, (4) to collect the first morning specimen (approximately 60 ml.) in a clean glass container, and (5) to keep urine cold and take it to the laboratory the same morning.

## Clinical signs and symptoms noted by the doctor or the mother

In addition to clinical tests the diagnosis of pregnancy may be based on signs and symptoms experienced by the mother and on others noted by the doctor during the examination.

**Presumptive signs**

These are signs and symptoms usually noted by the patient
↓

1. Cessation of menses
2. Tenderness and enlargement of the breasts
3. Nausea and vomiting
4. Quickening (18 to 20 weeks)
5. Frequency of micturition

**Probable signs**

These are usually signs noted by the doctor on examination
↓

1. Enlargement of the abdomen
2. Changes in size, shape, and consistency of the uterus
3. Softening of the lower uterine segment (Hegar's sign)
4. Softening of the cervix (Goodell's sign)
5. Discoloration of mucous membrane of the vagina (Chadwick's sign)
6. Enlargement and softening of fundus at site of implantation (von Fernwald's sign)
7. Uterine souffle (after sixteenth week)
8. Braxton Hicks's contractions may be felt (fourth month)
9. Pigmentation line on abdomen (linea nigra) and of the face (chloasma of pregnancy)
10. Positive pregnancy tests

**Positive signs**
↓

1. Audibility of fetal heart beat
2. Fetal movements
3. X-ray outline of fetal skeleton
4. Palpation of fetal parts by the doctor

| | |
|---|---|
| **GRAVIDA** | A pregnancy regardless of its duration. |
| **PARA** | Past pregnancies continued to the period of viability. |
| **PRIMIGRAVIDA** | A woman pregnant for the first time. She is a gravida i, a nullipara, or para O. |
| **NULLIPARA** | A woman who has not given birth. |
| **PRIMIPARA** | A woman who had one pregnancy and delivered after the period of viability. Para refers to pregnancies, not to fetuses. Therefore, if the delivery was multiple, she is still a primipara or para i. The primipara, para i (who had a multiple birth), during her second pregnancy is referred to as a gravida ii. After delivery she will be a multipara or para ii, even though she now has three children. |
| | If a woman has had an abortion and then becomes pregnant again, she is a gravida ii, para O. |
| **MULTIPARA** | A woman who has delivered two or more viable infants. |
| **MULTIGRAVIDA** | A woman during her second and subsequent pregnancies. |

## STUDY QUESTIONS
### Multiple choice

1. The immunodiagnostic test with Pregnosticon can be used when early diagnosis of pregnancy is important. Diagnosis can be made:
   (a) the eighth day after a missed period.
   (b) 4 weeks after ovulation.
   (c) 2 weeks after a missed period.
2. When instructing a woman in use of the charts for determining her period of ovulation, you would tell her that is necessary to continue the chart:
   (a) for at least 6 months.
   (b) for several months.
   (c) for a full menstrual cycle.
3. The elevation of temperature at ovulation and this sustained level for 2 weeks after ovulation is due to:
   (a) high levels of estrogen and progesterone during this time.
   (b) high levels of chorionic gonadotropic hormone.
   (c) decrease in progesterone.
4. The hormone sometimes referred to as a uterine tranquilizer is:
   (a) estrogen.
   (b) chorionic gonadotropin.
   (c) corpus luteum.
   (d) progesterone.

### Matching

Match the terms in the first column with their appropriate definitions in the second column:

(a) Chadwick's sign     __*Probable* sign of pregnancy

(b) Frequency     __Perception of fetal movements

(c) Linea nigra     __Discoloration of mucus membrane of the vagina

(d) Changes in size and shape of the uterus     __Softening of the lower uterine segment

(e) Quickening     __Line of pigmentation extending from umbilicus to symphysis pubis

(f) Goodell's sign — *Presumptive* sign of pregnancy

(g) Hegar's sign — May be caused by increased vascularity of pelvic organs

(h) Nausea and vomiting — Softening of the cervix

## SELECTED READINGS

*Pregnancy tests*

Bell, George H., Davidson, J. Norman, and Scarborough, Harold: Textbook of physiology and biochemistry, ed. 6, Baltimore, 1965, The Williams & Wilkins Co., p. 1043.

Brown, J. H., and Barker, S. B.: Basic endocrinology, Philadelphia, 1962, F. A. Davis Co., p. 41.

Grollman, Arthur: Clinical endocrinology and its physiological basis, Philadelphia, 1964, J. B. Lippincott Co., p. 408.

Keele, Cyril A., and Neil, Eric, editors: Samson Wright's applied physiology, ed. 11, New York, 1965, Oxford University Press, p. 499.

Prem, Donald A.: Temperature method in the practice of rhythm, Child Family 7:311, Fall, 1968.

*Diagnosis and duration*

Beck, A. C., and Taylor, E. Stewart: Obstetrical practice, ed. 8, Baltimore, 1966, The Williams & Wilkins Co., chap. 8.

Benson, Ralph: Handbook of obstetrics and gynecology, Los Altos, Calif., 1964, Lange Medical Publications, chap. 2.

Davidsohn, Israel, editor: Clinical diagnosis by laboratory methods, ed. 13, Philadelphia, 1962, W. B. Saunders Co., chap. 27.

Eastman, Nicholson J., and Hellman, Louis M., editors: Williams' obstetrics, ed. 13, New York, 1966, Appleton-Century-Crofts, p. 260.

Greenhill, J. P., editor: Obstetrics, ed. 13, Philadelphia, 1965, W. B. Saunders Co., chap. 10.

**For student's quick notes:**

# Chapter 4

# Fetology—period of the unborn

This chapter deals with conception and embryonic and fetal development. You will read about the interplay of heredity and environment. In addition to biological processes you will learn about the repercussions of prenatal environment to which the fetus is subjected and how these factors are believed to influence its intrauterine environment.

## Fulfillment of biological processes

The maturation of a minute sphere of cells into tissues, into specific organs evolving into human form; all governed by a power unseen; this is the story to learn and tell, second to none.

### Ovum transport

The greatest of nature's miracles is the conception, development, and birth of the infant. You have learned that the ovum is very tiny, barely visible to the naked eye, suspended in fluid called *cytoplasm,* and surrounded by a mass of cells for nourishment and protection called the *zona pellucida.* As the ovum leaves the graafian follicle, it is propelled into the fallopian tube by the fimbriated end of the tube. The cilia and musculature of the tube probably aid in directing the ovum's course to the upper third of the tube, where it awaits the sperm.

### Sperm transport

Sperm are the smallest of body cells. During coitus sperm are ejaculated in seminal fluid into the vagina. This deposit is called *semination.* Nature is ever so free with the production of sperm; millions are deposited at an ejaculation. Nature probably produces them in such abundance because the passage toward the tube is hazardous and slow, and many perish along the way. It is believed that this journey may be aided by action of uterine musculature. The sperm are ejaculated into a hostile environment—from a pH of 7.5 of the seminal fluid to a pH of 4.5—in the vaginal secretions; but lured by the rich glycogen content of the cervical secretions, especially at ovulatory time, sperm thrive in this favorable environment.

### Conception

As the sperm clusters around the ovum, they release the enzyme hyaluronidase to act on the zona pellucida (protective covering surrounding the ovum), which makes the penetration possible. Many sperm reach the ovum, but only one is successful in penetrating it. After this has occurred, the male and female pronuclei fuse, each contributing 23 chromosomes; thus the fertilized ovum, now a zygote with its 46 chromosomes and thousands of genes, each with its element of inheritance, has started its development into a human being.

The fusion of the nuclei is called fertilization, fecundation, conception, or impregnation. Cell division and redivision start immediately in geometric progression by forming a cell mass called the *morula.* After a journey of about 3 days through the tube, the morula (about a 25-cell mass) arrives in the uterus. This process is believed to be aided by cilia and the peristaltic motion of the tube. As these cells multiply, they arrange themselves around the periphery of the ovum in such a way that a cavity forms; the outer mass of cells is called the *trophectoderm,* and the inner is called the *embryonic cell mass.* The outer layer secretes a semifluid substance that nourishes the embryonic cells. The mass of cells is now called a *blastocyst* (Gr. *kystis,* sprouting bladder), or *blastodermic vesicle* (hollow sphere of cells). Another 3 to 4 days pass before the blastocyst attaches itself to the epithelial lining of the uterus. A structure called the *body stalk* connects the developing embryo with the wall of the vesicle; this is actually the rudimentary umbilical cord.

*Nidation*

The cells of the trophectoderm secrete proteolytic and cytolytic enzymes to help them burrow their way into the compact layer of the endometrium. This process of burrowing its way into the endometrium is called *nidation,* or *implantation,* and may cause slight bleeding, called *implantation bleeding.* The blastocyst usually nidates at a high level in the uterus on either the front or back wall. (See Fig. 4-1.)

During the first few weeks after nidation, trophoblasts (primary villi) appear over the entire blastodermic vesicle. They are vascular processes that have the power of cytolysis and are able to tap maternal blood vessels as a source of nourishment and oxygen for the embryo. These villi are the first stage of the developing *chorionic villi* (secondary villi) that secrete the chorionic gonadotropic hormone and synthesize proteins and glucose for approximately 12 weeks; by this time the fetal liver is capable of supplying glucose. The chorionic villi that invade the endometrium are called *chorion frondosum* and are exposed to a rich source of blood; they multiply rapidly and finally develop into the *placenta.*

The villi around the blastodermic vesicle

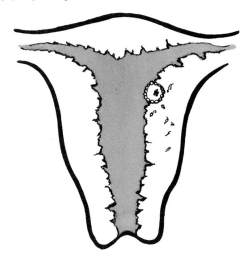

**Fig. 4-1.** Nidation of zygote into endometrial lining of uterus.

that do not invade the endometrium, that is, those that extend toward the uterine cavity, are called the *chorion laeve.* As the embryo grows, its sac protrudes into the uterine cavity and these chorion laeve stretch and become atrophic.

*The decidua*

If you recall the morphological changes that take place in the endometrium during the secretive phase of the cycle, you will remember that the blood vessels increase in size and the entire lining becomes more succulent and rich in glycogen. When conception occurs, the vascularity of the uterine wall increases greatly; this development is under the influence of the ovarian hormones, principally progesterone.

The endometrium at this time is given the name of *decidua,* the word meaning "to cast off," or discard, and this is actually what happens after the infant is born because the prepared lining of the endometrium *is* cast off.

This decidua is divided into three areas:

1. *Decidua vera (parietalis)* is the uterine lining exclusive of the area engrossed by the embryo or that part of the endometrium not directly associated with the development of the embryo.

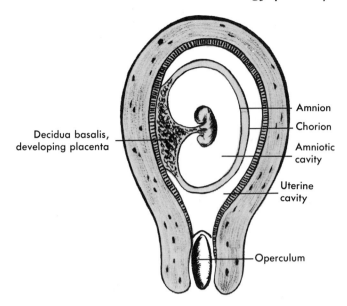

Decidua basalis, developing placenta

Amnion
Chorion
Amniotic cavity
Uterine cavity
Operculum

**Fig. 4-2.** Early development of embryo with fetal membranes and developing placenta. Operculum forms to prevent migration of bacteria into uterine cavity.

2. *Decidua basalis* is the portion of the decidua vera where nidation takes place; that is, the area where chorionic villi (frondosum) invade the maternal blood vessels and develop into the placenta (Fig. 4-2).

3. *Decidua capsularis* is the portion of the decidua vera that covers the blastocyst after it nidates, isolating it from the other portions of the uterus. It disappears as pregnancy advances.

### The funis[2]

The embryo is connected to the chorion frondosum (embryo's placenta) by the umbilical cord. This "cable line" between the fetus and placenta develops from the original body stalk and is a continuation of the chorion. It extends from the umbilicus to the fetal portion of the placenta and is attached either eccentrically or centrally. The average length of the cord is 55 cm. A short cord may cause delay in descent of the fetus; an excessively long cord is more likely to prolapse and become tangled during labor and delivery. The cord is made up of two arteries and one vein originating from chorionic villi, and the cord is covered with a layer of stratified squamous epithelium. An abnormal number of blood vessels in the cord may be associated with congenital anomalies in the fetus. The blood vessels are surounded by a mucoid substance, Wharton's jelly.

Approximately one half pint of blood flows through the cord every minute. This pressure causes the cord to be relatively erectile, or stiff, and not flexible as we view it after birth. If fetal movements cause looping of the cord, the turgor prevents the loops from knotting tightly. It is during the fetal sojourn through the birth canal, when the amount of blood in the cord is decreased, that flexibility occurs, with consequent tightening or knotting of any loops that might be in the cord.

### The yolk sac

Two cavities appear in the *inner embryonic cell mass;* the one is called the *amniotic cavity* and the other the *yolk sac.* The latter is a single layer of entodermal and mesodermal cells that are filled with albuminous matter. The first blood vessels to appear develop on this sac and communicate with vessels of the embryo. Just as soon as circulation is established between the chorionic villi and embryonic vessels, the growth of the yolk sac ceases.

### Embryonic-fetal membranes

*Chorion.* As the chorionic villi (frondosum) invade the endometrium, they grow and develop into the *chorion* that becomes the outer layer of the embryonic sac. This membrane extends out from the margin of the placenta to envelope the embryo. It is composed of two layers of tissue, an outer *ectoderm* (trophoderm) and an inner mesoderm. Chorionic circulation becomes established between the third and fourth week. (See Fig. 4-2.)

*Amnion.* While the chorion is developing, another auxiliary, transparent tissue called the *amnion* forms from the *inner embryonic cell mass* and is adherent, but not fused, to the chorion. These two, the amnion and the chorion, make up the embryonic-fetal sac. Amniotic fluid is secreted within this sac and serves as an important medium in the uterine life of the fetus.

### Amniotic fluid[4]

*Physiology.* The embryo-fetus is submerged in approximately 1,500 ml. of amniotic fluid during intrauterine existence; that is, up to about the seventh month when this fluid gradually diminishes to about 700 ml. at term. To the fetus this fluid is a "river of living waters" because it supplies just about its every need. To the biochemist this fluid is still a mystery and there are different opinions as to its sources; most authorities believe it is derived from fetal membranes (amniotic epithelium), lungs, and kidneys.

We know the amniotic fluid does function for the fetus's benefit by acting as a protective cushion, equalizing jolts and pressures, and preventing adhesions between the embryo and the sac, and it certainly allows for change in fetal position and posture. Finally, when the time to be born has arrived, the bag acts as a hydrostatic wedge, easing the way for the fetus through the birth canal. It is known that the fetus swallows the fluid and excretes it; so perhaps it may be a source of nourishment for it, containing protein, glucose, calcium, sodium, potassium, and chlorides. About 35% of the fluid is replaced every hour.

By examination of the fluid, it is possible to determine the sex of the fetus (p. 35). Fetal maturity can be estimated by examination of pigments in the fluid when done prior to the thirty-fifth week of gestation. The chromosome structure of fetal cells obtained from amniotic fluid may also be determined. This may lead to prediction of certain intrauterine inherited anomalies.

*Oligohydramnios.* When less than 300 ml. of amniotic fluid is secreted, it is termed oligohydramnios. This small amount of fluid allows the amnion to adhere to the fetus and it is believed to be a causative factor in some congenital abnormalities such as deformities in the legs and feet. Fetuses in this environment are often born postmature and have fetal renal agenesis.

*Polyhydramnios.* When there is more than 2,000 ml. of amniotic fluid at term, it is called polyhydramnios and is also believed to be associated with abnormalities such as congenital heart disease, esopha-

**Chemistry of amniotic fluid**

1. Slightly alkaline, pH 7.2
2. Contents: epithelial cells, leukocytes, serum, albumin, globulin, urates, minute particles of vernix caseosa, and various enzymes and organic and inorganic salts; normally no bacteria are present

geal atresia, or any abnormality of the alimentary tract. It is also found in mothers who are known cardiac patients.

## Development and physiology of the placenta

The placenta, a highly specialized organ with a most intricate and marvelous mechanism, functions in transmitting metabolic products between the mother and the fetus. This organ is a discoid mass, measuring about 3 cm. thick and 15 to 20 cm. in diameter and weighing about 600 grams. It grows more rapidly during the first trimester; up until the fifteenth week, it is heavier than the fetus. At term it is said to be approximately one sixth of the weight of the fetus.

The placenta is composed of two distinct portions; one is the *fetal portion,* developing from the chorionic villi (frondosum), and the other is the *maternal portion,* composed of decidua basalis (Figs. 4-3 and 4-4). Therefore, we will say that it is formed by chorionic villi and decidua basalis. The placenta becomes a distinct organ about the third month.

Two layers of trophoblastic cells, syncytial and Langhans' (cytotrophoblastic), function as semipermeable membranes and separate fetal from maternal blood flow. It is the syncytial cells of the trophoblasts that produce progesterone.

The *fetal surface is* covered by adherent amnion; many branching vessels course their way beneath this amnion. The *maternal surface* is divided into irregular-shaped segments called *cotyledons;* within these are many blood sinuses and intervillous spaces. (See Fig. 4-3.)

The maternal portion weighs about one sixth of the total weight. The surface area continues to increase throughout pregnancy, but the membrane between the maternal and fetal portions becomes very thin as pregnancy approaches term. This may permit permeability of certain substances such as drugs from the maternal to the fetal portion. Some women believe their blood flows through the veins of their off-

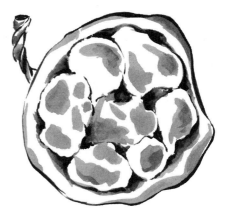

**Fig. 4-3.** Maternal surface of placenta.

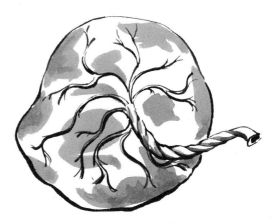

**Fig. 4-4.** Fetal surface of placenta.

spring, but now you know that this is not so, since the flow of blood is separate as is the mechanism of circulation.

### Placenta-embryo function

The placenta begins to function about the third week, that is, blood vessels pass from the embryo into chorionic villi, and nutritive substances pass from the mother's blood to the fetus. This is called hemotrophic nutrition. The placenta regulates the body temperature of the fetus, which is 0.5° F. warmer than that of the mother.

### Placenta transfer

During the latter part of pregnancy about 500 ml. of blood flows through the maternal circulation of the placenta per minute, and nearly 4 liters of water diffuse its cells each hour. As the maternal blood flows in and out of the sinuses, there is a constant selective interchange between intervillous spaces and fetal capillaries, which supply substances needed for growth and development of the fetus in exchange for waste products of fetal metabolism.

Fetal capillaries have "selective power"; some capillaries permit passage of waste products from fetal metabolism into the maternal portion to be excreted by the maternal metabolic processes. Other capillaries permit transfer of substances of small molecular weight, such as dextrose, amino acids, oxygen, minerals, vitamins, gamma globulin, and some red blood cells, from the maternal portion by dialysis. Some substances are transferred by pinocytosis, that is, particles are engulfed by the cells. As these capillaries extend into the fetal portion they enlarge to form veins, and finally converge at the umbilical vein. The fetus synthesizes more complex proteins and carbohydrates. Various other substances present in the fetal blood are possibly synthesized by some metabolic function not yet explainable.

The selective power of the placenta also serves as an effective barrier against passage of certain bacteria. "A number of antibodies are present in the maternal and neonatal circulations in approximately equal concentrations; antitoxins of diphtheria, tetanus, and scarlet fever are examples. Antibodies against pertussis, rickettsial organisms, rubella, measles, mumps, herpes simplex, unfluenza, syphilis, and toxoplasmosis are also among those transferred across the placenta."[*] Just how they cross over is still a mystery, as is the high degree of immunity the newborn acquires in utero.

### Transfer of oxygen

Fetal cells are not 100% oxygenated; this may be compensated for by the fact that the fetus has more blood cells while in utero. The uptake of oxygen by the fetus is high. (Uterine blood flow is increased during pregnancy by 500 ml. per minute.) Therefore, the *proportion* of oxygen the fetus uses is higher than that used by the mother. However, it does not require as great oxygen *concentration* in utero as it does after birth. Its hemoglobin has a greater affinity for oxygen than does adult hemoglobin and its red blood count is very high at birth.

Approximately 3 hours after birth the fetus has complete oxygenation of blood cells, and by the second week its count drops from 6 million to 5 million. This reduction in red blood cells (RBCs) is managed in a natural manner by the liver; hemoglobin is broken down into its components and passed off through the biliary system. Should this "natural" degeneration of RBCs occur at too rapid a pace, jaundice occurs. This is the so-called icterus neonatorum, or physiological jaundice. However, the bilirubin index readily falls and a Coombs' test is negative, in contrast to the pathological jaundice of erythroblastosis fetalis, which is caused by pathological destruction of RBCs, with resultant progressively rising bilirubin and with an associated diagnostic positive Coombs' test.

### Secretion, synthesis, and transfer of hormones and enzymes

By the end of the second month the placenta governs the endocrine mechanism of pregnancy by regulating the hormone transfer between mother and fetus. The placenta produces estrogens, corpus luteum, progesterone, relaxin, and its specific hormone, chorionic gonadotropin. You will recall that this is the chorionic gonadotropic hormone that provides the basis for pregnancy tests (p. 22). Placenta hormones also contribute to changes in the ducts and glandular tissues in preparation for lactation.

### Functional capacity of the placenta

Functional capacity of the placenta decreases as pregnancy approaches term. Whether this degenerative phenomenon is of clinical importance is debatable.

---

[*]From Hughes, James J.: Synopsis of pediatrics, St. Louis, 1967, The C. V. Mosby Co., p. 217.

Infectious agents, protozoan, and viruses known to transfer from placenta to fetus

| 1. Chicken pox | 8. Rubella |
|---|---|
| 2. Diphtheria | 9. Pertussis |
| 3. Herpes simplex | 10. Smallpox |
| 4. Influenza | 11. Syphilis |
| 5. Measles | 12. Toxoplasmosis |
| 6. Poliomyelitis | 13. Typhoid |
| 7. Rabies | |

*Placenta dysfunction syndrome*

When the placenta fails to perform its normal metabolic functions, fetal growth and development are jeopardized. This may be caused by some abnormality occurring during the early development of the placenta (trophoblastic stage), by toxemia (hypertension) during pregnancy, or by a postmature placenta.

*Placenta dysfunction syndrome with postmaturity*

From clinical observation it is evident that prolonged gestation has been, in some instances, detrimental to the fetus. The postmature infant may show clinical signs that lead us to believe that its nourishment and oxygen supply were interfered with. What the physiological reserve of the placenta is, and how much aging and damage it can tolerate and still maintain its functioning powers, are questions not yet answered. Much of the physiology of this versatile organ is still a mystery. See p. 287 for clinical symptoms of the postmature infant.

## Development and physiology of the fetus
### Determination of sex

Parents are usually so interested in the sex of the developing fetus that the first question many of them ask after delivery of the infant is, "What is it, a boy or a girl?" Scientists are able to predict the sex of the fetus by examination of the sex chromatin pattern in the cells that float freely in the amniotic fluid because the female cells contain distinctive chromatin bodies. The amniotic fluid is obtained by aspiration, but the procedure can be dangerous and is usually done only for medical reasons.

The human being has 23 pairs of chromosomes; 22 pairs are known as *autosomes*, and the remaining pair are *sex chromosomes*. The sex chromosomal pattern of the

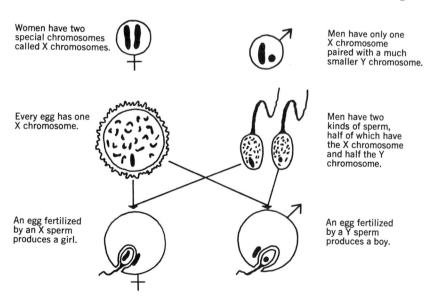

Fig. 4-5. Sex determination. (From Morgan, Clifford: Introduction to psychology, ed. 2, New York, 1961, McGraw-Hill Book Co.; with permission of McGraw-Hill Book Co.)

female is XX and the male XY. Whether the new individual will be a male or female is determined by the sperm. If the male contributes 22 autosomes plus the X (sex-determining chromosome), the offspring will be a female. If he contributes the Y (sex-determining chromosome), the offspring will be a male. (See Fig. 4-5.)

Scientists have long known that the sperm heads vary in size; some are round and small and others are large and elongated. The sperm with the small, round heads seem to travel faster and consequently reach the ovum before the sperm with the larger heads. It has been hypothesized that those with the small, round heads may carry the Y chromosome, and those with the larger head may carry the X chromosome. This just might explain why there are more males conceived than females.

*Period of the ovum—first 2 weeks*

During the first 2 weeks the sperm penetrates the ovum and the nuclei of the two gametes fuse. The union of the sperm and ovum restores the chromosome number to

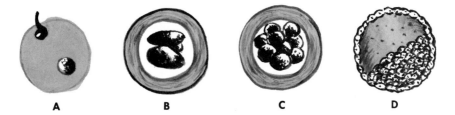

Fig. 4-6. A, Sperm penetration with fusion of nuclei of two gametes. B, Union of sperm and ovum restores chromosome number to 46; now a zygote. C, Rapid cell division (mitosis) results in mass of cells; morula stage. D, About the ninth day cells of the morula form a hollow ball of cells, a blastocyst, 2/100 inch in diameter.

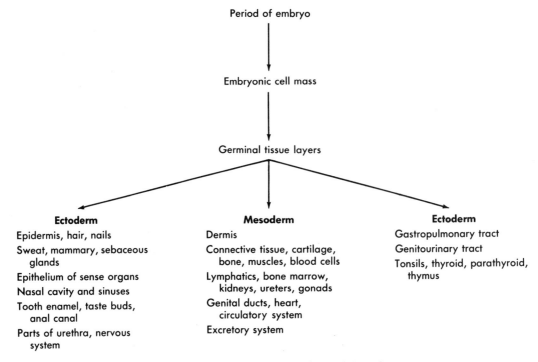

Fig. 4-7. Period of embryo, second to eighth week.

46 and the fused gametes are called a zygote. Rapid cell division (mitosis) results in a mass of cells, and this is called the morula stage. About the ninth day the cells of the morula form a hollow ball of cells, a blastocyst, which is $\frac{2}{100}$ inch in diameter. (See Fig. 4-6.)

*Period of the embryo—second to eighth week*

Each cell in this "mighty army of cells," by some unknown but marvelous power, is destined to take its specific place to complete the features of human form (Fig. 4-7).

Cells of the blastocyst give rise to the three primary germ layers from which develop all body systems.

*Period of the fetus*

The product of conception is called an *embryo* from implantation until the eighth week, at which time it resembles a human being and the "fetal state" is said to have been attained.

The student is not expected to study embryology during her course in maternity nursing; however, the mothers occasionally ask questions about the development of their baby. The developments about which most mothers seem interested are listed on the following pages; for a more detailed list see Fig. 4-8.

*First to fourth week*

The baby's heart begins to beat and its pulsation starts about the twenty-fourth day (Fig. 4-8, *A*).

*Fifth to eighth week*

The embryo begins to stir and by the end of the eighth week it resembles a human being. It is now called a *fetus* and is on the threshold of humanity (Fig. 4-8, *B*).

*Ninth to twelfth week*

Nail beds form on fingers and toes and sex can be determined by the twelfth week (Fig. 4-8, *C*).

*Thirteenth to sixteenth week*

Downy lanugo appears on the head, and blood vessels are visible beneath transparent skin. Some women experience "quickening" as early as the sixteenth week (Fig. 4-8, *D*).

*Seventeenth to twentieth week*

The fetus moves around enough for the mother to experience the wonderful feeling of "quickening." Many women who have negative feelings about their pregnancy tend to have a change of attitude when they experience movement of the fetus. It is also during this time that the doctor can hear the fetal heart tones (Fig. 4-8, *E*).

*Twenty-first to twenty-fourth week*

If the fetus is born at this time, it may make feeble attempts to breathe, but it does not survive more than a few hours (Fig. 4-8, *F*).

*Twenty-fifth to twenty-eighth week*

The fetus now gives the appearance of a "little old man," that is, its skin is wrinkled with very little deposit of fat. At the twenty-eighth week the fetus is considered viable and it may live with excellent nursing care (Fig. 4-8, *G*).

*Twenty-ninth to thirty-second week*

The fetus stores deposits of fat and minerals during this time, probably in preparation for its journey into separate existence (Fig. 4-8, *H*).

*Thirty-third to thirty-sixth week*

During this time the fetus continues to deposit fat and loses the wrinkled appearance of the skin (Fig. 4-8, *I*).

*Thirty-seventh to fortieth week*

The fetus is considered full term at 38 weeks. It gains approximately 2 pounds and grows 2 inches during these last weeks of intrauterine existence. The eyes are uniformly of a slate hue. It continues to store minerals and fat and adds the last finishing touches to its beauty, for the nurse who enjoys the newborn has the gift of seeing beauty in each one (Fig. 4-8, *J*).

**Fig. 4-8**

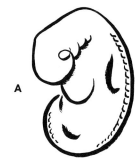

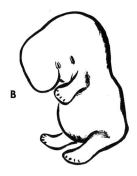

### Week 4
### End of first lunar month

Length: ¼ inch
Weight:
Development:

Embryo curled upon itself in such a position that head touches tail, and it does have a tail in this primitive state.

Heart is prominent and bulging; begins to pulsate about twenty-fourth day.

Arm and leg buds show primitive signs of formation.

Liver is formed and primitive blood cells are present.

First structures to develop are precursors of brain and heart.

### Weeks 5 to 8
### Second lunar month

1 inch
⅟₃₀ ounce

Organogenesis completed.

Heart assumes definite form. Face develops; structure of eye, ear, and nose appears, as does cardiac pulsation.

Head disproportionately large due to rapid brain development.

External genitalia appear but not discernible except by histological study of gonads.

Limbs recognized (in rudimentary form). Large muscles develop and are capable of contracting.

Scattered "blood islands" (hemopoiesis in fetal tissues).

Circulatory system between embryo and chorion completed. Begins to stir.

Brain is largest organ of body during this month. Resembles human being. Attains fetal state—on threshold of humanity by end of second month.

Meconium forms in intestines.

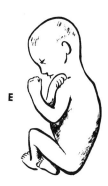

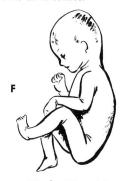

### Weeks 17 to 20
### Fifth lunar month

Length: 10 inches
Weight: 8 to 10 ounces

Lanugo more prominent, especially on shoulders.

Skin is less transparent.

Some deposits of fat.

Fingernails and toenails distinguishable.

Majority of mothers recognize movement (quickening) during this month.

### Weeks 21 to 24
### Sixth lunar month

12 inches
1½ pounds

Eyebrows and eyelashes defined.

Skin wrinkled.

May attempt to breathe, but if born, does not survive more than a few hours.

Vernix caseosa present on body.

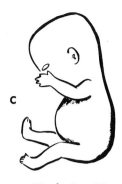

**Weeks 9 to 12**
**Third lunar month**
3 inches
1 ounce

Head disproportionately large, comprises ⅓ of entire fetus. Brain shows structural features.
Eyelids fused. Intestines contain bile. Nail beds form on fingers and toes.
Spontaneous movements occur.
Ossification centers appear in bones.
Sex may be determined by twelfth week.
Enamel-forming cells and dentin begin to form.
Kidney secretion by tenth week.
Blood formation begins in bone marrow.
Distinguishing sexual traits evolve.
Exhibits respiratory-like movements (reflex activity).

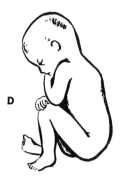

**Weeks 13 to 16**
**Fourth lunar month**
6 to 7 inches
4 ounces

Active movements of muscles. Downy lanugo on head. Blood vessels visible beneath transparent skin.
Fetal heart sounds can be heard.
Mother may feel fetus move (quicken) as early as the sixteenth week.
Ptyalin and pepsin are being secreted.
Liver assumes some of placenta's function.
Synthesizes fats from carbohydrates. Stores carbohydrates and iron.

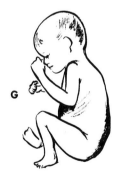

**Weeks 25 to 28**
**Seventh lunar month**
15 inches
2½ pounds

Appearance of little old man; skin red, wrinkled, and covered with vernix caseosa.
Membranes disappear from eyes and eyelids reopen.
May survive with excellent nursing care.
Respiratory and circulatory system developed sufficiently at this time that twenty-eighth week is considered period of extrauterine viability.

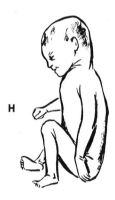

**Weeks 29 to 32**
**Eighth lunar month**
15 to 17 inches
3½ to 4 pounds

Deposits of subcutaneous fat.
Stores minerals, iron, calcium, phosphorus, nitrogen.
Testicles may be in scrotal sac.
Can be conditioned to respond to sounds outside mother's body.

*Continued.*

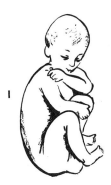

| **Weeks 33 to 36** | **Weeks 37 to 40** |
|---|---|
| **Ninth lunar month** | **Tenth lunar month** |
| Length: 19 inches | 20 inches |
| Weight: 5 to 6 pounds | 7 to 7½ pounds |
| Body and limb more rounded due to increased deposits of fat. | Considered full term at 38 weeks. |
| Skin loses wrinkled appearance. | Body is plump. |
| | Amount of vernix varies. |
| | Uniform color to eyes; are a slate hue. |
| | Storage of minerals continues. |
| | Testes may or may not be in scrotal sac. |
| | Acquires finishing touches to his beauty. |

*Fetal physiology* (Fig. 4-9)

Respirations ⟶ Rhythmic respiratory movements can occur in the latter months of pregnancy. Respirations at birth are thought to be a continuation of intrauterine respiratory activity, rather than an abrupt transition from an apneic state.

Responsiveness of the fetus ⟶ The fetus begins to stir in utero between the eighth and tenth week and is capable of responding to sounds outside the mother's body at about the thirtieth week.

Gastrointestinal function ⟶ The liver secretes bile, stores carbohydrates, iron, glycogen, and calcium during the last trimester, and begins to play a part in hematopoiesis during the second month.

The fetus synthesizes fat from glucose rather than absorbing it from the mother's blood.

Meconium, the end product of fetal metabolism, consists of vernix, cellular waste, and bile pigments that give it the characteristic black color. Meconium forms during the second trimester but is not excreted until after birth, unless the fetus is in distress or presenting as a breech.

Renal function ⟶ The kidneys function in utero but are not essential for fetal physiology.

| Formation of blood cells[8] ──────────→ | Nucleated red blood cells first form in the yolk sac and then in the placenta about the third week of development.<br>At 6 weeks the liver begins to form blood cells and by the twelfth week, the spleen and lymph tissue aid. Later on the bone marrow contributes. |

| Endocrine function ──────────→ | Secretions of the fetal thyroid may support inadequate maternal thyroid function.<br>Function of the fetal pancreas is greatly accelerated if the mother is a diabetic. |

## Multiple gestations

The frequency of twins varies in different countries and is greater among Negroes of our population, 14 per 1,000, as compared with American whites, 10 per 1,000. Two percent of the births in the United States are plural; these births account for approximately 6% of the fetal deaths.

It has been cited that multiple pregnancies account for more premature infants than any other known cause.[1] Diagnosis may be made on the following: (1) x-ray examination by the fourth month, (2) auscultation, and (3) considerable fetal activity.

## Physiology of fetuses in multiple gestations

The fetuses of a multiple gestation are certainly exposed to greater hazards during their development. If they are monozygotic and share a single placenta, it is possible that one does not receive adequate nutrition or oxygen; hence the differences in weights and immediate response to extrauterine existence. Where one has an inadequate oxygen supply, there is always the possibility of some effect on the intelligence potential. The fetus born last is more likely to be mentally retarded or stillborn. (See Fig. 4-10.)

### TYPES OF TWINS

| Identical | Fraternal |
|---|---|
| Develop from a single fertilized ovum that divides very early in its development. | Develop from fertilization of two separate ova; may occur by ripening of two graafian follicles or the development of two ova in a single follicle. |
| Synonyms: monozygotic, uniovular, homologous. | Synonyms: dizygotic, binovular, heterologous. |
| May be a genetic trait carried by either parent. | Approximately 67% are of this type. |
| Approximately 33% are of identical type. | May have two placentas, two chorions and two amnions; placentas sometimes fuse (Fig. 4-10). |
| May have one chorion, and a single or double amnion (rarely, a single amnion). | Race, age, parity do play a part. |
| May have two chorions and fused or separate placentas. | Occurs in later pregnancies of older women, up to age 37 to 38, then declines in frequency. |
| Occurs in equal frequency in every age group. | Are five times as common as identical twins. |
| Independent of race, age, parity. | May be of the same or opposite sex; differ as siblings do. |
| Are smaller, perhaps due to competition for nutrition. | Fare better than identical twins. |
| Have triple the perinatal mortality of dizygotic and a greater chance of congenital malformations in one of the pair.[1] | Heredity is prominent determining factor. |

In instances of dizygotic fetuses, one may nidate at a more favorable site for placental circulation, and consequently the other may be deprived of sufficient nutrition and oxygen. When there is a single amnion, there is also the possibility of intertwining of the cords.

The fetal mortality rate is especially high among those infants born to (1) very young mothers, (2) mothers delivering their first child, that is, born to a primagravida, and (3) mothers at age 45 and over.

For maternal complications see p. 111, and for complications during labor see p. 192.

### Distinctive features of fetal circulation

Fetal blood via the *umbilical arteries* flows into capillaries of the chorionic villi where waste products of metabolism are exchanged for oxygen and nutrients. The capillaries converge to form the *umbilical vein* that carries most of the blood directly to the fetal liver, which has already assumed its important role in metabolism. From the liver sinusoids and the hepatic veins, this blood reaches the *inferior vena cava*. The liver, however, cannot accommodate all the returning blood so that some is bypassed directly from the *um-*

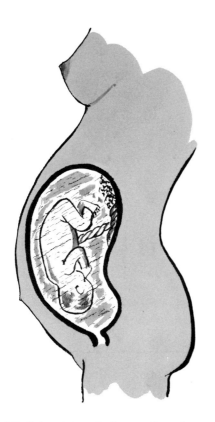

**Fig. 4-9.** Fetus at term in its aquatic environment.

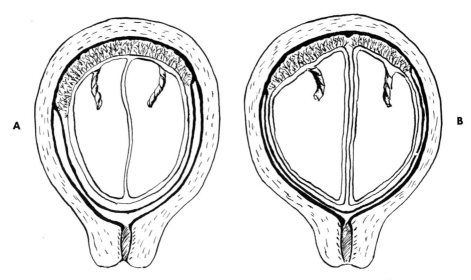

**Fig. 4-10.** Placentas with twins. **A,** Fused placentas. **B,** Two separate placentas.

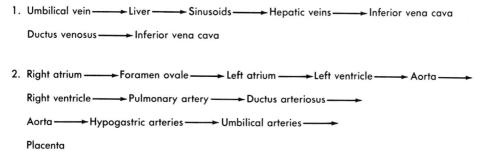

1. Umbilical vein ──────▶ Liver ──────▶ Sinusoids ──────▶ Hepatic veins ──────▶ Inferior vena cava

   Ductus venosus ──────▶ Inferior vena cava

2. Right atrium ──────▶ Foramen ovale ──────▶ Left atrium ──────▶ Left ventricle ──────▶ Aorta ──────▶

   Right ventricle ──────▶ Pulmonary artery ──────▶ Ductus arteriosus ──────▶

   Aorta ──────▶ Hypogastric arteries ──────▶ Umbilical arteries ──────▶

   Placenta

**Fig. 4-11.** Fetal circulation.

*bilical vein* into the inferior vena cava by way of the *ductus venosus.*

In contrast to the liver, the right heart has little to do, for the lungs do not function in fetal life and therefore need only a small amount of blood for nourishment. Two ways are therefore provided for blood to bypass the lungs—the *foramen ovale* and the *ductus arteriosus.*

The foramen ovale is an opening between the *right* and *left atria* with a small structure, the *eustachian valve,* to direct some of the blood through the foramen into the *left heart,* thus reaching the *aorta* more quickly. Blood that flows into the *pulmonary artery* via the *right ventricle* is shunted to the aorta by way of the ductus arteriosus that connects these two vessels. The aorta actually carries a mixture of oxygenated blood from the placenta and true venous blood from the fetal structures.

Where the aorta divides and branches into the hypogastric arteries, the umbilical arteries arise to complete fetal circulation by returning the blood to the placenta. Thus the umbilical *vein* carries oxygenated blood and the *two umbilical arteries* carry *venous* blood.

*Transition to extrauterine environment.* You should now be ready to ask the question: "What happens to these structures after birth?"

When the fetus is born and starts breathing, pulmonary circulation, of course, changes because all the blood must now flow to the lungs for oxygenation. The increased return of blood to the left ventricle brings about functional closure of the fora-

men ovale. In only about 50% of infants will this closure be permanent by the end of the first year. This closure is believed to be aided by placing the infant on his right side when he is put in the incubator. (See Fig. 4-11 and p. 167.)

The ductus arteriosus (about the third month) and the ductus venosus (about the fifth month) become ligaments, as does the umbilical vein. The rising oxygen saturation of the blood stimulates the respiratory center and closure of the ductus arteriosus.

## Hereditary and environmental influences on the developing embryo
### Hereditary factors

Scientists have presented evidence showing that ordinarily chromosomes transmitted to the offspring are not altered. Nevertheless (with further study and many advances in science), there is strong evidence to support the hypothesis that unfortunate circumstances (such as x-radiation exposure and certain drugs) can alter gene structure and result in interference with the normal development of embryonic tissues.

Prenatal uterine environment supports normal physiological processes of the embryo and fetus. Heredity guides this physiological development in that the genes control cell metabolism. (See Fig. 4-12.)

The *nature* of embryonic tissue is determined by gene structure. When a parent transmits a defective gene (mutation), it is called a *hereditary defect.* Normal genes may also be made defective by contributory factors such as certain dietary deficiencies,

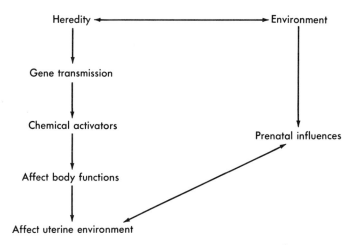

**Fig. 4-12.** Hereditary and environmental influences on the developing embryo.

infection, or toxic effect of drugs. These are called *acquired defects.*

### Environmental factors

The hypothesis is that an unfavorable uterine environment may be responsible for alterations in genes, that is, capable of producing cell changes. These mutations cause "tissue arrests" that in embryonic development occur during the period of organogenesis (eighteenth to thirty-eighth day).

Stress factors are also thought to bring about chemical changes affecting normal maternal metabolic processes. Reports from numerous sources are reviewed and studied by geneticists to determine just how much stress can interfere with the normal functioning of the embryo's gene activity. Not only does the fetus require nourishment and oxygen, but it also requires a peaceful environment during its sojourn in the mother's uterus.

Before we read about the various "stress" factors believed to contribute to an unfavorable uterine environment and to alter genetic physiology (cell chemistry), we must nevertheless remember that their conclusions are mostly based on experimentation with animals. With reference to human embryology the reports are conceptual and fragmentary, and it would be fallacious to ascribe any one factor as being the absolute contributor. However, they may provide clues for further research.

*Nutrition.* That the nutritional status of the mother affects fetal environment is not questionable. But do severe nutritional deficiencies contribute insults to organogenesis? Based on animal experimentations, the answer is yes. Rats fed a diet deficient in vitamin D invariably produce offspring that are stunted and malformed. Likewise, excess as well as deficiency has been found to have a wide variety of deleterious effects.

That nutritional deficiencies contribute to adverse effects on human organogenesis is still highly speculative. Reports show tissues during stages of differentiation appear to be sensitive to lack of certain vitamins, especially vitamin $B_{12}$. Rickets (as an example), largely a disorder of nutrition, affects bone development in infants, but we cannot ignore the fact that this may have begun during uterine environment or that many interacting factors other than nutrition may have contributed. The relationship between the mother's diet and its effect on fetal development is clearly evidenced in endemic cretinism when the offspring's mental deficiency is the result of the mother's iodine deficiency.

It is known that fetal malformations are more common in women with deficiencies of folic acid or errors in folic acid metabolism. Folic acid plays a vital part in human cell formation and tissue growth; the defects from this deficiency are usually those involving errors in fusion, such as anencephaly or cleft lip.[3,5]

*X-radiation.* The teratogenic effects of radiation on embryonic tissues when used for therapeutic measures is well established; this effect depends in part on the gestational stage and the dosage administerd. Most malformations are believed to occur between the second and seventh week, since this is the interval of major organogenesis; an exception is the central nervous system, which develops continually during fetal life and for a few weeks postnatally. The central nervous system is highly susceptible, and defects are likely to be hydrocephaly and microcephaly. Records show that these conditions occur in infants born of mothers who were irradiated after the fifth month. The opinion has been expressed that the pregnant uterus should never be subjected to radiotherapy, because even low doses may cause cancer and leukemia in the infant.[6]

Experiments with animals indicate that radiation may also damage the germ cells. Effects of radiation are cumulative; therefore, long-term radiation might result in mutant genes.

When the doctor orders roentgen pelvimetry during labor, and the mother shows concern, the nurse can assure her that any fears she may have are unjustified and that there is no evidence that roentgenography used for diagnostic examinations late in pregnancy or during labor have any effect on the fetus.

*Maternal age.* The incidence of congenital anomalies with relation to maternal age has been of wide interest and study. The conclusions drawn from many studies reveal that very young parents (15- to 17-year age group) and those in their late reproductive phase (late 40s) are more likely to have offspring with congenital abnormalities.

How this exerts its effect in not understood, but the opinion has been expressed that perhaps the germ cells are either too young (underdeveloped) or too old to participate normally in gametogenesis and result in chromosomal aberrations. Since genes interact with their environment, it may be that variations in a woman's endocrine balance produce an unfavorable environment for gene activity at these ages.

Of the various congenital abnormalities, the incidence of Down's syndrome, hydrocephalus, and anencephalus seem to be related to the increasing age of the mother. There are also reports on the relationship between age of the father and abnormalities of the offspring, although maternal age is said to be more important than paternal age in Down's syndrome. Age is a factor related not only to abnormalities but also to a higher incidence of abortions, stillbirths, and premature deliveries.

### Transplacental transmission of infectious and contagious diseases

Today it is known that many virulent agents, such as bacteria, protozoa, and viruses, are capable of traversing the placenta and consequently of damaging embryonic tissues. It is also known that in some instances damage occurs not by transfer of the virus or bacteria, but as the result of their toxic effects on the mother.

As the result of a major epidemic of German measles in Australia in 1940, Dr. N. McAlister Gregg, an Australian ophthalmologist, observed a definite relationship between congenital cataract and maternal rubella. This stirred the interest of scientists and biochemists and through their research much has been learned about the permeability of the placenta to these virulent agents. Gregg's findings not only confirmed theories that these viruses were etiological factors in abortions, that is, death of the fetus, but also added knowledge concerning various teratogenic effects. Between 10% and 30% of those mothers exposed delivered infants with congenital abnormalities; organs usually involved are the ear, heart, and eye. The greatest risks to the embryo from the German measles virus is during the period of organogenesis.

Rubella occurring weeks before conception may still leave its tragic consequences on the fetus (congenital rubella). If the mother has been infected, the virus can traverse the placenta before onset of the rash and may not even manifest any deleterious effects on the mother (subclinical rubella). This transplacenta rubella infection appears to continue as a contagious disease in the neonatal period, since the virus has been isolated from urine and throat swabs of some of these infants at birth. Deliberate infection of young girls by exposing them to associates with rubella may induce natural immunity to the disease, but this is not without risk when considering the complications of rubella.

Until the present time, gamma globulin was used as a preventive measure, that is, to prevent transmission of the disease, but the value of this was questionable since transmission probably occurs before the mother is even aware of her exposure.

Today another link of achievement can be added to the chain of medical progress due to the work of Dr. Harry M. Meyer, Jr., and Dr. Paul D. Parkman, who in April of 1966 announced the development of a live, attenuated rubella-virus vaccine, HPV77. This HPV77 strain has been extensively tested to date. Who will be included in the immunizations program is one of the main issues. Authorities agree that there is a risk in giving the vaccine to women of childbearing age because she might be pregnant or become pregnant within a few months after the inoculation and the vaccine might cross the placenta and attack the fetus. It seems logical that immunizing children would reduce the risk of exposure of pregnant women. Also vaccinating the woman immediately after she completes a childbearing cycle, that is, during the early puerperium when another pregnancy is highly improbable, would protect her from this danger.

*Measles (rubeola).* Measles, when transferred to the embryo, usually results in abortion or fetal death. The teratogenic effects do not compare in severity to those caused by rubella virus. If the mother is immune as the result of a previous attack, the infant remains immune for approximately the first 6 months of life.

*Smallpox.* Smallpox, when transferred to the embryo, results in abortion in about 50% of the cases. Congenital smallpox may occur; in such cases the infant may be born with pockmarks.

*Mumps.* When transferred to the embryo, mumps usually results in abortion or fetal death. In some cases, congenital abnormalities have been attributed to this infection.

*Varicella.* No evidence is available to indicate a teratogenic effect from varicella.

*Influenza.* There is no substantial evidence that the human embryo can be infected with an influenza virus.

• • •

The causative agents of herpes simplex, poliomyelitis, toxoplasmosis, malaria, typhoid, and pertussis can be transmitted to the fetus. Toxoplasmosis is known to be associated with mental deficiency.

*Syphilis.* Prenatal care is indeed preventive care! If there were sufficient time to make the diagnosis of syphilis and institute immediate treatment, there would be no more stillbirths or congenital abnormalities due to syphilis.

Syphilis is transmitted to the fetus after the eighteenth week. It is believed that prior to this time the Langhans' layer of chorion forms a barrier and prevents passage of the *Treponema pallidum.* (This layer is no longer present in the placenta after this time.) Adequate treatment prior to the fifth month constitutes prevention of infection of the fetus. Adequate treatment after this time will affect a cure but with, perhaps, osseous stigmata. When the disease is of many years duration, the danger to the fetus is not as great.

Syphilis in the fetus causes interstitial changes in the lungs, liver, spleen, and pancreas and causes osteochondritis in the long bones. The fetus may die in utero, be stillborn, be premature, or be born with congenital abnormalities. The placentas in such cases are abnormally large and pale in color. If syphilis is acquired shortly before delivery, the infant will be normal but must be protected by inoculation from local lesions in the birth canal.

*Gonorrhea.* It is not known with certainty whether the gonococcus causes intrauterine infection of the fetus. During pregnancy the infection is usually confined to the lower genital tract, the urethra, Skene's glands, Bartholin's glands, or the cervical glands. However, during delivery it can be spread up into the uterus, the peritoneum, and the blood.

The woman has a profuse, green-colored discharge that causes pain and burning on urination. This discharge is highly infectious, and if it gets into the infant's eyes during the birth process, blindness may result.

Penicillin, 600,000 units daily for 1 week, usually effects a cure. Condylomata acuminata (skin warts) may be associated with gonorrhea.

### Transplacental transmission of drugs

The discovery that the drug thalidomide produces teratogenic effects on embryonic tissues opened many avenues for implications of other drugs. It has been implied that all drugs may be potential hazards to fetal tissue. This may be pure conjecture.

It was previously stated on p. 34 that

**Table 4-1.** Possible effects of drugs on the embryo, fetus, and neonate

| Drug | Effect |
| --- | --- |
| Estrogens, progestins, androgens | Virilization |
| Analgesics and certain tranquilizers | May reduce thermal stability of newborn |
| Iodides | Stimulate development of goiter and possible mental retardation |
| Dicumarol, Coumadin | Hemorrhage, fetal death |
| Salicylates (excess) | Neonatal bleeding |
| Barbiturates (excess) | Neonatal bleeding |
| Tetracyclines | Inhibits bone growth; abnormal formation and discoloration of teeth |
| Sulfonamides | Kernicterus |
| Vitamin K analogues | Hyperbilirubinemia |
| Reserpine | Slows heart rate; may be responsible for nasal congestion and respiratory distress |
| Quinine | Thrombocytopenia |
| Diuretics | Electrolyte imbalance |
| Nitrofuratoin (Furadantin) | Hemolysis |
| Aminopterin | Anencephaly |
| Amethopterin | Anomalies and abortions |
| Thalidomide | Phocomelia |
| Atropine sulfate | Fetal tachycardia |

the passage of substances to the fetal portion of the placenta and on into fetal circulation is largely related to their molecular weight. Since most drugs are of low molecular weight, it is assumed that the majority may get into fetal circulation.

Drugs known to be definitely teratogenic to fetal tissue, in addition to thalidomide, are certain antifolic acid compounds (aminopterin) and synthetic progestational compounds; the latter result in external genital virilization (Table 4-1).

Since it is not known which drugs are teratogenic to the embryo, nor whether damage is done during preimplantation period or during organogenesis, doctors are cautious about ordering drugs for the pregnant woman unless they are indispensable to maternal health. Much of the damage is believed to take place so early in pregnancy that the woman in all probability is not even aware that she has conceived. Many facets need to be weighed, such as the chemistry of the drug, the quantity taken, the rate and mechanism of transfer, and the genotype of the mother and fetus.

The nurse needs to keep herself informed regarding scientific progress in drugs and her function is to advise women against self-medication. If the woman is taking medication and has reason to suspect that she is pregnant, the nurse should advise her to consult the physician before continuing with the drug.

**Drug addiction.** When the drug addict becomes pregnant and carries the fetus to term, it will invariably manifest symptoms of drug addiction. Fortunately, studies show that these women are more likely to deliver prematurely or deliver stillborn infants, but if carried to term, the infant usually has no clinical signs at birth, but after about 24 to 48 hours he exhibits symptoms of drug withdrawal. These symptoms are twitching of extremities, a sharp shrill cry, marked irritability, diarrhea, and vomiting.

### Tobacco and smoking

One of the most frequently asked questions by the pregnant woman is, "Does smoking have any effect on the fetus?" Or, "How many cigarettes may I smoke each day?" This subject has received much attention, especially since studies have been done and reports furnished on the incidence of lung cancer and cigarette smoking.

There is some evidence that low birth weight and the incidence of prematurity are related to excessive cigarette smoking. One concept is that smoking may cause vasoconstriction of the placental vessels and may limit the blood supply to the fetus, and this in turn retards growth. Other studies show a relation between the number of cigarettes smoked daily and the incidence of prematurity.

### Emotional stress phenomenon

What effect do maternal emotions have on the embryo and fetus? This question is open for wide discussion. One hypothesis is as follows: stressor agents stimulate the anterior pituitary to secrete increased amounts of adrenocorticotropic hormone (ACTH). This in turn stimulates the adrenal cortex to release cortisone. Cortisone can be catabolic and interfere with development of embryonic tissues.

When the mother reacts to emotional tension, physiological changes take place in her body and chemical agents such as epinephrine and adrenaline are released into the blood and are shortly transmitted to fetal circulation (neurohumoral transfer) via the placenta. Opinions as to how this transference affects the embryo and fetus are controversial. It is known that (1) maternal hormonal stimulation may affect glandular function of the fetus and (2) maternal fatigue causes more frequent and stronger fetal movements. Observation of these infants shows a persistence of disturbance during postnatal life, such as feeding and sleep problems. These observations prove nothing, since numerous other factors may have contributed, but they open avenues for research.

It has been cited that the umbilical cord and placenta are not nerve-free structures. For further study of these structures see reference 7 (network of nerves found in the placenta).

## Blood incompatibilities and maternal sensitization

You have been reading in this chapter about various factors in the mother that may adversely affect the fetus. The mother may also be sensitive to substances reaching her from the fetus. She reacts to these substances, which, if they in turn reach the fetus, may affect its normal development. Maternal sensitization to blood incompatibilities is an example.

Pregnant women are, of course, especially interested in blood incompatibilities, since they know that somehow the infant is involved. When they visit with their obstetrician, they have every opportunity to talk with him and have their various questions answered at the level of their understanding. But the mothers in the prenatal clinic are not always this fortunate, especially if clinics are understaffed. She senses the pressures and even though she may have questions in mind, she hesitates asking anyone to discuss them with her. Here is where the nurse can prove her worth, since she has opportunities to talk with the patients. To do this, she must have basic knowledge of her subjects; she must have a pool of resourceful knowledge from which she can draw worthwhile information and she must be able to interpret this at the patient's level of understanding.

Prerequisite to understanding Rh sensitization, the nurse needs to know about blood group factors in man and the antigen-antibody reactions that result in red blood cell destruction. Most red blood cells of man contains antigens, agglutinable substances that cause the red cells to clump when they come in contact with serum containing specific antibodies (isoagglutinins). Blood groups are named according to the antigen content: A, B, AB if the cells contain both A and B, or O if the cells contain neither A nor B. Serum, likewise, may contain an anti-A or anti-B agglutinin; group O serum contains both, and

group AB serum contains neither or its cells would clump. Blood containing cells with A antigen and blood with serum containing anti-A agglutinins are said to be incompatible. When cells containing A antigen are injected into an animal (or man), they stimulate the recipient to form anti-A antibodies, and the serum becomes able to agglutinate group A cells.

There is, however, another group of factors called Rh antigens because they are found in cells of the rhesus monkey. Rh factors are found also in the cells of 85% of white people and these are designated as Rh positive. Rabbits inoculated with rhesus monkey blood cells develop an anti-Rh immune serum that does not agglutinate the other 15% of white people, and these are called Rh negative. An Rh-negative person injected with Rh blood will become sensitized to the antigen and be stimulated to develop anti-Rh agglutinins. Similarly an Rh-negative woman carrying an Rh-positive fetus may become sensitized.

*Fetomaternal transfusion and maternal isoimmunization.* You learned previously that fetal and maternal blood circulate independently, with the placenta serving as the exchange center. Through experimentation it is known that fetal Rh-positive cells can be identified in maternal Rh-negative blood during the last trimester of pregnancy.

Placental damage can occur during an amniocentesis, when fluid is withdrawn for diagnostic purposes. Other investigators report transfer associated with manual removal of the placenta. In this manner (transplacental passage) the mother is being sensitized (maternal isoimmunization) to the Rh factor and in subsequent pregnancies the Rh-positive fetus is affected by the presence of these antibodies.

If the woman does not have the Rh factor in her red blood cells, but the fetus does (acquiring this from the father's genes), and the fetal red blood cells gain access into maternal circulation, the mother will then develop anti-Rh antibodies against this antigen. The anti-Rh antibodies return to fetal circulation, unite with the antigen in the fetal red cells, and cause an antigen-antibody reaction with hemolysis and destruction of the cells with a resultant inadequate transfer of oxygen to the fetus. This disorder is called erythroblastosis (Gr. *erythros,* red; *-blastos,* germ; *-osis,* increase) fetalis. The infant may be stillborn or born with such severe anemia that death is inevitable. See Fig. 4-13 and the discussion on hydrops fetalis, p. 290. Maternal complications associated with carrying a severely affected fetus are polyhydramnios and preeclamptic toxemia.

The occurrence of erythroblastosis is about once in every 200 pregnancies, yet about one in twelve pregnancies involve a mother who is Rh negative and a fetus that is Rh positive. This deviation is attributed to the infrequency with which this reaction occurs in first pregnancies, and in other cases the antigens from the fetus may not traverse the placenta. The clinical manifestations in the infant will be discussed in Chapter 26.

Today many geneticists and technicians use the letter D instead of the original Rh. So that this may not be confusing to you in your reading, a "D" cell is an Rh-positive cell.

Blood incompatibilities can also occur between the mother and the fetus from A or B antigens. About two thirds of the blood incompatibilities are due to ABO and about one third are due to Rh, but the incompatibility caused by the Rh is more severe than the ABO.

The various factors contributing to unfavorable uterine environment are at the present time uncontrollable. As our geneticists and biochemists delve into the intricate forces involved, the picture, we hope, may change and with proper prenatal care many of these factors may in time be controllable.

### Amniocentesis and intrauterine transfusion

At intervals throughout pregnancy, an indirect Coombs' test is performed to determine the titer of anti-Rh isoagglutinins. This maternal antibody may not always reflect the severity of the disease. Therefore, the amniocentesis for a study of amniotic fluid (Fig. 4-14) enables the doctor to determine the severity of the hemolytic process in the fetus and indicates whether the pregnancy need be interrupted prior to 36 or 38 weeks' gestation.

If there is a hemolysis of fetal cells, there will be a concentration of hemoglobin breakdown products (yellow pigment) in the fluid. Analysis of the fluid is by a spectrophotometer.

The amniocentesis is usually initiated between the twenty-eighth and thirty-second week of pregnancy. The nurse instructs the patient to empty her bladder and then assists her in assuming comfort in a supine position. The patient is sedated before the procedure is started. The nurse prepares the abdominal wall for local anesthesia. The doctor determines the fetal position and usually withdraws the fluid in the area between the fetal head and shoulders. At least 5 ml. of amniotic fluid is removed. When the titer goes above a critical level, the intrauterine blood transfusion may follow to overcome fetal anemia caused by rapid destruction of red cells.

In 1964 Dr. A. William Liley of New Zealand performed the first successful, dramatic procedure in treatment of erythro-

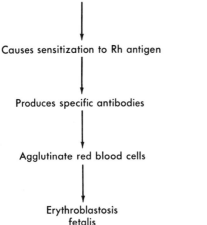

Rh antigen introduced into tissues of Rh-negative individual

↓

Causes sensitization to Rh antigen

↓

Produces specific antibodies

↓

Agglutinate red blood cells

↓

Erythroblastosis
fetalis

**Fig. 4-13.** Erythroblastosis fetalis.

blastosis by prenatal transfusion for rhesus isoimmunization. The transfusion of blood into the peritoneal cavity of the fetus becomes absorbed by the lymphatic system and thereby enters fetal circulation. This absorption takes about 3 days. (See Fig. 4-15.)

A Tuohy needle is introduced through the mother's abdomen into the abdomen of the fetus. This procedure is usually per-

formed in the x-ray department some 12 hours after a radiopaque fluid is injected into the amniotic sac to outline the fetus. This provides visualization of fetal position on an x-ray television screen and guides the doctor in directing the needle into the lower abdomen of the fetus. Usually about 300 to 400 ml. of O, Rh-negative packed red cells are given, but this varies with duration of the pregnancy and size of the fetus. With

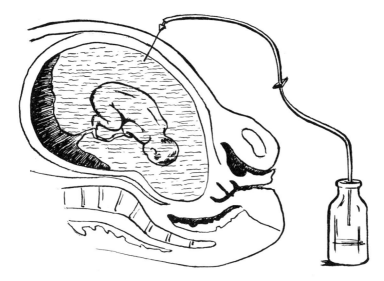

**Fig. 4-14.** Amniocentesis.

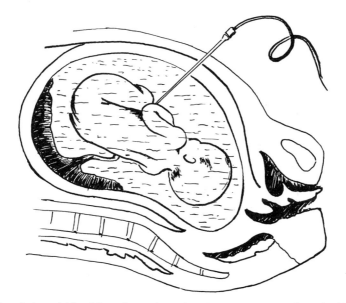

**Fig. 4-15.** Transfusion of blood into the peritoneal cavity in treatment of erythroblastosis fetalis.

this procedure the fetus may be carried closer to term, reducing risks of prematurity and associated respiratory syndromes.

The danger involved is the possibility of needle puncturing a placenta vessel with subsequent hemorrhage and fetal anemia. The doctor explains the procedures to both the husband and the patient, tactfully presenting possible complications. The nurse in attendance can reinforce the doctor's explanation by showing warm, genuine interest.

Intrauterine transfusion has also been attempted by "open method," that is, opening the uterus and introducing the blood through the saphenous vein. In most of these experimental cases the procedure induced a premature onset of labor.

*Rh$_0$ (D) immune globulin (human) Rh$_0$-Gam*[*]—*for the prevention of Rh isoimmunization.* Another dramatic advance in medical progress has been the preparation of anti-D gamma globulin for Rh prophylaxis. This Rh$_0$ (D) immune globulin (human) Rh$_0$Gam was developed by Dr. Wm. Pollack, Dr. Vincent J. Freda, and Dr. John G. Gorman.

The globulin is prepared from the blood plasma of Rh-negative individuals who have been sensitized during a previous pregnancy and thereby have the specific antibody against Rh-positive blood cells. The globulin can be effective only in women who have not previously been sensitized by blood of an Rh-positive baby.

By injecting the Rh-negative mother with this preparation, all circulating Rh antigens that have entered maternal circulation are destroyed. This injection is given to the woman delivering an Rh-positive, direct Coombs' negative baby, ABO compatible with the mother. Rh$_0$Gam is given to all Rh-negative primigravidas who up to time of delivery have had normal negative Coombs' titers. This is to neutralize the possible sensitization of the mother that could have occurred during the third stage of labor. This is also given to all Rh-negative

multigravidas who up to the time of delivery have had normal negative Coombs' titers. The idea is that even though the titers have been negative *prior* to *present* delivery, the present delivery *possibly could* sensitize her by fetal reflux into maternal circulation during the third stage. It has been cited that Rh$_0$Gam can be effectively administered as late as a week after delivery.[9]

Rh$_0$Gam administered after each Rh incompatible pregnancy is a specific prophylaxis against Rh$_0$ (D) immunization. This, then, should reduce, if not eliminate, hemolytic disease of the newborn.

**STUDY QUESTIONS**
*True and false*

(T)  (F)  1. The fetus stirs in utero and resembles a human being between the eighth and tenth week of gestation.

(T)  (F)  2. Sex of the fetus can be determined by the twelfth week of gestation.

(T)  (F)  3. Most mothers-to-be feel the fetus "quicken" by the end of the third month of gestation.

(T)  (F)  4. With good nursing care the fetus can live outside the uterus after the twentieth week of gestation.

(T)  (F)  5. The outer layer of the embryonic sac is called the chorion.

(T)  (F)  6. Syphilis is transmitted to the fetus after the eighteenth week of gestation.

(T)  (F)  7. Folic acid plays a vital part in human cell formation and tissue growth.

(T)  (F)  8. A fetus is considered full term by the thirty-eighth week of gestation.

*Multiple choice*

1. Anti-D gamma globulin for Rh prophylaxis (Rh$_0$Gam) is administered to the mother:
   (a) immediately after delivery.
   (b) within 24 hours of delivery.
   (c) within 72 hours of delivery.

2. Complete oxygenation of blood cells in the newborn takes place in approximately:
   (a) 1 week after birth.
   (b) 12 hours after birth.
   (c) 3 hours after birth.

3. By the end of the first trimester of pregnancy the endocrine mechanism of pregnancy is controlled by the:
   (a) ovaries.
   (b) uterus.
   (c) placenta.

---

[*]Available from Ortho Pharmaceutical Corp., Raritan, N. J.

4. Studies show that the drug addict is likely to:
   (a) deliver prematurely.
   (b) deliver a stillborn infant.
   (c) carry the fetus beyond a 40-week gestation.
   1. c only   2. a only   3. a and b
5. In preparing a patient for an amniocentesis, one of the duties of the nurse is to:
   (a) see that the patient empties her bladder.
   (b) assist the patient in assuming Sims' position.
   (c) assist the patient in assuming Fowler's position.

## Matching

Match the terms in the first column with their appropriate definitions in the second column:

(a) Ductus arteriosus — Portion of decidua in which nidation takes place

(b) Fraternal twins — Amniotic fluid secreted by cells of this sac

(c) Chorionic villi — Opening between right and left atria

(d) Capsularis — Portion of decidua covering the blastocyst

(e) Placenta — Protective covering surrounding the ovum

(f) Amnion — Heredity a prominent determining factor in this type of twin

(g) Zona pellucida — Term used for attachment of fertilized ovum to endometrium

(h) Basalis — Blood that flows into the pulmonary artery via right ventricle shunted to the aorta by this structure

(i) Nidation — Regulates body temperature of the fetus

(j) Ductus venosus — Endometrium during pregnancy

(k) Chorionic gonadotropin — Primary villi develop over blastodermic vesicle

(l) Decidua — Independence of age, race, parity in this type of twin

(m) Trophoblasts — Hormone present in the blood, amniotic fluid, colostrum, and human milk

(n) Identical twins — Some of the blood that traverses the umbilical vein passes directly into the inferior vena cava through this structure

(o) Foramen ovale — Outer layer of embryonic sac

(p) Chorion — Secretes chorionic gonadotropic hormone

## REFERENCES

1. Babson, Gorham S., and Benson, Ralph C.: Primer on prematurity and high-risk pregnancy, St. Louis, 1966, The C. V. Mosby Co., p. 35.
2. Benirschke, Kurt: Abnormal cord insertion in placenta, J.A.M.A. **204**:279, April 15, 1968.
3. Hibbard, Bryan M.: Folic acid and reproduction, Nurs. Mirror **123**:305, Jan. 6, 1967.
4. Huntingford, Peter J.: Detection of genetic defects, Nurs. Mirror **127**:23, Aug. 2, 1968.
5. Kitay, D. Z.: Folic acid in pregnancy, J.A.M.A. **204**:79, April, 1968.
6. Montagu, M. F., Ashley: Prenatal influences, Springfield, Ill., 1962, Charles C Thomas, Publisher, p. 456.
7. Page, Ernest W.: Some evolutionary concepts of human reproduction, Obstet. Gynec. **30**: 318, Sept., 1967.
8. Schaffer, Alexander: Diseases of the newborn, Philadelphia, 1965, W. B. Saunders Co., p. 549.
9. Rh immune globulin: an answer which leaves a few questions, Medical news section, J.A.M.A. **210**:1843, Dec., 1969.

## SELECTED READINGS
### Nutrition

Excess vitamin D in pregnancy, Nurs. Mirror **126**: 42, April 5, 1968.
14 institutions keep tract of 60,000 infants: poorly nourished mothers major birth defect focus, J.A.M.A. **204**:24, May 20, 1968.

### Smoking and tobacco

Douglas, C. O.: Gestation and concurrent disease, Nurs. Mirror **126**:38, May 31, 1968.
Hytten, Frank E., and Leitsch, Isabella: The physiology of human pregnancy, Oxford, 1964, Blackwell Scientific Publications, Ltd., p. 260.
Montagu, M. F. Ashley: Life before birth, New York, 1964, New American Library, Inc., pp. 100-116.
Smoking interferes with ability to utilize vitamin C, J.A.M.A. **208**:626, April 28, 1969.

### Maternal age

Bender, S.: The senior primigravida, Nurs. Mirror **124**:555, Sept. 15, 1967.
Illingworth, R. S.: The development of the infant and young child, ed. 3, Baltimore, 1966, The Williams & Wilkins Co., p. 33.
Mitchell, James: Over 35 and pregnant—really a risk? Consultant **6**:16, Oct., 1966.

### X-rays

Little, Wm. A.: Weighing the risk of fetal damage, x-rays in pregnancy, Amer. J. Nurs. **66**: 1308, June, 1966.
Nundy, T. D.: X-rays in obstetrics, Nurs. Mirror **124**:21, Aug. 25, 1967.
Raventos, Antolin: X-ray in pregnancy, Amer. J. Nurs. **66**:1308, June, 1966.

*Fetal physiology*

Assali, N. S.: Some aspects of fetal life in utero and changes at birth, Amer. J. Obstet. Gynec. 97:324, Feb. 1, 1967.

Bakwin, Harry, and Bakwin, Ruth: Clinical management of behavior disorders in children, ed. 3, Philadelphia, 1966, W. B. Saunders Co., p. 6.

Beck, A. C., and Taylor, E. Stewart: Obstetrical practice, ed. 8., Baltimore, 1966, The Williams & Wilkins Co., chap. 6.

Flanagan, Geraldine: The first nine months of life, New York, 1962, Simon & Schuster, Inc.

Horger, E. O., and Hutchinson, Donald: Diagnostic use of amniotic fluid, J. Pediat. 75:503, Sept., 1969.

Howell, Doris A.: Identification of problems in fetal physiology, Hosp. Top. 46:87, March, 1968.

Lanman, Jonathan: Delays during reproduction and their effects on the embryo and fetus, New Eng. J. Med. 278:993, May 2, 1968.

Munford, R. S.: Care of the infant in utero, Maryland Med. J. 17:56, Aug., 1968.

Smith, Carl: Blood diseases of infancy and childhood, ed. 2, St. Louis, 1966, The C. V. Mosby Co., chaps. 1 and 5.

*Placenta physiology*

Dancis, Joseph: Symposium on homeostasis of the intrauterine patient, Bull. Sloane Hosp. Women 14:108, Fall, 1968.

McKay, R. J., Jr., and Smith, Clement: Postmaturity and placenta dysfunction. In Nelson, Waldo E., editors: Textbook of pediatrics, ed. 8, Philadelphia, 1964, W. B. Saunders Co., p. 358.

Schaffer, Alexander: Diseases of the newborn, Philadelphia, 1965, W. B. Saunders Co., chap. 2.

Villee, Dorothy B.: Development of endocrine function in the human placenta and fetus, New Eng. J. Med. 281:473, Aug. 28, 1969.

Villee, Dorothy B.: Development of endocrine function in the human placenta and fetus, New Eng. J. Med. 281:588, Sept. 4, 1969.

Watson, E. H., and Lowrey, G. H.: Growth and development of children, ed. 2, Chicago, 1967, Year Book Medical Publishers, Inc., chap. 3.

*Multiple gestation*

Abraham, J. M.: Character of placentation in twins, as related to hemoglobin levels, Clin. Pediat. 8:526, Sept., 1969.

Dunkley, P. A.: Premature and plural-being prepared, Nurs. Mirror 126:15, Feb. 2, 1968.

Green, G. H.: Multiple pregnancy, Nurs. Mirror 126:13, Feb. 2, 1968.

Kaelber, Charles T., and Pugh, Thomas: Influence of intrauterine relations on the intelligence of twins, New Eng. J. Med. 1280:1030, May, 1969.

Strudwick, Rose, Uniovular premature twins, Nurs. Mirror 124:346, July 14, 1967.

*Infectious and contagious diseases*

Buynak, Eugene B., Hilleman, Maurice R., Weibel, Robert E., and Stokes, Joseph, Jr.: Live attenuated rubella virus vaccines, J.A.M.A. 204:195, April 15, 1968.

Cherry, James D., Bobinski, John E., and Comerci, George D.: A clinical trial with live attenuated rubella virus vaccine (Cendehill 51 strain), J. Pediat. 75:79, July, 1969.

Grayston, J. T., Detels, R., Chen, K. P., Gutman, L., Kin, K. S. W., Gale, J. L., and Beasley, R. P.: Field trial of attenuated rubella virus vaccine, J.A.M.A. 207:1107, Feb. 10, 1969.

Hardy, Janet B.: Adverse fetal outcome following maternal rubella after the first trimester of pregnancy, J.A.M.A. 207:2414, March 31, 1969.

Katz, Richard, White, L. R., and Sever, J. L.: Maternal and congenital rubella, Clin. Pediat. 7:323, June, 1968.

Larsen, Grace: What every nurse should know about congenital syphilis, Nurs. Outlook 13:86, March, 1965.

The new rubella virus vaccine, Clin. Pediat. 8:410, July, 1969.

Rawls, Wm. E.: Serologic diagnosis and fetal involvement in maternal rubella, J.A.M.A. 203:623, Feb. 26, 1968.

*Drugs*

Babson, Gorham S., and Benson, Ralph C.: Primer on prematurity and high-risk pregnancy, St. Louis, 1966, The C. V. Mosby Co., p. 105.

DiPalma, Joseph: The drugs used in pregnancy, RN 31:51, April, 1968.

Kahn, Eric J., Neumann, Lois D., and Polk, Gene-Ann: The course of the heroin withdrawal syndrome in newborn infants treated with phenobarbital or chlorpromazine, J. Pediat. 75:495, Sept., 1969.

Little, Wm. A.: Weighing the risk of fetal damage: drugs in pregnancy, Amer. J. Nurs. 66:1302, June, 1966.

Lord, J. Myron: Hazards of antimicrobial therapy to mother and fetus, Hosp. Top. 46:83, Jan., 1968.

*Determination of sex*

Amarose, Anthony, Wallingford, A. J., Jr., and Plotz, E. J.: Prediction of fetal sex from cytologic examination of amniotic fluid, New Eng. J. Med. 279:715, Sept. 29, 1966.

Valentine, G. H.: The mechanism of genetics, Clin. Pediat. 7:263, May, 1968.

Valentine, G. H.: The chromosome disorders, Philadelphia, 1966, J. B. Lippincott Co., pp. 5-6.

*Blood incompatibilities—fetomaternal sensitization*

Allen, Donald M.: Prevention of Rh isoimmunization, Clin. Pediat. **7**:643, Nov., 1968.

Ascaria, Wm. Q., Allen, A. E., Baker, W. J., and Pollack, W.: Evaluation in women at risk of Rh immunization, J.A.M.A. **205**:71, July 1, 1968.

Clarke, C. A.: The prevention of rhesus babies, Sci. Amer. **219**:46, Nov., 1968.

Diamond, Louis K.: Protection against Rh sensitization and prevention of erythroblastosis fetalis, Pediatrics **41**:1, Jan., 1968.

Gunn, Alexander: The prevention of haemolytic disease of the newborn—the final step, Nurs. Times **65**:907, July 17, 1969.

Golub, Sharon: Now: a new weapon against Rh hemolytic disease, RN **31**:38, Aug., 1968.

Lin-Fu, Jane S.: New hope for babies of Rh-negative mothers, Children **16**:23, Jan.-Feb., 1969.

Stratton, F., and Renton, P. H.: Serologic tests in relation to prenatal and postnatal diagnosis of hemolytic disease of the newborn, Clin. Pediat. **6**:330, June, 1967.

*Intrauterine transfusion*

Abraham, J. M.: Intrauterine feto-fetal transfusion syndrome, Clin. Pediat. **6**:405, July, 1967.

Bowman, John M., Friesen, R. F., Bowman, W. D., McInnis, A. C., Barnes, P. H., and Grewar, D.: Fetal transfusion in severe Rh isoimmunization, J.A.M.A. **207**:1101, Feb. 10, 1969.

Fairweather, D. V. I.: Intra-uterine transfusion of the fetus, Nurs. Mirror **126**:19, May 3, 1968.

Gregg, Grace, and Hutchinson, Donald: Developmental characteristics of infants surviving fetal transfusion, J.A.M.A. **209**:1059, Aug. 18, 1969.

Karnicki, Jadwiga: Prenatal transfusion, Nurs. Times **63**:445, April 7, 1967.

*The amniocentesis*

Creasman, W. T.: Fetal complications of amniocentesis, J.A.M.A. **204**:949, June 10, 1968.

Weber, Lennard L.: Amniocentesis, a valuable parameter in obstetric management, Hosp. Top. **44**:93, Dec., 1966.

*Drug addiction*

Montagu, M. F. Ashley: Prenatal influences, Springfield, Ill., 1962, Charles C Thomas, Publisher, pp. 325-326.

Scheinfeld, Amram: Your heredity and environment, ed. 4, Philadelphia, 1965, J. B. Lippincott Co., p. 35.

Smith, Felicia Oliver: Number of babies born to addicts increases, RN **29**:31, Oct., 1966.

*Emotional stress phenomenon*

Downs, Florence S.: Maternal stress in primigravidas: a factor in the production of neonatal pathology, Nurs. Sci. **2**:348, Oct., 1964.

Liley, H. M. I.: Modern motherhood, New York, 1966, Random House, Inc., p. 32.

Montagu, M. F. Ashley: Life before birth, New York, 1964, New American Library, Inc., pp. 156-171.

**For student's quick notes:**

# Chapter 5

# Physiological and psychological adjustments

In this chapter you will learn of the physiological changes incident to pregnancy and of the marvelous forces that propel these transitions. You will acquire knowledge concerning the various emotional reactions toward pregnancy and the environmental factors that contribute to parents' acceptance or rejection of pregnancy. This chapter also discusses the importance of sound physical and emotional fitness as a contributory factor toward a happier, healthier period of pregnancy.

## Physiological adjustments

In order that growth and development of the fetus may proceed according to nature's pattern, the maternal organism is subjected to manifold physiological adjustments. All of a woman's feminizing influences come into play!

The physiological needs that must be met are (1) to provide a bountiful source of oxygen and nutrients for both the fetus and her own metabolism, (2) to supply the demands on her physical resources necessary for the mechanism of labor and delivery, and (3) to provide for metabolic adjustments of her body for its new role, motherhood.

The adjustments involving the generative organs are more pronounced, and those involving the uterus the most extensive. This is understandable when one considers the size of the average fetus at term, the placenta, and the sac of amniotic fluid.

### The vagina

Throughout pregnancy there is progressive hypertrophy of the vaginal epithelium and elastic tissues in preparation for distension of the birth canal. Due to this increased activity, there is a heavy desquamation of the vaginal, glycogen-rich cells. This contributes to the vaginal discharge, which at times becomes quite profuse and annoying and is a common and not infrequent complaint of the pregnant woman. It is in the acid medium of vaginal secretions (lactic acid from the glycogen), pH 4 to 5, that Döderlein's bacilli flourish and contribute to preventing the invasion of pathogenic organisms that grow only in an alkaline medium. However, this change in pH of the vaginal secretions favors the growth of the monilial (yeastlike) organism and results in monilial infection. If the woman contracts this monilial infection during pregnancy and is not treated, it is likely that her infant may develop thrush.

The color of the vaginal mucosa changes due to an increase in vascularity of the vaginal canal, and during the early months it takes on a purple hue. This change may be observed by the doctor during the pelvic examination, and it may be used as an early clinical diagnostic sign, Chadwick's.

## The uterus

*Enlargement.* A number of factors contribute to uterine enlargement: (1) the endocrine system, since enlargement of the uterus will occur even in the event of an ectopic pregnancy, (2) augmentation of the uterine musculature, (3) development of the decidua, (4) hypertrophy and hyperplasia of connective tissues, (5) increase in vascularity of preexistent fibers, and (6) formation of new muscle cells. The uterus enlarges more rapidly at the site of implantation, von Fernwald's sign, and the uterus grows more rapidly during the third, fourth, and fifth months of gestation.

Early in pregnancy the uterine walls are thick, but the muscle fibers stretch and the uterine wall thins out to accommodate growth. Approaching term, the thickness of the uterine wall is reduced considerably and averages 0.5 cm. As the uterus increases in size, it also changes in weight, shape, and position (Table 5-1). Changes in the uterine lining were described in Chapter 2.

*Arrangement of muscle fibers.* The outer layer of muscles forms a hoodlike arrangement over the fundus and assists in exerting a downward force during a uterine contraction. The middle layer consists of interlacing fibers arranged to contract down on blood vessels after placental separation from the uterine wall and thus prevent hemorrhage. It is also this middle stratum that provides a great deal of force derived during a uterine contraction. (See Fig. 5-1.)

*Shape and consistency.* As the uterus increases in size, it also changes in weight, shape, and position. It becomes spherical during the second trimester. As the fetus lengthens, the contour changes to a more ovoid shape. Then as term approaches, the transverse diameter of the fundus increases and assumes a piriform shape.

During the early weeks of pregnancy there is a definite and progressive softening of the uterus. This is attributed to changes in the vascular system. As early as the fifth week, during a pelvic examination,

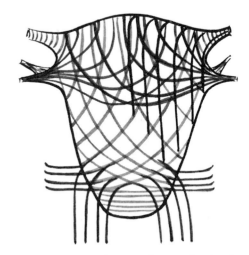

**Fig. 5-1.** Schematic drawing of uterus showing interlacing of muscle fibers.

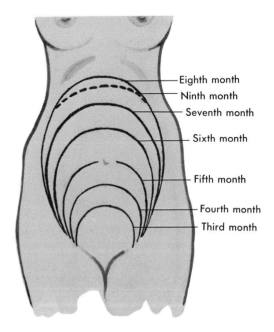

Eighth month
Ninth month
Seventh month
Sixth month
Fifth month
Fourth month
Third month

**Fig. 5-2.** Fundus height at various months of pregnancy.

Table 5-1

|  | Nonpregnant uterus | Pregnant uterus |
|---|---|---|
| Length | 2¾ inches | 11 inches |
| Width | 1¾ inches | 9½ inches |
| Depth | 1 inch | 8¼ inches |
| Weight | 1 ounce | 2.2 pounds |
| Capacity | 2 ml. | 4,000 ml. |

the doctor may note a soft spot anteriorly in the midline of the uterus. As the isthmus of the uterus lengthens, compressibility can be felt at the lower uterine segment. These are referred to as Ladin's and Hegar's signs, respectively. There is also a softening and enlarging of that area where the zygote nidates, von Fernwald's sign.

*Position.* The position of the uterus is normally one of antiflexion. As the uterus rises out of the pelvic cavity (about the fourth month), it tends to vary its position slightly because the upper portion is mobile. However, there is extensive hypertrophy of the round ligaments and they keep the uterus in line. As the uterus continues to rise, the intestines are displaced laterally, and as the fundus reaches its greatest height, it may even tip the liver. (See Fig. 5-2.)

*Contractility.* Early in pregnancy the uterus contracts at irregular intervals. These are painless, infrequent contractions, but as pregnancy advances they assume a more rhythmic pattern. This increased contractility is attributed to increased concentration of actomyosin in the uterine muscles.

These contractions may be felt through the abdominal wall soon after the fourth month and are referred to as Braxton Hicks's contractions. The purpose of these contractions is to facilitate return of venous blood to the placenta and so aid the oxygenation of fetal blood. Although they do not ordinarily cause pain, some women do complain that they are annoying. They may become sufficiently strong during the last few weeks to be confused with commencing labor. If this happens, the contractions are referred to as "false labor."

If the doctor places the stethoscope just above the symphysis, to the right or left, he can detect a rushing sound, called "uterine souffle," as the blood courses through the large uterine vessels. This is audible at about the sixteenth week and is decreased during a uterine contraction. The doctor may also be able to hear the sound of the blood as it courses through the umbilical arteries. This is referred to as "funic souffle."

Quickening, "feeling life," is experienced by the mother first as an indistinct fluttering, then as quite vigorous movements of the fetus. Perception of these movements occurs about the sixteenth week.

### The cervix

The cervix also undergoes softening due to rapid proliferation of cervical mucosa. This softening can be felt about the sixth week and is referred to as Goodell's sign. Under the influence of hormone stimulation, the secretions from the glands of the endocervix contribute to the increased vaginal discharge. Mucus accumulates in the cervical canal from these secretions and forms a mucus plug to seal off the cervical canal and to prevent bacteria from entering the uterine cavity. This mucus plug is referred to as the "operculum." The increased vascularity of the vagina and cervix during pregnancy is one of nature's ways of preparing the birth canal for the fetal journey.

### The pride of pregnancy

When the woman is standing, much of the uterus rests on the anterior abdominal wall. This alters her center of gravity.

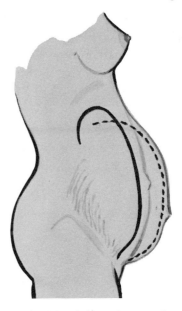

**Fig. 5-3.** As fetal head descends into pelvic cavity, fundus sinks downward and forward—phenomenon known as "lightening."

To compensate for this increased pressure on the abdomen, the woman walks with head and shoulders thrust backward and with the chest protruding. This gives her a characteristic stride in walking called "pride of pregnancy."

Within approximately 2 weeks of term (in primigravidae) the uterus gradually sinks downward and forward as a result of the fetus's head descending into the true pelvis. This settling is referred to as "lightening" and usually occurs gradually. Now the mother-to-be feels less congested and breathing becomes easier. In the multipara this phenomenon may not occur until uterine contractions are established and true labor is in progress. The height of the fundus and "lightening" provide a rough estimate of the duration of pregnancy. (See Fig. 5-3.)

### Fallopian tubes and ovaries

The lining cells of the fallopian tubes also undergo changes. As the uterus grows the position of the tubes is altered so that they lie parallel to its long axis.

The ovaries enlarge, especially the one containing the corpus luteum, which by the end of the second month is recognized as "corpus luteum of pregnancy." After the first month of pregnancy the ovaries may be removed, yet the pregnancy continues to successful termination; the placenta functions as an endocrine gland and secretes the essential hormones.

### Circulatory system

***The blood.*** A marked increase in the maternal blood and plasma volume starts at the end of the first trimester and increases to a level of 40% to 50% above normal by the end of the second trimester. There is a slight decline after the thirty-fourth week. This hypervolemia is designed to meet the demands of the vascular system throughout pregnancy. Because of this increase in volume, the concentration of hemoglobin and erythrocytes decreases, as does the hematocrit value, and this condition is often referred to as "pseudoane-

mia" of pregnancy. The values return to normal during the early postpartum period.

The hemoglobin concentration at term averages about the same as for the nonpregnant woman (12.5 to 14 grams), and the hematocrit is 35%. When the hemoglobin concentration is less than 10.5 grams per 100 ml. and the hematocrit value is below 30%, this condition may be considered as a true anemia rather than as the effect of hypervolemia. Toward the end of term, bone marrow function increases and the concentration of red blood cells reaches a normal average again.

There are obstetricians who do not accept pseudoanemia as normal. They are of the opinion that the hematological value of 12 grams for the nonpregnant woman should be maintained during pregnancy and that there should be an increase in total hemoglobin mass after the twenty-fourth week of gestation.

The white blood cells average 10,000 to 11,000 per cubic millimeter during pregnancy, but in some women may average 15,000 white blood cells (physiologic leukocytosis). A further increase occurs when the woman has a prolonged labor. This physiologic leukocytosis continues for the first few days of the puerperium.

The circulatory adjustments are adequate even though there is a greater amount of fluid circulating and the metabolism is increased during the latter half of pregnancy to approximately 13% above normal, but a strain is placed on the heart when circulatory diseases are complicated by pregnancy.

Blood flow in the lower extremities is slower during the latter part of gestation because the weight of the uterus presses on the pelvic brim and may even constrict flow of blood in the veins of the legs (impairing circulation). This increased venous pressure contributes to edema, to development of varicosities in the legs, vulva, and rectum, as well as to constipation.

***The heart.*** As the uterus rises the diaphragm is elevated, displacing the heart upward and to the left; by the end of the second trimester the cardiac output of the pregnant woman is augmented as much as 40% above that of the normal nonpregnant woman. It then decreases to near average at term.

**Blood pressure.** These physiological changes in the circulatory system influence the blood pressure. During normal pregnancy, particularly during midtrimester, both the systolic and diastolic pressures tend to drop, but toward term rise again to prepregnant levels.

**Blood clotting.** Fibrin, the constituent of the blood associated with clotting, and plasma fibrinogen are increased during pregnancy. Nature's plan is visible again in augmenting this clotting factor at the time of delivery when the danger of hemorrhage is greatest.

## Abdominal wall

It is understandable that as the uterus enlarges the abdominal wall will be distended. It becomes thinner and relaxes as pregnancy advances. Cutaneous striae, called "striae gravidarum" (Fig. 5-4), appear as irregularly curved, reddish streaks in the skin of the abdomen, the upper thighs, and buttocks in the latter months of pregnancy. After pregnancy, the reddish color changes to a glistening silvery line

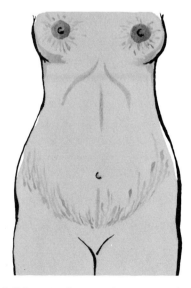

**Fig. 5-4.** Schematic drawing of striae gravidarum.

and resembles scar tissue. In subsequent pregnancies new striae appear in addition to the silvery white markings of the previous pregnancy. These are attributed not only to breaks in elastic fibers in deep layers of the skin but are also believed to have their origin in the glandular mechanism, perhaps increased activity of the adrenal cortex.

In some women the recti muscles separate in the midline due to the pressure exerted against the abdominal walls, forming a "diastasis" of the recti muscles.

## Skin changes

In addition to striae gravidarum, pigment deposits (melanocytes) appear in other areas of the body. A thin line of pigmentation occurs along the midline from above the umbilicus to the symphysis, forming the "linea nigra of pregnancy." Accentuated pigmentations occur about the nipples. A facial pigment may appear over the cheeks, bridge of the nose, and forehead, which is known as "chloasma gravidarum," or mask of pregnancy. These pigmentations are attributed to a hormone, MSH (melanocyte-stimulting hormone), secreted by the intermediate lobe of the hypophysis. Melanin (Gk. *melas,* black) ordinarily produces a tan to brown color. This hormone level drops after pregnancy and those areas affected become lighter again.

## Gastrointestinal system

As with the other organs the stomach and intestines are displaced by the enlarging uterus. The relaxin hormone is believed to contribute to decreased gastric motility. Secretions of hydrochloric acid and pepsin are slowed and there is a slight fall in blood sugar level.

Decreased motility and altered position prolong emptying time of the stomach. This, along with decrease in secretions, is believed to contribute to heartburn, a common complaint. The nurse should instruct women to avoid fatty, fried foods, especially if they experience episodes of heartburn.

*Urinary tract*

There are normal physiological changes in both renal function and structure of the urinary tract during pregnancy. Since there is an increased volume of blood filtered through the kidneys, their physiology or work is increased. Pituitrin influences reabsorption of water; aldosterone influences the reabsorption of sodium chloride. There is ureteral and kidney pelvis dilatation, particularly of the right ureter. This is attributed to the fact that the enlarging uterus compresses the ureters as they pass over the pelvic rim, and the uterus has a tendency to rotate slightly to the right (the large descending colon and rectum are in the left side of the pelvis). Frequently, these factors cause stasis of urinary drainage and the development of pyelitis.

Hypoperistalsis occurs as early as the second month. Implications have been made that this could be due to the relaxin hormone. As the presenting part settles in the mother's pelvis, there is also a displacement of the base of the bladder, which causes the area to become edematous. All of these factors add to susceptibility to infection. Dilatation of the kidney pelvis may predispose to development of pyelonephritis. Some mothers show transient albumin in their urine. This is thought to be due to congestion of the renal capillaries. For some women the frequency of micturition subsists throughout pregnancy due to increased vascularity of all pelvic organs. Other women experience this "frequency" during the early weeks of pregnancy because of bladder compression as the uterus rises out of the pelvis, and then again during the latter weeks as the presenting part settles in the pelvis.

Glycosuria and lactosuria may be present due to lowered renal threshold. The latter is attributed to secretions from the mammary gland in preparation for lactation. Small amounts of lactose are found in the urine of about 50% of all pregnant women. When this occurs, a blood sugar determination may be ordered by the doctor to differentiate nondiabetic glycosuria from true diabetic glycosuria.

Glycosuria occurs particularly in the latter months of pregnancy and more often in the primigravidae than in the multigravidae.

*Respiratory system*

Even though the pressure of the rising uterus elevates the diaphragm, the thoracic cage is enlarged and the total oxygen consumption increases progressively. The mucous membranes of the nasopharynx and accessory sinuses are congested and edematous. This may cause nosebleed at intervals during pregnancy.

*Temperature*

There is a slight rise in temperature early in pregnancy due to increased activity of the corpus luteum. About the fourth month of gestation there is a gradual fall, and as parturition approaches, the temperature returns to normal levels.

Comparison studies done on pregnant and nonpregnant women show that as early as the first month the temperature of the breasts will also be elevated on an average of 1° F.

*Endocrine glands*

Thyroid ⟶ The size of this gland increases during pregnancy as does the iodine content of the blood. There is an average of 50% increase of thyroxine, which promotes galactopoiesis, helping restore declining milk flow.

Adenohypophysis ⟶ This gland enlarges to twice its normal size. It secretes a number of hormones conducive to normal physiology of pregnancy, such as prolactin and the gonadotropins.

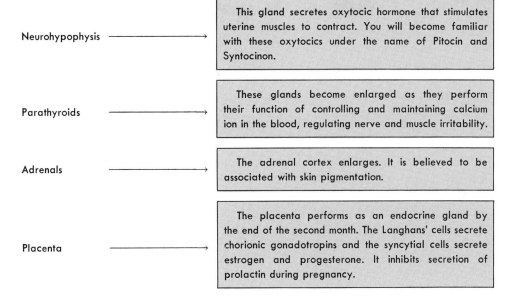

Neurohypophysis ——————→ This gland secretes oxytocic hormone that stimulates uterine muscles to contract. You will become familiar with these oxytocics under the name of Pitocin and Syntocinon.

Parathyroids ——————→ These glands become enlarged as they perform their function of controlling and maintaining calcium ion in the blood, regulating nerve and muscle irritability.

Adrenals ——————→ The adrenal cortex enlarges. It is believed to be associated with skin pigmentation.

Placenta ——————→ The placenta performs as an endocrine gland by the end of the second month. The Langhans' cells secrete chorionic gonadotropins and the syncytial cells secrete estrogen and progesterone. It inhibits secretion of prolactin during pregnancy.

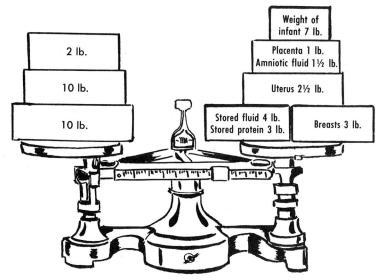

**Fig. 5-5.** Approximate weight distribution during pregnancy.

## Weight

During the first few months of pregnancy, some women may lose a few pounds, others gain on an average of 3 pounds. Although individual rates of weight gain vary widely, surveys show an average gain of 20 to 25 pounds—10 pounds the second trimester and 11 pounds the third. Much of the weight increase is due to retention of water, which is a phenomenon in all preg-

**Table 5-2.** Average weight distribution

|  | Pounds |
|---|---|
| Fetus | 7 |
| Plancenta | 1 |
| Fluid | 1½ |
| Uterus | 2½ |
| Breasts | 3 |
| Stored fluid, including blood volume | 4 |
| Fat and protein | 3 |

nant women. An average of 7 liters is retained during pregnancy. About half of this is accounted for in the fetus, placenta, and amniotic sac. A clinical sign of general retention of water is noted with weight gain and associated with one of the principal complications of pregnancy—preeclampsia. (See Fig. 5-5 and Table 5-2.)

### The breasts

Before the woman may surmise that she is pregnant, she may be aware of a tenderness in her breasts. Other women may "presume" that they are pregnant because of this change. As the weeks go by, the breasts increase in size due to hypertrophy and hyperplasia of the mammary alveoli and to an increase in fat. The diameter of the blood vessels enlarges and bluish veins become visible beneath the skin. By the end of the second month, the nipples become erectile and deeply prominent; the areola also becomes broader and more pigmented. This pigmentation varies in women; the pigment does not become as dark in blondes as in brunettes. About the fourth month a yellowish fluid may be expressed from the breasts. This is called colostrum and may serve as the first nourishment for the newborn. Scattered about the areola are numerous sebaceous glands (follicles) called tubercles of Montgomery. These are not usually obvious in the nonpregnant woman, but become distended and quite evident as pregnancy progresses. (See Fig. 1-6.)

*Physiology.* As stated on p. 8, the lobules of the breasts contain numerous acini. The function of the acini is the secretion of milk that forms in their epithelial lining. This function is inhibited during pregnancy by the action of estrogens and progesterone in the circulation. The decrease in the amount of these hormones in the blood after delivery allows the luteotropic hormone (LTH), prolactin, to act on the alveolar epithelium. (See p. 218.)

Despite the intricate physiological processes of these remarkable structures, women invariably suppress this marvelous function in preference for scientific, artificial methods of feeding.

## Psychological adjustments
### Factors contributing toward acceptance or rejection

Now that you have completed your study of the physical adjustments that occur in the woman's body during pregnancy, do not permit your interest in the somatic to outweigh your attention to the psychological. For although good physical health is conducive to the woman's feelings of well-being and contributes to a positive emotional response to her pregnancy, other factors, influenced by her past environment, also play a part in making the experience rich and rewarding. It is not just the woman's reproductive organs that are involved, but her adjustment includes her total personality. The woman who is happy in her marriage is more likely to adjust well to the preparatory adventures into motherhood and to appreciate the three greatest joys of motherhood: (1) life within, (2) giving birth (self-participation), and (3) the infant at her breast. Too often in today's world families are no longer a closely knit unit, and the average young girl does not approach motherhood with the basic stable standards as did her elders. Her cultural image of motherhood may be a very vague concept and she may find herself in a situation that she is not nearly ready to accept.

Her attitudes when the diagnosis of pregnancy is established are related to (1) emotional maturity, (2) marital compatibility, (3) relationship with her mother, and (4) acceptance of her femininity and maternal role. The relationship with her mother is often a powerful, motivating force. She may lean constantly on her mother, turning to her for all the answers regardless of what the doctor or nurse may try to teach her. On the other hand, it may be the occasion of the first dynamic disengagement from her mother. It may even mark a transition in relationship when, for the first time, she accepts her mother instead of expressing an attitude of belligerent defiance.

In studying changes of attitudes, one finds they may follow a pattern of rejection changed to acceptance. During the early months of pregnancy a woman is more likely to show resentment or ambivalent feelings; she may be coated with doubts, indifferent toward her family and friends, and lacking in inner participation, that is, she attends to her family needs because she has no other choice. Most women experience a change in attitude and a feeling of well-being during the second trimester, especially when she feels the fetus "quicken" within her. She now becomes more outgoing, her attitudes toward her family are again those of concern, and her willingness to administer to their needs is foremost in importance. Then, again, toward the end of the period of pregnancy, she becomes irritable, doubts return, and her one desire is to have it all over with. Thereafter she may experience intervals of guilt feelings because of her early rejection of pregnancy. Rejections are, to a certain extent, considered normal emotional reactions. They may be expressed by both partners, directly or indirectly, and motivated by environmental factors.

The announcement of pregnancy may also create anxieties in the husband. It may come at a time when he is least contemplating an addition to the family. There are numerous reasons why a man might show attitudes of rejection toward his wife's pregnancy. He is bound to have added responsibilities, including financial demands. He, too, experiences emotional pressures, sensing changes in his wife, especially her rejection of his attention. He may wonder if her love for him will persist or whether it will be replaced by devotion for the infant. Fatherhood may be as upsetting to him as motherhood is to the woman. Men have even been known to experience episodes of morning nausea and vomiting. Every woman wants her husband's approval. Therefore, his attitudes are especially important because of the impact they have on her. Women need support and pro-

tection, that is, to be "mothered." The one to do this is the husband. His devotion communicates a manifestation of his love that is so vital to her feeling of well-being. His importance cannot be overemphasized.

We accept doubts and fears as a normal accompaniment of all new adventures. Doctors understand that women have mixed feelings about motherhood and they understand how they respond to these feelings. Their fears may be multiple, but we will mention only a few of the most common ones.

Years ago woman's greatest fears centered around how she would get through the delivery and whether the infant would be alive; they were also filled with culturally instilled fears, with superstitious beliefs showered on them by well-wishers.

Today, woman's greatest fear concerns the ability to cope with the demands of motherhood. Does she possess the attributes to make a good mother? Can she meet the patterns her husband may have set for the rearing of his children? Unfortunately the homemade psychologists are still in our midst and she is easily disturbed by their "do's" and "don't's." Information from current literature is not always interpreted correctly and can play havoc with her thoughts so that she becomes anxious about the imperfections in physical characteristics of the baby. Here both the doctor and the nurse can help her turn a deaf ear.

Alterations in her figure are of great concern, especially to the primigravida. Day-by-day her figure becomes more grotesque, a physical change with many emotional impacts. All sorts of phobias (usually voiced by the well-wishers) play havoc with her thoughts. She worries because her relationships with her husband have changed. Her sexual responses frighten her as they reach extremes from desire to repulsiveness. Her breasts, one of her cherished characteristics of her femininity, appear to lose their beauty. When she feels the movement of life within her, she may laugh or she may cry; her mood swings alarm her. As she approaches the fulfillment of her "phase of pregnancy," she becomes clumsy, stumbles, loses self-confidence, and feels foolishly out of proportion.

Doctors are aware of these responses. This is one of the many reasons why the "family" should put complete trust in her obstetrician. The obstetrician usually arranges an appointment early in her pregnancy, when both the woman and her husband can be present, to give them a better insight into the biopsychological changes accompanying pregnancy. The husband needs to have both his own and his wife's emotional responses interpreted to him. He is then more likely to tolerate her reactions and it certainly helps him fulfill his wife's needs as they vary from day to day. Pregnancy may then be a period of harmony instead of discord.

### Pseudocyesis or psychogenic pregnancy

Pseudocyesis is a condition in which a woman resorts to an imaginary pregnancy instead of a real one. Pseudocyesis occurs about once in 1,000 obstetrical cases. More often, perhaps, this occurs in infertile, married women for whom the desire to have a baby becomes an obsession, but it has also occurred in women who had persistent secretions of corpus luteum and progesterone.

Of course the probable signs of pregnancy do not exist, but psychic forces bring about physiological changes—amenorrhea, nausea and vomiting, and an increase in size of the abdomen. These add to the patient's illogical insistence that she is pregnant.

The patient needs an environment where she will find kindly explanations, and the nurse's function is to direct her to a doctor who will help her face reality instead of denial.

### STUDY QUESTIONS
*Multiple choice*

1. The uterus grows more rapidly during the:
   (a) first and second month of gestation.
   (b) third, fourth, and fifth month of gestation.
   (c) sixth and seventh month of gestation.

2. The blood plasma volume increases 40% to 50% above normal levels:
   (a) by term.
   (b) by end of second trimester.
   (c) during the first trimester.

3. The pregnant woman is said to have a true anemia when:
   (a) the hemoglobin is below 12 grams and hematocrit below 35%.
   (b) the hemoglobin is below 13 grams and hematocrit below 30%.
   (c) the hemoglobin is below 10.5 grams and hematocrit below 30%.

4. Normally there is:
   (a) an increase in basal metabolism during the first trimester, with a decline during the last trimester.
   (b) a decline in the basal metabolism during the first trimester, with an increase during the last trimester.
   (c) a decline in basal metabolism during the last trimester.

5. Cardiac output is increased as much as 40% during:
   (a) the first trimester.
   (b) by the end of the second trimester.
   (c) by the end of the third trimester.

6. The uterus:
   (a) contracts irregularly throughout pregnancy, but causes no discomfort to the mother.
   (b) starts to contract between 16 and 20 weeks' gestation.
   (c) contracts throughout pregnancy but the mother-to-be is usually not aware of this before 16 to 20 weeks' gestation.

7. The nurse knows:
   (a) when a mother-to-be is overfatigued, she can expect the fetus to be much less active.
   (b) when a mother-to-be is overfatigued, she can expect the fetus to exhibit stronger and more frequent movements.
   (c) there is no relation between maternal fatigue and fetal activity.

### Matching
Match the terms in the first column with their appropriate definitions in the second column:

(a) Diastasis of recti muscles — __Hypervolemia during pregnancy

(b) Estrogen — __Contributes to edema of vulva and rectum

(c) Thyroxine — __Weight gain may be a clinical sign of retention of water; associated with a complication of pregnancy

(d) Lactosuria — __Glands that enlarge during pregnancy and control and maintain calcium ions

(e) Toxemia — _Sebaceous glands about the areola

(f) Adrenals — _Due to pressure exerted against the abdominal wall

(g) Transient albumin — _Inhibits secretion of prolactin

(h) Colostrum — _Lobe of gland releasing oxytocin

(i) Neurohypophysis — _Ducts in the breast serving as reservoirs for milk

(j) Pseudoanemia — _First source of nourishment for the infant

(k) Glucosuria — _Due to congestion of renal capillaries

(l) Parathyroids — _Stasis of urinary drainage may result in this complication

(m) Tubercles of Montgomery — _Enlargement of these glands during pregnancy is believed to be associated with skin pigmentation

(n) Prolactin — _May be due to lowered renal threshold

(o) Pyelitis — _Attributed to secretions from mammary glands

(p) Lactiferous — _Helps promote galactopoiesis

(q) Increased venous pressure — _Adenohypophysis secretes this hormone

## SELECTED READINGS

*Physiological aspects*

Beck, A. C., and Taylor, E. Stewart: Obstetrical practice, ed. 8, Baltimore, 1966, The Williams & Wilkins Co., chap. 7.

Eastman, Nicholson J., and Hellman, Louis M., editors: Williams' obstetrics, ed. 13, New York, 1966, Appleton-Century-Crofts, chap. 8.

Guyton, Arthur: Textbook of medical physiology, Philadelphia, 1966, W. B. Saunders Co., chap. 78.

Hytten, Frank, and Leitch, Isabelle: The physiology of human pregnancy, Oxford, 1964, Blackwell Scientific Publications, Ltd., chaps. 9 and 11.

Linde, Shirley: Common problems of pregnancy and what to do about them, Today's Health 46:40, April, 1968.

*Psychological aspects*

Bakwin, Harry, and Bakwin, Ruth: Clinical management of behavior disorders in children, ed. 3, Philadelphia, 1966, W. B. Saunders Co., chap. 24.

Bibring, Grete L.: Recognition of psychological stress often neglected in obstetric care, Hosp. Top. 44:103, Sept., 1966.

Coleman, Arthur D.: Psychological state during first pregnancy, Amer. J. Orthopsychiat. 39:788, Oct., 1969.

Gillman, Robert D.: The dreams of pregnant women and maternal adaptation, Amer. J. Orthopsychiat. 38:688, July, 1968.

Grimm, Elaine: Relationship of personality variables to psychological and physiological reactions throughout pregnancy. In Richardson, Stephen A., and Guttmacher, Alan F., editors: Childbirth—Its social and psychological aspects, Baltimore, 1967, The Williams & Wilkins Co., pp. 21-24.

Horsley, J. Stephen: Psychology of normal pregnancy, Nurs. Times 62:400, March 25, 1966.

Newton, Niles: Maternal emotions, New York, 1955, Paul B. Hoeber, Inc., chap. 4.

Stone, Anthony: Cues to interpersonal distress due to pregnancy, Amer. J. Nurs. 65:88, Nov., 1965.

*Pseudocyesis*

Beck, A. C., and Taylor, E. Stewart: Obstetrical practice, ed. 8, Baltimore, 1966, The Williams &. Wilkins Co., p. 122.

Benson, Ralph: Handbook of obstetrics and gynecology, Los Altos, Calif., 1964, Lange Medical Publications, p. 621.

Davis, M. Edward, and Rubin, Reva: DeLee's obstetrics for nurses, ed. 18, Philadelphia, 1966, W. B. Saunders Co., p. 92.

Grimm, Elaine: Pseudocyesis. In Richardson, Stephen A., and Guttmacher, Alan F., editors: Childbirth: its social and psychological aspects, Baltimore, 1967, The Williams & Wilkins Co., p. 8.

**For student's quick notes:**

Chapter 6

# Nutrition during the period of pregnancy

Every infant has the right to be born healthy. Adequate nutrition contributes to an ideal uterine environment for the developing embryo and fetus. This chapter will aid you in teaching pregnant women how good nutrition influences the outcome of pregnancy, labor, delivery, the puerperium, and the health of the baby. You will learn the nursing responsibilities in counseling women who have problems associated with nutrition and diet planning.

### Results of nutritional studies

1. Growth and development of the infant is influenced by the mother's preconceptional nutrition.
2. Low-protein intake increases the incidence of abortions.
3. A relationship exists between poor nutrition and the occurrence of complications during pregnancy and parturition and the condition of the infant.
4. Good nutrition does have a favorable influence on the outcome of pregnancy.
5. Supplementing the diet with protein and vitamins reduces the incidence of toxemia.

## Nutritional needs during the period of pregnancy

The period of pregnancy demands few changes in the dietary pattern of the woman whose body is well nourished prior to her reproductive age; her body is already prepared to meet the increased physiological requirements during pregnancy and lactation. Her status of preconceptional nutrition is as important for a healthy pregnancy, parturition, and a normal, healthy infant as is her diet during gestation. "In fact, it is believed that the birth weight of the infant is more closely correlated with the weight of the mother at conception than to the weight gain of the mother during pregnancy."* The metabolic adjustments for some women may require simple modifications, but this poses no problem.

Eating for two may be an old wives' adage, depending on how one interprets it; she certainly needs more of the basic foods in *proper proportions*.

### First trimester

What are the pregnant woman's energy requirements during this trimester?

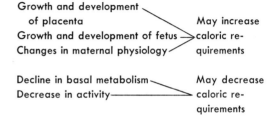

Growth and development of placenta
Growth and development of fetus → May increase caloric requirements
Changes in maternal physiology

Decline in basal metabolism
Decrease in activity → May decrease caloric requirements

*From Guthrie, Helen Andrews: Introductory nutrition, St. Louis, 1967, The C. V. Mosby Co., p. 319.

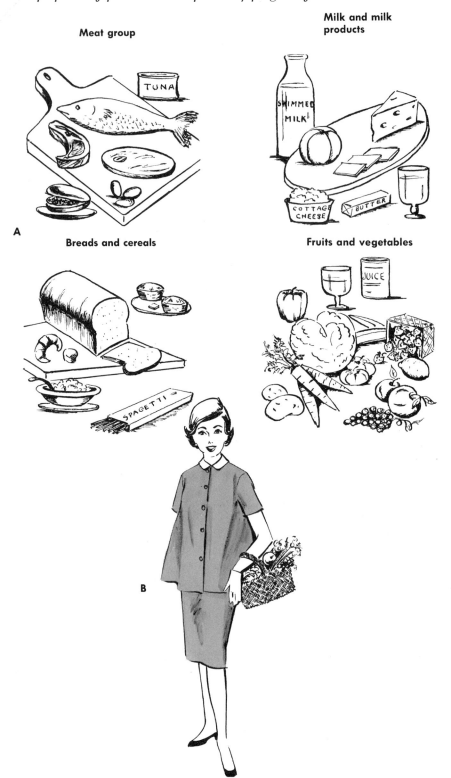

Meat group

Milk and milk products

Breads and cereals

Fruits and vegetables

A

B

**Fig. 6-1. A,** A guide to the wise selection of foods. **B,** A wise selection of food means better health for mother and baby.

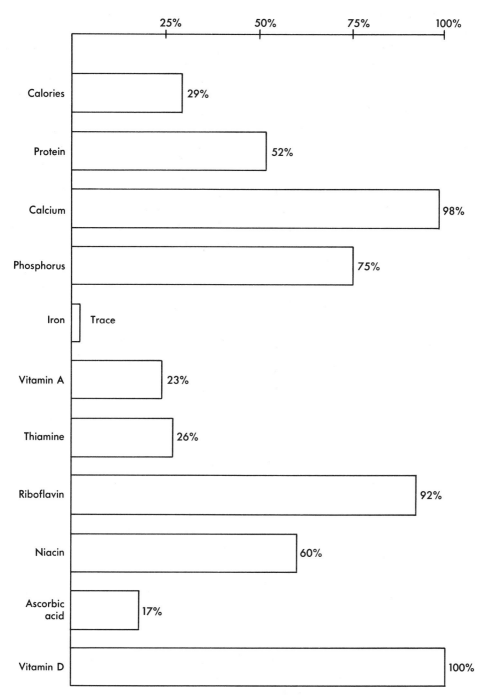

**Fig. 6-2.** Contribution of one quart of fortified milk to nutritive requirements of pregnancy. (Based on Bowes, A, and Church, C.: Food values of portions commonly used, ed. 10, revised by Church, C., and Church, H., Philadelphia, 1966, J. B. Lippincott Co. and on Recommended dietary allowances, 1968 revision, National Academy of Sciences–National Research Council.)

A variety of basic foods and close attention to quality instead of quantity aid the woman in adjusting to the metabolic changes during this trimester. The National Research Council recommends 2,000 calories for the woman between the age of 18 and 35. (See Figs. 6-1 and 6-2.)

### Second trimester

Since two thirds of fetal growth occurs during the second half of pregnancy, the woman needs extra nutrients for the building of fetal tissues and for meeting the increased metabolic needs of her body. Calories should be increased by 10% and proteins increased by 10 grams daily. A daily serving of foods from the meat group, in addition to one or two eggs and selecting liver frequently as the meat of choice, will meet these increased demands. From the vegetable group, leafy vegetables, of course, are excellent sources of vitamins and minerals, especially if eaten raw. They lose some of their vitamins and minerals during long cooking, so a pressure cooker is ideal and might be suggested by the nurse. Citrus fruits, cabbage, turnips, and peppers are abundant in vitamin C, if eaten raw. From the bread group, white enriched bread and whole grain cereals are valuable sources of proteins, minerals, and vitamins. Since the calcium should be increased by 10% and proteins by 10 grams during this trimester, the nurse should review the milk products group with the woman.

### Third trimester

About one half of the total weight increase occurs during this trimester. Extra calories, usually about 200, are permitted. The doctor determines this according to individual energy requirements, age, and weight gain. It must be remembered that although the metabolic rate increases, the mother's activity is somewhat restricted, and that this is the time when the fetus accumulates fat. Care must be taken so that she does not gain too heavily. Protein requirements are the same as in the second

trimester and the calcium requirement is 1,200 mg. daily. Although the calcium requirement of the fetus is greater during the third trimester, the dietary requirement is still 1,200 mg. because as the need increases, the body utilizes the supply more efficiently. (See Fig. 6-3.)

If she does overeat, superfluous fat accumulates and in many instances contributes to a difficult delivery. This is the time when the in-between-meal snacks should consist of raw vegetables and fresh citrus fruits. These supply vitamins without greatly increasing the calories, and they may also aid in relieving constipation, a common complaint during this trimester. Shortly before the end of gestation, many women lose from 1 to 2 pounds.

Some doctors reduce the sodium intake to 0.8 to 1.5 grams daily during pregnancy to help avoid edema. When salt is restricted, the nurse should review with the woman foods to be avoided, such as packaged and canned soups, bacon, packaged lunch meats, and peanut butter. The nurse might also suggest that she check labels on packages of food to note the salt content. If the nurse counsels the woman in the selection of foods low in salt, she is more likely to adhere to the doctor's instructions.

The woman can receive vitamin C in abundance from fresh fruits (citrus). Other fruits, such as bananas and figs, are also good, but when calories are being counted, the nurse needs to counsel the woman as to which fruits are high in carbohydrates.

Beverages are, of course, important; plain water ought certainly to be included. Advise the woman to distribute her fluids throughout the day, rather than after the evening meal, to avoid interrupting her night's sleep. The nurse also needs to remind the woman of the high caloric value of cocoa and malted milk shakes and the high sugar and sodium content in soft-drink beverages.

Alcohol readily crosses the placenta but it is not known to have any deleterious effects on the fetus. The nurse should advise the patient to discuss the use of alcoholic beverages with her doctor because their high caloric content must be considered.

## Problems associated with weight control[2,3]

The woman who is underweight when she conceives or who fails to gain weight during pregnancy is just as great a concern to the doctor as is the obese woman. The nurse need only ask herself, "How can the woman inadequately nourished supply ample nutrients for growth and development of a healthy infant?" One or both suffer!

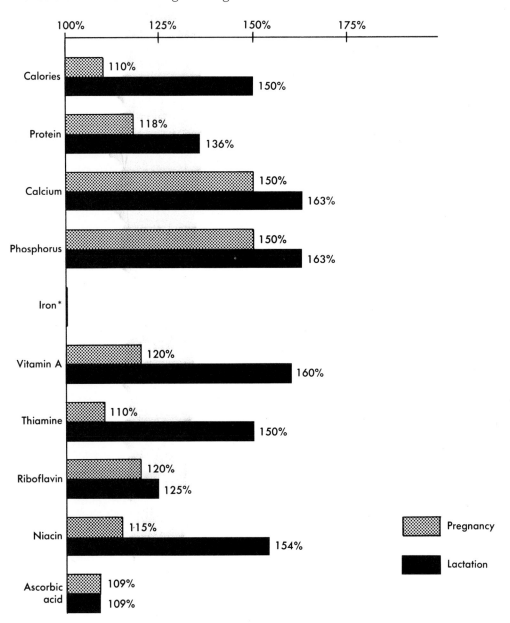

*Iron RDA remains at same high level of 18 mg. during pregnancy and lactation.

**Fig. 6-3.** Nutritive needs during pregnancy and lactation with reference to normal nutritive requirements.

The doctor determines the underlying cause that might be pathological, psychological (women withholding food intentionally), or economical. The woman who is underweight readily experiences fatigue and is more likely to succumb to infections, especially tuberculosis. If the appetite is depressed, the nurse should encourage the woman to try frequent, small meals high in carbohydrates, ample fats, vitamins, and minerals and point out sources of energy foods such as jellies, butter, and mayonnaise. When the nurse points out to the mother that a healthy start in life for her baby depends on her good nutrition, she is more willing to cooperate.

The woman who is overweight at conception will be faced with the problem of

*Text continued on p. 77.*

## PROTEINS

| Function | Food sources |
| --- | --- |
| Protein is the most essential element in the mother's diet. The woman with a healthy body has a better retention of nitrogen in her tissues, and consequently fetal nitrogen demands, which are essential in the formation of healthy tissues and strong bones and in the development of tooth structure, are met. Proteins also influence the length of the fetus, are essential for hormone and enzyme synthesis, and are building blocks for successful lactation. | Proteins are most adequately found in animal sources, whole grains, and legumes. Proteins of animal sources are more efficiently utilized and are excellent sources of iron that aid in the formation of hemoglobin. |

## FATS

| Function | Food sources |
| --- | --- |
| Fats furnish fuel for metabolism, are a good source of calories for the underweight woman, and are essential for absorption of fat-soluble vitamins. Approximately 25% of the total caloric intake should consist of fats. They are needed to meet fat requirements of the fetus; fat deposition takes place during the last trimester. | Fats are mainly found in meats, butter, cream, vegetable oils, egg yolk, and nuts. |

## CARBOHYDRATES

| Function | Food sources |
| --- | --- |
| Carbohydrates are a source of energy for body metabolism. When eaten in excess, they are stored as adipose tissue. | Carbohydrates are found in sugars, starches, all fruits, vegetables, and grains. |

## MINERALS

| Function | Food sources |
|---|---|
| **Calcium** and **phosphorus**[4] are essential for calcification and formation of teeth and for good bone structure and contribute to maintenance of heart beat.<br><br>If the mother knows that the infant's teeth are formed during fetal life and how essential these minerals are in the formation of strong bones, she is more likely to include foods rich in these minerals.<br><br>Extra calcium is essential so that she has rich sources from which the fetus can draw during the latter part of pregnancy. Ingestion of 1.2 grams of calcium daily will allow for adequate storage. Next to protein, calcium and phosphorus have the important function of new tissue formation. Ingestion of 1.2 grams of phosphorus daily will supply ample amount for fetal needs. | One quart of milk furnishes over three fourths of the day's calcium requirement. The recommended daily amount is 1.2 grams when vitamin D intake is adequate; remember that this vitamin is essential for absorption of calcium and phosphorus.<br><br>Milk, cheddar cheese, and green leafy vegetables are the main sources of calcium.<br><br>Organ meats are the richest sources of phosphorus; other sources are whole grain products, legumes, nuts, milk, and eggs. |
| **Iron** enables our red blood cells to carry oxygen. Most women start pregnancy with limited stores of iron, and it is the belief of many doctors that all pregnant women should be advised to take iron supplements, especially when there are signs of anemia, for women who have closely spaced pregnancies, or where the woman has a multiple pregnancy. Absorption is higher during the last trimester, attributed to increased transferrin. Recommended daily allowance is 18 mg. per day. | Iron is found in organ meats (liver and kidney), leafy vegetables, dried fruits, egg yolk, and whole grains. Iron is stored in the liver of the newborn during the last trimester. If the mother's diet contains sufficient iron, the fetus will have enough to supply his needs until foods other than milk are ingested. |
| **Sodium** and **potassium** aid in the maintenance of fluid balance. | Sodium and potassium are found in vegetables, milk, and meats. |
| Dietary **iodine** needs to be increased during pregnancy for added demands of the thyroid gland. Inadequate intake may result in simple goiter in the mother and baby. | Iodized salt and seafoods are sources for iodine. |

## FAT-SOLUBLE VITAMINS

| Function | Food sources |
|---|---|
| **Provitamins A** (carotenes) are converted in the body to vitamin A and are essential for growth, maintenance of epithelial tissues, and tooth development. An additional 1,000 I. U. daily is the recommended amount for the second and third trimesters. | The A group is found in both dark green and yellow vegetables. One quart of whole milk furnishes one fourth of the woman's dietary allowance. Preformed vitamin A is found in egg yolk, butter, and oleo. |
| The **D group** promotes growth and proper mineralization of bones and teeth; 400 I. U. are recommended daily to promote utilization of calcium and phosphorus. These vitamins are passed from mother's body and stored in fetus and are also stored in breasts in preparation for lactation; this protects infant against rickets. | The D group is found only sparsely in foods such as fish, liver, and eggs. One quart of fortified milk supplies recommended amount and vitamin D is generated by sunlight. Synthetic supplements are available. |
| The relation of **vitamin E** to nutrition has not been clearly defined; the requirements are believed to be adequately met by a normal diet. | Wheat germ, nuts, legumes, and eggs are rich in vitamin E. |
| The **K group** is essential for formation of the proteins, prothrombin, and fibrin and for normal clotting of the blood. | The K group is found in green leafy vegetables, egg yolk, soybean, liver, lettuce, kale, and spinach. |

## WATER-SOLUBLE VITAMINS

| Function | Food sources |
|---|---|
| The **B complex group** is essential for chemical changes in the tissues, red blood cell formation, and nerve stability and is an active constituent of enzyme system. | Vitamin B complex is found in liver, yeast, wheat germ, legumes, whole grains, cereals, and milk. |
| **Ascorbic acid** influences the formation of hemoglobin, healthy bones, and connective tissues and promotes resistance to infection. | Ascorbic acid is found in citrus fruits and green leafy vegetables, preferably uncooked. |

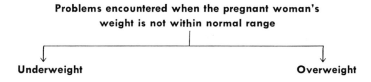

**Problems encountered when the pregnant woman's weight is not within normal range**

**Underweight**

Failure to gain an average amount of weight, especially during the first and second trimesters, is believed to be one factor contributing to premature births. The woman is usually anemic and complains of fatigue. She is less likely to develop toxemia, but if it does occur, it tends to be more severe.

**Overweight**

The woman is more likely to show glycosemia, hypertension, and increased incidence of toxemia and to have difficult labors.

keeping her weight stable or losing excess pounds. The doctor decides whether the patient is overweight and restricts her caloric intake as he sees fit. Seldom is the restriction less than a 1,500 calorie diet. With a greater restriction there is the danger of inadequate retention of proteins. The nurse must remember that for the obese woman it is not just the fats that must be reduced; carbohydrates and proteins in excess of body needs can be stored as fat deposition. Her function is to reinforce the doctor's instructions and to counsel the woman in selection of foods to best meet the doctor's recommendations.

### The nurse counsels on nutrition[5,8]

In counseling women on nutrition and diet planning, the nurse needs to take the following into account: (1) preferences in cooking, (2) the budget, and (3) the multiplicity of factors contributing to family food habits.

Persons who have strong feelings about food are not going to be flexible to suggestions. If the woman was forced to eat certain foods as a child, she very likely has an aversion for them now and should never be made to feel guilty about her food habits.

As nurses, we are all too familiar with advice such as "limit your salt intake," "cut down on fats," "add vitamins," "drink more milk, it is the most nearly perfect food," and "milk contains protein and you do need protein." Mothers must get tired of our dietary advice because at times it is repetitious and often confusing. While one nurse tells her to drink plenty of milk, another informs her that large quantities of milk may predispose to muscle tetany due to increased amounts of phosphorus absorbed from the milk.

Handing the woman a sheet of printed instructions that include a list of certain foods and telling her that she needs to add extra vitamins and minerals to her diet has little meaning for her and is certainly not the answer. If it is important to discuss calories, then we should be able to define the meaning and function of them for her; if we use a printed form for a particular diet, then we take time to explain and interpret the information so that she may fit it into her customary food patterns. Otherwise the back of the form will likely be used for the *usual* weekly grocery list.

Most of your opportunity for teaching and counseling will take place in the prenatal clinic. It is with this group of women that you can offer guidance in wise spending, which will perhaps result in a better selection of foods while still maintaining the minimum daily requirements.

We learn from mothers that their chief stumbling block in trying to better their nutrition is convincing their husbands that there is a need to change the selection and

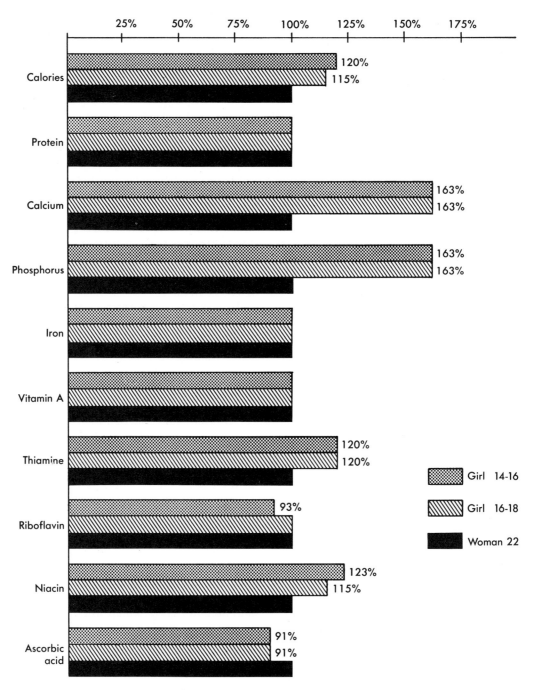

**Fig. 6-4.** Nutritive needs of teen-age girl as compared with needs of adult woman.

perhaps the preparation of foods. He, too, has his cherished foods and is accustomed to having his wife prepare them for him in a certain way. The manner in which the nurse relates the importance of the qualitative aspects of the diet in balanced proportions and how it is related to the growth and development of his unborn child may be the deciding factor that convinces the prospective father to follow the doctor's suggestions.

The nurse should counsel the woman to supplement her diet with vitamins only as prescribed by the doctor. One can take too many vitamins, such as an excess of vitamin D that causes abnormal calcium deposits in fetal bones.[1]

One of the outstanding concerns of all young mothers during pregnancy is weight control. She no longer accepts obesity as the price for having a baby and consequently has a conflict between increased appetite and weight control. The pregnant woman need not "starve" herself or go hungry if she knows how to plan the proper distribution of quality foods. Here is where she may need counseling on nutrition because she must practice moderation.

There is particular concern for the young, immature woman undergoing her first pregnancy. The girl who conceives during her early and midteens is likely to be poorly nourished because of erratic diets and therefore is not prepared to meet the demands involved in the physiological adjustments her body must make.[6,7] (See Fig. 6-4.)

Dietary habits of families tend to remain relatively constant. If the adolescent girl does break from this tradition, it is to conform to patterns of her group, and in the United States this means popularity and a slender figure at almost any price. This occurs at a time when nutritional requirements are high.

We cannot ignore the fact that a healthy body contributes to emotional adjustments. The emotional instability of this age group, plus the tremendous emotional adjustment that must be made to a pregnancy, may

contribute to the low retention levels of the essential nutrients, especially calcium, vitamin C, and iron. There is danger, too, that the proteins will be used for energy rather than for growth. Even though the adolescent group is least amenable to nutrition education, if what we have to offer is well presented, it is more likely to be understood, and if understood, accepted.

## Pica

Pica practice means that one ingests quantities of nonfood substances such as laundry starch, clay, plaster, toothpaste, and coal. Pica tends to be a cultural habit found almost exclusively among Negro women. Superstitious beliefs that ingestion of large amounts of starch or clay during pregnancy will reduce nausea and vomiting and produce beautiful babies are passed from mothers to their daughters. Ingestion of large amounts of dry starch blocks the absorption of iron. Studies show that there is a relation between anemia and pica; the hemoglobin level is considerably lower in those women who engage in this practice.

**STUDY QUESTIONS**

*Multiple choice*

1. The nurse knows that:
   (a) half of the fetal calcium deposits are made during the last month of gestation.
   (b) the fetus stores calcium equally during the second and third trimesters.
   (c) provided the woman is in good health at the beginning of pregnancy, her calcium stores will be adequate for fetal demands.
2. Women in poor nutritional status at the time of conception are likely:
   (a) to develop symptoms as pregnancy progresses.
   (b) to deliver prematurely.
   (c) to deliver postmaturely.
      1. a and c    2. a and b    3. c only
3. Approximately 25% of the pregnant woman's caloric intake should be made up of:
   (a) fats.
   (b) proteins.
   (c) carbohydrates.
   (d) minerals and vitamins.
4. When caloric intake is restricted to less than 1,500 calories per day, there is the danger of:
   (a) loss of too much weight.
   (b) inadequate retention of proteins.
   (c) inadequate utilization of carbohydrates.

5. Protein requirements during the third trimester are:
   (a) the same as in the second trimester.
   (b) increased by 10%.
   (c) increased by 10 grams daily.

## Matching

Match the terms in the first column with their appropriate definitions in the second column:

(a) Abortions —— Necessary for folic acid metabolism

(b) Fats —— Protein intake should be increased by 10 grams daily during this trimester

(c) Phosphorus —— About one half of the total weight increase occurs during this trimester

(d) Vitamin D —— Essential for absorption of fat-soluble vitamins

(e) Third trimester —— Low-protein intake is said to increase incidence of this complication

(f) Toxemia —— Essential for synthesis of hormones and enzymes

(g) Proteins —— A too high content of this mineral in the tissues may cause neuromuscular irritability

(h) Vitamin C —— Excessive gain in weight increases incidence of this complication

(i) Second trimester —— Essential for absorption of calcium

## REFERENCES

1. Excess vitamin D in pregnancy, Nurs. Mirror **126**:42, April 5, 1968.
2. Flowers, Charles: How to persuade pregnant women to diet, Consultant **7**:20, July-Aug., 1967.
3. Glenn, Morton: A new look at dieting, weight control: safety "must" for all mothers-to-be, Family Circle **70**:19, May, 1967.
4. Grollman, Arthur: Clinical endocrinology and its physiologic basis, Philadelphia, 1964, J. B. Lippincott Co., chap. 10.
5. Heap, Beth: Sodium restricted diets. In Brennan, Ruth, editor: Nutrition, Dubuque, Iowa, 1967, William C. Brown Co., pp. 174-179.
6. Leverton, R. M.: The paradox of teen-age nutrition, J. Amer. Diet. Ass. **53**:13, July, 1968.
7. Mitchell, Barbara, Huenemann, Ruth L., Shapiro, Leona R., and Hampton, Mary C.: Food and eating practices of teen-agers, J. Amer. Diet. Ass. **53**:17, July, 1968.
8. Morris, Ena: How does a nurse teach nutrition to patients. In Brennan, Ruth, editor: Nutrition, Dubuque, Iowa, 1967, William C. Brown Co., pp. 42-49.

## SELECTED READINGS

Bogert, L. Jean, Briggs, George M., and Calloway, Doris Howes: Nutrition and physical fitness, ed. 8, Philadelphia, 1966, W. B. Saunders Co., chap. 21.

Brandt, M. Bertha: Nutrition in pregnancy. In Lytle, Nancy, editor: Maternal health nursing, Dubuque, Iowa, 1967, William C. Brown Co., pp. 66-80.

Brewer, Thomas H.: Worry less about total weight gain in pregnancy—more about malnutrition, Consultant **7**:18, Nov.-Dec., 1967.

Eastman, Nicholson J., and Jackson, Esther: Weight relationships in pregnancy, Obstet. Gynec. Survey **23**:1003, Nov., 1968.

Greenhill, J. P., editor: Obstetrics, ed. 13, Philadelphia, 1965, W. B. Saunders Co., chap. 8.

Hillman, Robert W., and Hall, J. Edward: Nutrition in pregnancy. In Wohl, Michael G., and Goodhart, Robert S., editors: Modern nutrition in health and disease, ed. 3, Philadelphia, 1964, Lea & Febiger, part 3, chap. 36.

Hytten, Frank E.: The physiology of human pregnancy, Oxford, 1964, Blackwell Scientific Publications, Ltd., chaps. 9 and 14.

Illsley, Raymond: Maternal nutrition. In Richardson, Stephen, and Guttmacher, Alan, editors: Childbearing: its social and psychological aspects, Baltimore, 1967, The Williams & Wilkins Co., pp. 122-125.

Keele, Cyril A., and Neil, Eric, editors: Samson Wright's applied physiology, ed. 11, New York, 1965, Oxford University Press, Inc., pp. 415-434.

Mayer, Jean: Some aspects of the relation of nutrition and pregnancy. In Brennan, Ruth, editor: Nutrition, Dubuque, Iowa, 1967, William C. Brown Co., pp. 56-64.

Montagu, M. F. Ashley: Life before birth, New York, 1964, New American Library, Inc., p. 32.

Montagu, M. F. Ashley: Prenatal influences, Springfield, Ill., 1962, Charles C Thomas, Publisher, pp. 57-112.

Rubin, Alan: Nutrition during pregnancy and lactation, Child Family **5**:3, Summer, 1966.

Scrimshaw, Nevin: Nutrition functions of maternal and child health programs in technically underdeveloped areas. In Brennan, Ruth, editor: Nutrition, Dubuque, Iowa, 1967, William C. Brown Co., pp. 50-55.

Smith, Moyna E.: Less nonsense about nutrition, Nurs. Times **63**:345, March 17, 1967.

Stevens, Harriet: Nutritive value of the diets of medically indigent pregnant women, J. Amer. Diet Ass. **50**:290, April, 1967.

White, Hilda S.: Inorganic elements in weighed diets of girls and young women. Minerals in young women's diets, J. Amer. Diet. Ass. **55**:38, July, 1969.

Williams, Sue Rodwell: Nutrition and diet therapy, St. Louis, 1969, The C. V. Mosby Co., chap. 17.

*Pica practices*

Coltman, Charles A. Jr.: Pagophagia and iron lack, J.A.M.A. **207**:513, Jan. 20, 1969.

Dunston, Beverly: Pica practices, Nurs. Sci. **1**:32, April, 1963.

Elliott, Jane: Pica and pregnancy. In Rains, Pearl, editor: The nursing clinics of North America, Philadelphia, 1968, W. B. Saunders Co., p. 299.

Misenhimer, Harold R.: Food cravings during pregnancy, Redbook **131**:47, Aug., 1968.

Pica and iron deficiency, J.A.M.A. **207**:552, Jan. 20, 1969.

Pregnant women find white clay a delicacy, Today's Health **47**:19, Jan., 1969.

**For student's quick notes:**

# Chapter 7

# Minor discomforts and complications associated with the period of pregnancy

Although one of our nursing objectives is to see the woman through her pregnancy in good health, minor discomforts do occur. This chapter discusses the etiology and management of these discomforts.

Many women relate that they go through pregnancy feeling "just fine" or that they "never enjoyed better health." If the woman understands something about the various physiological changes and practices good daily health habits, most of the discomforts can be kept at a minimum. The opinion has been expressed, however, that discomforts tend to be exaggerated among women who are carrying "unplanned" babies.

## Mild nausea and vomiting[1]

Mild nausea with vomiting is one of the most common disturbances during early pregnancy. Many theories of its etiology have been offered: (1) allergy to the high gonadotropin level produced by the trophoblasts, (2) decreased liver glycogen reserve, (3) lack of pyridoxine, (4) diminished gastric motility, and (5) nausea aggravated by emotional disturbances, called "psychological" morning sickness.

Nausea usually occurs early in the first trimester and subsides by the end of 12 weeks. The nausea is usually bothersome when the stomach is empty, that is, in the mornings as the woman awakens. Occasionally it persists throughout the day. She is usually advised to keep dry crackers by her bedside and to nibble on them before arising. Acidosis tends to develop at night when the sugar intake is low. Sucking on a piece of hard candy before arising may counteract the acidosis. She is then usually able to tolerate a light breakfast. If the nausea occurs during the day, frequent small meals, eaten slowly, are more likely to be tolerated. She should avoid foods distasteful to her during this time.

If the nausea and vomiting continue, normal metabolic processes may be disturbed and a serious complication, *hyperemesis gravidarum*, may result. You will learn about this in Chapter 9.

From reports of some obstetricians it would seem that the incidence of nausea and vomiting is declining. Women have more knowledge concerning pregnancy, and through prenatal care many of the psychogenic stimuli have been eliminated. Women are not as fearful of labor and delivery; thus they can approach childbirth with relatively less fear than did their mothers.

## Backache

Backache is usually due to muscle strain because of alterations in posture as the body maintains balance. The nurse can advise the woman early in her pregnancy about the importance of good posture, to squat when picking up objects from the floor, and of the proper way to position herself when sitting on a chair. A sagging mattress can cause prolonged flexion of the back and may also be a cause of early morning backache. Placing a long board directly beneath the mattress adds support so well-appreciated by the woman whose rest is disturbed because of backache. It should be remembered that backache is sometimes an early sympton of bladder infection. These "tips" can avoid added strain on back muscles and may prevent much of the discomfort. (See Fig. 7-1.)

### Constipation

Constipation is more likely to occur in women who do not have regular bowel habits. Pregnancy then intensifies the condition, since (1) activity is decreased, (2) muscles lose tonicity because the hormone relaxin slows peristalsis, and (3) during the latter weeks, pressure of the presenting part causes congestion of the lower bowel.

Measures that the nurse may suggest to the patient include (1) training the bowels

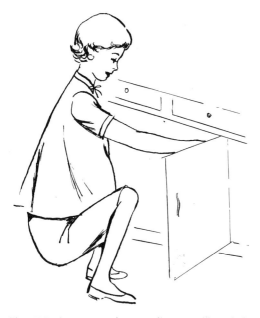

**Fig. 7-1.** Squatting relieves pull on muscles of the back and helps maintain balance.

to act regularly, (2) increasing roughage in the diet, (3) drinking a glass of fruit juice on arising in the morning, and (4) including fruits such as figs, dates, and prunes in the diet. The nurse should caution the woman against the use of laxatives or enemas without first consulting the doctor. Mineral oil is contraindicated, since it interferes with the absorption of vitamins and nutrients, unless taken at bedtime.

### Palpitation and dyspnea

Not infrequently some women become alarmed because they experience a sudden bounding palpitation of the heart and shortness of breath. This is usually the response of the heart and blood vessels to meeting the metabolic demands of the developing fetus. In most instances this does not mean that the adjustment is not efficient, but nevertheless the woman should be advised to mention it to her doctor. Since the gravid uterus fills most of the abdominal cavity, you can readily understand how this restricts easy breathing. This is bothersome until "lightening" occurs, when the patient feels some relief. Some women tell us they sleep better if propped up by pillows, others prefer lying flat or on their side in a Sims' position. The woman should, of course, assume the position most comfortable for her.

### Edema

There are a number of reasons why the pregnant woman experiences periods of edema: (1) adrenal and placental hormones tend to favor retention of sodium and water, (2) prolonged standing increases venous pressure, (3) circular garters constrict circulation, and (4) nutritional edema (deficiency in protein) may be a contributing factor. Edema is more frequent in the lower extremities, especially during the second and third trimesters. The woman should be advised to avoid any constricting clothing and to plan for frequent rest periods, during which the legs can be elevated. If the doctor orders diuretics for the patient and limits her intake of salt, the nurse should help the patient in planning her selection of foods and preparation of meals. See Chapter 8, edema associated with toxemia.

### Epistaxis

All the mucous membranes in the body become congested during pregnancy as the result of hormonal activity. Frequent or infrequent episodes of nosebleeds may occur. The woman needs to be assured that this is nothing to worry about but to mention it to her doctor.

### Faintness and syncope

A feeling of "lightheadedness" may be a sign of anemia or, perhaps, of hypoglycemia and should, of course, be reported to the doctor. Since emotions can influence circulation, it may be no more than a nervous manifestation.

### Fatigue[3,4,6]

When fatigue occurs early in pregnancy, it is believed to be related to release of hormones. Late in pregnancy the added weight, of course, would contribute to the tired feeling.

The tired, pregnant woman is not necessarily lazy; she needs more rest. Early to bed, late to rise may be a good pattern; however, sleep during the day might cause insomnia at night. For these women, periods of relaxation and quiet can do wonders to relieve fatigue. Be it sleep or rest, it should be planned according to each woman's needs.

If the nurse explains why her body requires more sleep and rest, the woman may be relieved of the guilt feelings she may have about being lazy or losing interest in her family. Fatigue or being sleepy during the day may also be a sign of anemia and heightens the risk of toxemia. The woman should certainly discuss this with her doctor. Rest may prevent premature labor!

### Gingivitis

Turgescence of the gums may cause irritation of the gingivae that, along with changes in salivary pH, may lead to bleeding gums and dental caries. Gingivitis is sometimes attributed to dietary deficiencies, particularly vitamin C.

### Hemorrhoids

Hemorrhoids are varicosities in the anal region; they are the result of increased pressure and dilatation of the hemorrhoidal veins and of pressure of the enlarging uterus obstructing venous return. Swelling or thrombosis of these veins causes pain and itching. They are certainly aggravated by constipation. The nurse might suggest that the woman rest in the Sims' position several times a day; this lessens pressure on the congested veins and does offer relief (Fig. 7-2). Treatment may be a sitz bath, witch hazel compresses, anal suppositories, or anesthetic ointments.

### Leukorrhea

Leukorrhea is an increase in normal physiological secretions from the vaginal canal, or it may be an indication of local disease. An increase of estrogen, of blood supply to the vaginal epithelium, and of secretions from the cervical glands all contribute to this annoying discharge. Women with leukorrhea do not usually have pruritus unless they have poor personal hygiene habits.

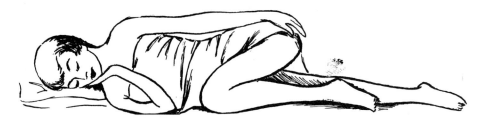

**Fig. 7-2.** Sims' position is comfortable for the pregnant woman to assume. Lessens pressure on congested veins.

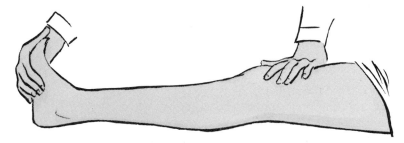

**Fig. 7-3.** Method of relieving leg cramps.

When such is the case, the nurse should certainly instruct the patient concerning vulval hygiene. The following complaints voiced by the patient should alert the nurse to refer the patient to the doctor: (1) pruritus, (2) purulent discharge with foul odor, (3) edema of the vulva, and (4) burning on urination. The doctor will take smears for the diagnosis of vaginal infections such as trichomoniasis or candidiasis. Metronidazole (Flagyl), nystatin (Mycostatin), and aqueous gentian violet have all been found to be dependable as therapeutic agents.

### Muscle cramps

Muscle cramps occur more in the lower extremities. The most probable cause has been attributed to a disturbed ratio of calcium and phosphorus, with serum calcium reduced and serum phosphorus increased. If the woman complains of leg cramps, the nurse can have her lie on her back and extend the affected leg, while the nurse places pressure on the patient's knee with her left hand, and with the right hand, forcing the toes upward; or she may knead the affected muscle. (See Fig. 7-3.)

Vitamins B and D are sometimes ordered by the doctor; aluminum hydroxide gel (Amphojel or Creamalin), a.c., is also ordered to remove phosphorus from the intestinal tract.

### Pruritus[5]

Pruritus is a disorder causing much distress due to intense itching sensation. The constant irritation from scratching causes areas of the skin to become excoriated. Abdominal pruritus may be due to stretching of the abdominal wall. Generalized pruritus is attributed to liver dysfunction or products of fetal metabolism that are foreign to the maternal organism. Pruritus usually starts during the last trimester and disappears soon after delivery. It is known that the same condition occurs in subsequent pregnancies. Methods of treatment are (1) ultraviolet irradiation, (2) antipruritic medications, and (3) a diet high in proteins and low in fats, with adequate B complex vitamins. The patient is usually instructed to avoid alcoholic beverages and highly seasoned foods.

### Ptyalism[2]

Ptyalism, or hypersalivation, is caused by hyperactivity of the parotid glands. It has been cited that the etiology involves an emotional factor. It may continue throughout pregnancy and then disappears during the early puerperium. It is likely to occur in subsequent pregnancies. Astringent mouthwashes are sometimes recommended by the doctor.

### Pyrosis or heartburn

Pyrosis is a burning sensation along the esophagus from the regurgitation of acidic gastric contents into the esophagus. The cause, it is believed, is decreased motility of the gastrointestinal tract and upward displacement of the stomach. It tends to occur about the third or fourth month, increases in severity as pregnancy advances, and is aggravated by lying down. Women

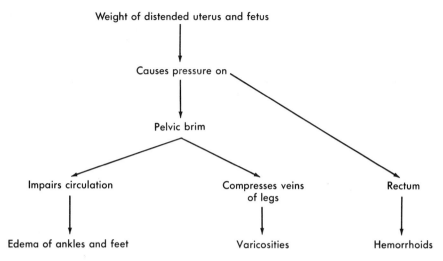

Weight of distended uterus and fetus

↓

Causes pressure on

↓

Pelvic brim

Impairs circulation          Compresses veins of legs          Rectum

↓                                    ↓                              ↓

Edema of ankles and feet          Varicosities                   Hemorrhoids

**Fig. 7-4.** Weight of distended uterus and fetus, causing edema of ankles and feet, varicosities, hemorrhoids.

with heartburn are advised to eat small, frequent meals slowly, to avoid fried foods, and not to lie down directly after eating. A "small" amount of fatty food, such as butter or cream, taken 15 to 30 minutes *before* the meal will stimulate the flow of gastric juices and inhibit secretion of acid in the stomach. The nurse should mention good posture, since it may contribute to relieving congestion of the organs. Drugs such as a mixture of aluminum hydroxide gel and magnesium hydroxide (Maalox) or aluminum hydroxide and magnesium trisilicate (Gelusil) may be ordered by the doctor to reduce gastric acidity.

### Varices

Varices may be congenital or acquired. During pregnancy they occur more in the lower extremities and in some women extend into the groin and affect the veins of the genitalia. They tend to become more extensive in succeeding pregnancies. Because of a weakness of the vascular walls, they cannot support the pressure from the increased intrapelvic flow of blood. The veins become inflamed and painful and the woman complains of fatigue and pressure. (See Fig. 7-4.)

Elastic Ace bandages may be ordered by the doctor to compress the varices. If the

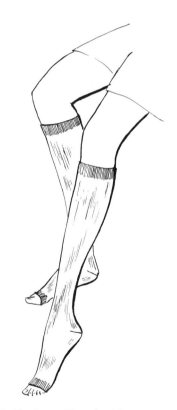

**Fig. 7-5.** Elastic stockings furnish support and comfort.

patient has edema along with the varices, the nurse should instruct her to apply the Ace bandages before she gets out of bed in the morning and at no time to wear circular garters. (See Fig. 7-5.)

Women with varices should avoid standing for long intervals and take frequent rest periods to elevate the legs. Placing the legs in an upright position for a few minutes several times a day facilitates drainage of blood from the lower extremities, since blood flow in the lower limbs is slowed as pregnancy progresses.

If the doctor orders leg exercises, the nurse should be prepared to reinforce his instructions by going over the exercises with the woman. If the patient has varices along the leg, the doctor may order the elastic Ace bandage or elastic stockings to be applied before the patient is taken to the delivery room to prevent trauma while the legs are in stirrups. Trauma to the veins predisposes to thrombophlebitis. Care and gentleness must be exercised while placing the legs in and out of the stirrups. The legs should be elevated and lowered together slowly.

Vitamin C is believed to reduce size of varicosities, to prevent bleeding, and to be concerned in formation of collagen and endothelium of the blood vessels.

**STUDY QUESTIONS**

*Multiple choice*

1. Good posture is a means of preventing and relieving backache. The nurse may suggest the following for relief of added strain on back muscles:
   (a) to pick up objects from the floor, advance one foot forward and then squat.
   (b) wear a girdle if you are accustomed to doing so.
   (c) distribute your weight evenly on both feet.
   (d) all of these.
2. Women with heartburn should be advised to:
   (a) lie down for 30 minutes after eating.
   (b) eat three substantial meals with no in-between-snacks.
   (c) take a small amount of fatty foods such as butter or cream 30 minutes a.c.
   (d) take small, frequent meals and avoid fried foods.
   1. a and b      2. c and d      3. d only

3. The doctor advised a mother-to-be to purchase elastic stockings because of her varices. You would tell her to:
   (a) put them on before getting out of bed in the morning.
   (b) put them on after she has walked around for awhile.
   (c) remove them for short intervals during the day.

*True or false*

(T) (F)  1. Carbohydrates are more easily retained by nauseated mothers-to-be than are proteins.
(T) (F)  2. Thoracic breathing predominates throughout pregnancy.
(T) (F)  3. Varices may be congenital.
(T) (F)  4. Trauma to varices predisposes to thrombophlebitis.
(T) (F)  5. Walking is the best and safest form of exercise.
(T) (F)  6. Fatigue early in pregnancy is normal and may be related to release of hormones.
(T) (F)  7. Body tone is improved by supervised prenatal exercises.
(T) (F)  8. Pressure edema is more marked in the mornings than in the evenings.
(T) (F)  9. Calcium deficiencies may contribute to edema.
(T) (F) 10. Palpitation of the heart occurring in healthy pregnant women is attributed to sympathetic nervous disturbance.
(T) (F) 11. The objective of prenatal exercises is to minimize pain and length of labor.

**REFERENCES**

1. Horsley, J. Stephen: The psychology of normal pregnancy, Nurs. Times **62:**400, March 25, 1966.
2. Jacobs, Walter H., and Janowitz, Henry D.: Ptyalism. In Rovinsky, Joseph, editor: Medical, surgical and gynecologic complications of pregnancy, Baltimore, 1965, The Williams & Wilkins Co., p. 177.
3. Montagu, M. F. Ashley: Prenatal influences, Springfield, Ill., 1962, Charles C Thomas, Publisher, pp. 217-223.
4. Norris, A. S.: The tired mother, Child Family **5:**11, Summer, 1966.
5. Rothman, Stephen, and Shapiro, Arthur: Pruritus during pregnancy. In MacBryde, Cyril, editor: Applied pathologic physiology and clinical interpretation, ed. 4, Philadelphia, 1964, J. B. Lippincott Co., p. 911.
6. Williams, Barbara: Sleep needs during the maternity cycle, Nurs. Outlook **15:**53, Feb., 1967.

**SELECTED READINGS**

Eastman, Nicholson J., and Hellman, Louis M., editors: Williams' obstetrics, ed. 13, New York, 1966, Appleton-Century-Crofts, chap. 12.

Greenhill, J. P., editor: Obstetrics, ed. 13, Philadelphia, 1965, W. B. Saunders Co., chap. 29.

Keith, Russel P.: The expectant mother, Redbook **127**:38, June, 1966.

Mercantini, Edward S.: Skin problems during pregnancy, Consultant **6**:24, June, 1966.

**For student's quick notes:**

# Chapter 8

# High-risk pregnancies

Despite the fact that much has been learned about the internal and external environment of both mother and fetus, which has greatly increased the likelihood of a successful outcome of pregnancy, complications do occur; some are avoidable through prenatal care, others are not.

## Metabolic complications
### Hyperemesis gravidarum

In Chapter 7 you studied about nausea and vomiting during pregnancy. Hyperemesis differs only in degree. Years ago this condition caused death; today curative methods are instituted when the condition is still incipient.

Hyperemesis gravidarum is defined as aggravated, excessive physiological nausea and vomiting. The cause is unknown but many theories have been advanced; for example, it has been thought (1) that high levels of chorionic gonadotropic hormone produced by the trophoblasts may contribute, since the incidence of nausea and vomiting occurs and disappears with the increase and decrease of this hormone between the sixth and twelfth week, (2) that degenerative products result from the function of the trophoblasts as they invade the endometrium, or (3) that psychic factors such as fear of the responsibilities involved in motherhood or loss of independence, which may cause conflicts within, may affect the normal function of endocrine and autonomic nervous system and result in the sensation of nausea and vomiting.

Excessive vomiting results in the disturbance of metabolites, dehydration, electrolyte depletion, and an unstable acid-base balance. Since the woman is unable to retain food or liquid, she may lose as much as 7 pounds in a week and the blood may show hemoconcentration; depletion of carbohydrates leads to ketosis. Diagnosis is usually made on the presence of acetone and diacetic acid in the urine and blood.

*Treatment and nursing responsibilities.* Hospitalization itself may be a therapeutic response; the change in atmosphere, the desire to "get away from it all," and the genuine interest of the nurse may all contribute toward recovery.

Treatment is to replace lost fluids and maintain electrolyte balance when oral feedings are not tolerated. The nurse should attach no importance to the woman's episodes of vomiting. She must handle the patient firmly, but with due sympathy. She can assure her that the doctor's regimen of therapy is certain to correct the condition. With continuous intravenous hydration along with sedatives, the woman is usually ready in a few days to tolerate oral feedings. The amount of intravenous fluids is determined by the amount of oral fluids retained and urine excreted. Accurate intake and output is important. The daily requirement is usually between 2,000 and 3,000 ml., supplemented with vitamins, especially the B complex. Included in the therapy is the aim to keep the patient quiet. Compazine, 10 mg., intramuscularly three times a day, or Compazine suppositories are sometimes ordered.

When the patient stops vomiting and develops the desire to eat, oral feedings are reinstituted. The nurse should encourage the patient to select foods palatable to her and see that they are served in small portions as frequently as she can tolerate them. Lukewarm liquids tend to be nauseating; therefore the nurse must see that hot foods are served piping hot and that cold liquids are iced.

### Toxemia

Toxemia is a "specific" hypertensive disease of pregnancy, arbitrarily divided into preeclampsia and eclampsia; the latter involves convulsions and coma. Toxemia is a disease of history; Hippocrates made reference to eclampsia, and Vassili Stroganoff, in 1897, introduced his treatment by means of quietude, sedatives, and purgatives. The onset may be insidious or abrupt. The major manifestations of toxemia are retention of salt and water. It is characterized by (1) hypertension, (2) edema, and (3) proteinuria. These manifestations develop during the last trimester (after the twenty-fourth week). An exception is that preeclampsia may occur early in pregnancy as a complicating disease in women with vascular or kidney disease or hydatidiform mole. It may occur during the early puerperium and is then called postpartum toxemia. Both preeclampsia and eclampsia are sometimes called eclamptogenic toxemia. The fact that it does occur with hydatidiform mole shows that the fetus is not essential for its development or progress. (See Figs. 8-1 and 8-2.)

*Etiology.* Although various hypotheses concerning the etiology of toxemia have evolved from years of research, it remains the baffling problem in obstetrics. Theories have been advanced such as (1) impairment of uteroplacental circulation; (2) hormonal mechanism (increased amounts of estrogen and progesterone secreted by the placenta may have adverse effects on kidney function and on edema); (3) stressful factors; (4) increased maternal-fetal corticosteroids; (5) maternal absorption of toxins from the placenta; (6) diet, especially one high in carbohydrates and salt and low in protein; and (7) deleterious substances in the blood.

*Preeclampsia and a psychogenic component.* One may read that emotional stress seems to have a predisposition to toxemia. Histories of many women with preeclampsia show emotional instability. This stress is believed to contribute to generalized arteriolar spasms.

*Incidence.* Factors known to influence the incidence of toxemia are (1) socioeconomic, (2) multiple gestation, (3) age, (4) parity, and (5) race.

Approximately 5% of all pregnant women become toxemic. It occurs more frequently in the primigravida (especially the very young) and in those over 30 years of age and is more frequent in the Negro. It is also higher in the economically underprivileged and the poorly nourished segment of population.

Six to 7% of pregnant women in the United States develop toxemia.

↓

In 5% of these women the preeclampsia progresses to eclampsia.

↓

In the United States 1.6% of the eclamptic patients die.

The complications known to predispose to toxemia are (1) diabetes, with vascular or renal involvement, (2) acute hydramnios, (3) hydatidiform mole, (4) obesity, and (5) essential hypertension.

### Criteria for diagnosis

*Hypertension.* Hypertension occurs in about 5% of all gravid women in our country. It is said to be present when the resting blood pressure is above 140/90. However, a blood pressure below this level may be associated with a toxemic process, and, on

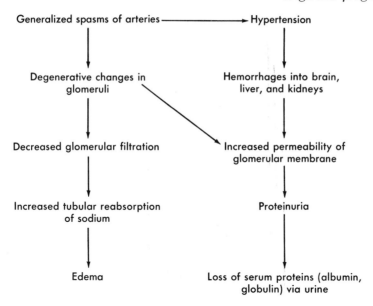

Generalized spasms of arteries ⟶ Hypertension

Degenerative changes in
glomeruli

Hemorrhages into brain,
liver, and kidneys

Decreased glomerular filtration

Increased permeability of
glomerular membrane

Increased tubular reabsorption
of sodium

Proteinuria

Edema

Loss of serum proteins (albumin,
globulin) via urine

**Fig. 8-1.** Pathology of preeclampsia. During the second half of gestation glomerular filtration rate is normally 50% above nonpregnant levels; in preeclampsia this rate falls.

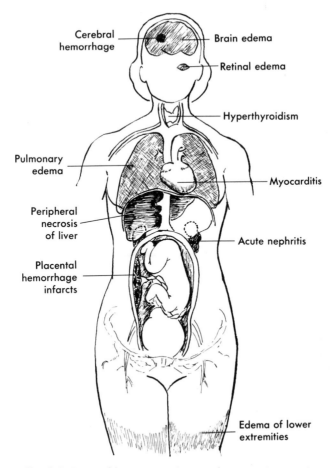

**Fig. 8-2.** Principal lesions occurring in eclamptogenic toxemia.

the other hand, one above this level is not necessarily significant of toxemia but may be the classical "essential" hypertension.

A more dependable prognostic sign of preeclampsia is a rise of 30 mm. or more in systolic pressure and 15 mm. or more diastolic, above the individual's usual level. The diastolic value is the more reliable because it indicates peripheral vascular spasms. When the diastolic pressure reaches 90 mm. of mercury or more, it is an absolute evidence of preeclampsia.

A single blood pressure reading is not a reliable guide, since there are various conditions contributing to inaccuracy—apprehension, tensions, and instances where the cuff is not fitted properly. The woman should be at rest and the reading taken on at least two separate occasions.

Essential hypertension complicating pregnancy may be coincident, that is, manifestations may occur before the twenty-fourth week, or may have been known to exist before pregnancy. Blood pressure levels may exceed 140/90 with no development of proteinuria. However, 15% to 30% of these women when they become pregnant will exhibit a true toxemia superimposed on their essential hypertension. It should be remembered that during midpregnancy the blood pressure tends to fall and then during the last trimester, returns to the previous levels. These latter readings, therefore, do not necessarily indicate hypertension of pregnancy. The most reliable criterion for diagnosing "specific hypertension" of pregnancy is persistent albuminuria and edema.

*Edema.* Although weight gain due to sodium and water retention is an important factor in predisposition to toxemia, caloric weight gain also contributes. About 40% of pregnant women have symptomatic edema; approximately 8% of these develop toxemia. Retention of fluids in the tissues may be accompanied by an abnormal gain in weight of over 1 pound per week. The swelling appears rapidly, begins in the lower extremities, and progresses upward.

Edema involving the upper part of the body is significant of preeclampsia; oliguria may accompany this edema. Edema may be the first sign of preeclampsia or it may follow hypertension. Tightness of the woman's rings is a significant sign.

*Proteinuria.* Proteinuria is due to renal vasospasms and implies damage to glomerular structures, which allows passage of proteins that the tubules cannot reabsorb. This excess protein, with albumin casts, is found in the urine. The amount varies from a trace to 8 or 10 grams in 24 hours. Proteinuria is usually coincident with hypertension, although it may precede or follow the elevation in blood pressure. When proteinuria continues longer than 2 or 3 weeks, the woman is frequently left with permanent vascular and renal damage.

***Program of treatment at home.*** When the woman's blood pressure is elevated to 140/90, the doctor usually gives her specific instructions for home care. The nurse's function is to review these instructions with the patient.

*Low salt diet* and ample fluids.* High protein is supplemented with pyridoxine and folic acid. The nurse should interpret a low salt diet with ample fluids for the woman to mean no salt used for cooking, no salt used at the table when eating, and the avoidance of foods known to be high in salt. The nurse also needs to impress upon the woman the importance of limiting her caloric intake. The ingestion of unlimited food will enhance her present condition.

The nurse should instruct the patient in recording her fluid intake and output. If her output is approximately 1,000 ml. or more daily, the doctor will usually want the patient to take about 2,500 ml. of salt-free fluids daily. The nurse can encourage her along this line.

*Ample rest.* Explain the importance of frequent periods of rest, especially after meals, and how rest contributes toward achieving loss of salt and water, and a decrease in blood pressure. Household work

---

*To reduce edema.

and social activities must be curtailed. If proteinuria appears, the patient is put on complete bed rest at home or admitted to the hospital.

*Medications.* The doctor may prescribe the following medications: (1) sedatives—phenobarbital, 30 mg. orally, three times daily; (2) diuretics—hydrochlorothiazide (HydroDiuril) or chlorthalidone (Hygroton), 50 mg. orally in the morning.

The nurse needs to be firm and stress the importance of the woman's adhering to dosage of medication prescribed. The doctor may want her to supplement the diuretic with potassium to avoid hypokalemia. The nurse may suggest that she include ample quantities of orange juice in her selection of fluids.

The nurse also instructs the woman to report at once headaches, blurred vision, or increased edema. If the patient does not respond to this plan of treatment within 48 hours, she is usually admitted to the hospital.

On admission, bed rest is mandatory and visitors restricted. The doctor's orders may include the following:

1. Daily weight, limiting gain to 8 ounces per week
2. Blood pressure and fetal heart sounds every 4 hours (when the patient is awake)
3. Diet—low sodium (less than 1 gram of salt per day), low fat, high carbohydrate, and high proteins to equal 1,500 to 1,800 calories
4. Accurate intake and output records with inlying catheter for determination of urinary excretion (If total urine is less than 800 ml. for 24 hours, 20% dextrose [I.V.] may be ordered to promote diuresis, to correct hemoconcentration, and to protect the liver.)
5. Vital signs every 4 hours (when patient is awake)
6. Medications including sedatives, diuretics, and antihypertensives (see specific medications below)
7. Daily urinary protein determinant

(excess of 0.3 gram in 24 hours is abnormal)
8. Retinoscopy[1]
9. Serial estriol levels to determine fetal jeopardy

Sedatives are ordered in adequate doses. Heavy sedations are usually undesirable, since it interferes with cerebral oxygenation and depresses fetal circulation.

The objectives of this treatment are (1) to prevent convulsions (eclampsia) by lowering blood pressure, (2) to establish diuresis, and (3) to preserve pregnancy to viability.

### Specific medication for preeclampsia and eclampsia
*Sedatives and anticonvulsants*

| | |
|---|---|
| Phenobarbital | 30 mg. orally, 3 times daily |
| Diphenylhydantoin (Dilantin) | 0.1 Gm. orally, 3 times daily |
| Methylphenylethylhydantoin (Mesantoin) | 0.1 Gm. orally, 3 times daily |
| Amobarbital sodium (Amytal) | 0.3 Gm. I.M., every 8 hours |
| Morphine sulfate | 15 to 30 mg., depending on size of patient |

(Morphine quiets the patient, but tends to reduce output and to have depressing effect on fetus.)

| | |
|---|---|
| Chlorpromazine (Thorazine, Largactil) | 50 mg. I.M., every 4 hours for 48 hours |

(Used for depressant effect on central nervous system and for hypotensive action.)

*For salt and water diuresis*

| | |
|---|---|
| Chlorothiazide (Diuril) | 250 to 500 mg. orally, daily |
| Hydrochlorothiazide (HydroDiuril) | 25 to 50 mg. orally, daily |
| Acetazolamide (Diamox) | 350 mg. daily |

*Antihypertensives*

| | |
|---|---|
| Magnesium sulfate (Epsom salt) | Initial dose usually 10 ml. of 25% aqueous solution, I.M. or I.V.; re- |

| | peated I.M. in doses of 5 Gm. every 4 to 6 hours if output is over 100 ml. per hour |
|---|---|
| Hydralazine (Apresoline) | 20 to 40 mg. in 250 ml. of 5% dextrose in water, I.V., stat. |
| | 100 to 150 mg. 4 times daily, gauged by blood pressure response |
| Cryptenamine tannate (Unitensen) | 2 mg. slowly, I.V. stat. 2 mg. orally, 3 times daily |

*Specific nursing responsibilities*

1. Observe carefully and constantly for signs and symptoms of developing eclampsia, which is characterized by generalized, intermittent, convulsive seizures. Marked hypertension precedes the convulsions, stertorous breathing, and frothing at the mouth, and then coma, hypotension during the coma, and usually a rise of temperature to 103° F. follow. In about one half the cases the convulsions occur before labor, one fourth during intrapartum, and one fourth within 24 hours of delivery.

The patient may give the following warning signs: (a) severe headache, (b) nervous irritability, (c) blurring of vision due to edema and hemorrhage, (d) sensation of constriction around the thorax, (e) epigastric pain and nausea, the result of congestion and vascular changes in the liver, and (f) fixed expression of the eyes that may be the sign of imminent eclampsia.

2. The patient should not be disturbed unnecessarily. Keep blood pressure cuff on the arm and padded tongue blade at hand, and a bulb syringe, suction machine, and oxygen available for immediate use.

3. Report a fluid output of less than 30 ml. per hour.

4. If the patient shows signs of nausea or vomiting, she should be turned on her side to prevent aspiration pneumonia.

5. The nurse would do well to keep at hand those medications that the doctor may need so that there be no delay in administration and no needless traffic to and from the room.

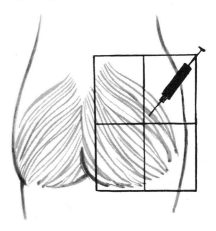

**Fig. 8-3.** Site of intramuscular injection.

6. Magnesium sulfate acts as a central nervous system depressant and lowers the blood pressure. It therefore protects the mother from convulsions and has the advantage of not causing fetal depression. If the order is to give this drug intramuscularly, the nurse must remember to inject it deep into the gluteal muscle and take care to avoid the sciatic nerve (Fig. 8-3). Do not repeat a magnesium sulfate injection if the fluid output is below 100 ml. per hour, if respirations are less than 16 per minute, and if the knee jerk reflex is absent. The nurse should always have at hand 20 ml. of a 10% aqueous calcium gluconate for the doctor's immediate use, if anuria or respiratory depression develops.

7. Apresoline is sometimes ordered to increase renal and coronary circulation. If the patient is receiving this drug, observe her for side effects such as nausea, vomiting, and palpitation.

8. Observe for signs of onset of labor and have the emergency delivery pack at hand.

9. Vascular spasms cause premature separation of the placenta; therefore the nurse should report any vaginal bleeding. However, separation may start centrally and the bleeding may be concealed; therefore changes in blood pressure and fetal heart sounds would be her clue. The nurse might also inquire as to the availability of dextran or whole blood, remembering that

hypofibrinogenemia may accompany an abruptio placentae. Dextran, a high molecular sugar, gives tone to the blood vessels.

Prior to 36 weeks' gestation, the doctor follows conservative treatment. After this period and when the patient has been stabilized by medical management, the doctor may induce labor, preferably by amniotomy alone, or he may choose to do a cesarean section.

Preventive care is truly appreciated when one realizes that early detection of the signs and symptoms allows time for appropriate treatment while the toxemia is in the incipient stage. This is one of the outstanding reasons why the nurse should stress antepartum supervision.

*Maternal mortality.* Preeclampsia and eclampsia have become one of the leading causes of maternal mortality in this country; the triad is hemorrhage, infections and other medical complications, and toxemia.

*Maternal prognosis.* The prognosis depends on adequate prenatal care, which is said to be good if eclampsia or the development of an abruptio placentae does not occur. The prognosis is grave if the patient is in prolonged coma, has rapid heart rate (over 150 per minute), a temperature of 103° F., pulse over 120, persistent elevation of blood pressure followed by a sudden drop, and less than 30 ml. fluid output per hour. If the pulse rate stays between 90 and 100 and is strong, it is a good sign, but a pulse over 120 is a poor prognostic sign.

Puerperal psychosis occurs in about 5% of those who do recover and there is also possible transient blindness from retinal detachment. The causes of death are (1) circulatory collapse, (2) cerebral hemorrhage, and (3) renal failure.

About one third of the women who have preeclampsia continue with persistent hypertension. However, some of these women had hypertensive disease prior to pregnancy. The others usually have a return of normal blood pressure, negative proteinuria, and the disappearance of the edema. Manifestations may last through the second week postpartum. About one third will

also have repetition of the toxemia in subsequent pregnancies.

*Fetal prognosis.* Fetal prognosis is poor in eclampsia, because this is the largest maternal cause of fetal mortality. The convulsions of eclampsia cause hypoxia and acidosis. Abruptio placentae and hypofibrinogenemia associated with eclampsia also lower the chances of survival. Premature termination of pregnancy with hyaline membrane disease as a sequel makes the perinatal mortality rates high. There is some evidence that preeclampsia and eclampsia may be factors in mental retardation or behavior problems of the offspring.

*Postpartum toxemia.* Physiologically the postpartum patient is still under the influence of pregnancy, and toxemia may occur 10 to 14 days after delivery. Eclampsia usually appears within the first 12 hours after delivery, but the nurse should observe the woman for at least 48 hours. During this time a valuable prognostic sign is diuresis.

### Diabetes mellitus

History reveals that the pregnant diabetic of a generation ago faced problems of infertility, repeated abortions, or deliveries of stillborn infants. Today pregnancy for the diabetic poses a much more favorable outlook. Important problems still confront the doctor, but with modern medical knowledge and full cooperation of the patient, the mortality rate is less than 1%. Diabetes still complicates one in every 300 to 400 pregnancies.

Diabetes (Gr. *diabeaniein*, running through), mellitus (L. *mellitus*, honeysweet) is the inability to metabolize glucose properly. Sugar in the urine during pregnancy may be due to (1) lactosuria, (2) renalglycosuria, or (3) diabetes. Fifty percent of pregnant women and even more of the primigravidas show small amounts of sugar in the urine. The findings of a fasting blood sugar reading of 130 mg. per 100 ml. or more and a glucose tolerance test reaching 170 mg. per 100 ml. or more are suspicious of diabetes. It has been stated that all pregnant women should have a 2-hour postprandial blood sugar determination during each trimester of pregnancy.

Transitory gestational diabetes may be difficult to diagnose in women not known to be diabetic because intermittent physiological glycosuria does occur normally during pregnancy, and the tests may give irregular results. Stress associated with pregnancy may cause an abnormal glucose tolerance. This "emotional glycosuria" is attributed to increased secretion of epinephrine.

Conditions alerting the doctor to the possibility of prediabetes are (1) hydramnios, (2) repeated abortions, (3) history of stillbirths, (3) abnormal glucose tolerance curve, and (5) babies with increasing birth weights. When a woman not known to have diabetes delivers a large baby (10 to 12 pounds), it is ground for further studies, that is, it may be indicative of diabetes.

*Management.* When the "known" diabetic suspects she is pregnant, she should place herself in the hands of an obstetrician. It is important that both an internist and the obstetrician follow her throughout her pregnancy and the puerperium. Women with a history of long-standing diabetes may be poor obstetric risks.

Acidosis, preeclampsia, and hydramnios are the major causes of intrauterine death, and the risk is increased in patients who have advanced vascular and renal changes. However, with adequate care, close supervision by both doctors, and the cooperation of the patient, these risks can be diminished.

The obstetrician needs a complete history of the patient, including previous pregnancies, complications such as preeclampsia, hypertension, and stillbirths, and insulin requirements. He needs data concerning her nutritional status—whether she is overweight, underweight, or of normal weight. For the overweight woman the caloric intake is usually kept at 1,500, but otherwise calories are allowed to 3,000, depending on height, present weight, and activity. The diet per day is usually one made up of 150 to 200 grams of carbohydrates, 2 grams of protein per kilogram of body weight, fat added to make up the prescribed calories, usually 1 gram salt (in absence of fluid retention), and vitamins, iron, and calcium the same as for the nondiabetic.

He also needs to know of any source of focal infection and her blood pressure. He orders a fasting blood sugar and a urinalysis for protein, glucose, ketone bodies, and presence of albuminuria. The urine needs to be kept free of acetone. He also orders a blood urea nitrogen and a regular examination by the ophthalmologist. These women are sometimes placed on chlorothiazide, 250 to 500 mg. daily, with potassium.

The woman is usually requested to report at 2- to 3-week intervals up to the twenty-eighth week and then weekly, depending on her intelligence, cooperation, and severity of the disease.

*Control of insulin.* She may require slightly less insulin during the first trimester (a decrease is noted in approximately two thirds of the patients). Insulin requirements usually increase (65% or more) during the latter half of pregnancy.

Ten percent require no change and 25% require less. Oral hypoglycemic agents are contraindicated, pending further studies. The sulfonylurea compounds pass the placenta barrier and may be related to potential teratogenesis in the fetus.

The woman is admitted to the hospital if she shows signs of toxicity, acidosis, or hydramnios. She is usually hospitalized at the thirty-fifth week for maximum control of the diabetes and to determine condition of the cervix and mode of delivery. Delivery is advocated at the thirty-sixth week because (1) the fetus tends to be large, especially if born to mothers with transitory gestational diabetes, and they often suffer damage in passing through the birth canal; (2) it has been stated that the placenta ages more rapidly; (3) these infants tend to have higher mortality rate if left in the uterus until term, and (4) there is greater possibility of cervical lacerations if the fetus is large.

*Mode of delivery.* The clinical judgment of the physician determines the time and mode of delivery; after the thirty-eighth week there is the likelihood of a stillbirth; before the optimal time, there is the likelihood of prematurity, when the doctor may order x-ray studies for distal femoral ossification for fetal maturity, and visualization of a severely edematous fetus (halo sign) to aid him in his decision.

Diabetes may be difficult to control during the early puerperium. Hypoglycemia is relatively common, and secretion of lactose in preparation for function of lactation and other metabolic changes that normally occur as the body adjusts to the prepregnant state all contribute.

*Nursing responsibilities.* The nurse can teach the woman to examine her urine daily for acetone bodies and to recognize signs and symptoms of acidosis, hypoglycemia, or hyperglycemia.

She should instruct her to report any infection, to get in touch with her doctor whenever she does not feel well, and not to become overfatigued, since this decreases carbohydrate tolerance. The nurse deals with both the uncooperative as well as the cooperative woman. There are those who ignore the disease and fail to heed instructions. Many times a reasonable explanation can change an uncooperative patient into a most willing one. The patient needs help in understanding why it is important that she adhere to the doctor's regimen, why complications must be prevented, and what may happen if she is lax in attention to her diet or to urine examination. She needs in-

### Effect of pregnancy on the diabetic

1. Insulin requirements usually increase.
2. Hypoglycemia is likely to occur during first half of pregnancy; acidosis, precoma, and coma occur during last trimester.
3. Pregnancy generally lowers carbohydrate metabolism.
4. Stress of pregnancy may produce an abnormal glucose tolerance.
5. Pregnancy is a stimulus to the pancreas; therefore the amount of circulating insulin increases.
6. High estrogen level of pregnancy may predispose to diabetes because estrogen affects glucose tolerance of the liver.

### Effect of diabetes on pregnancy

1. Increased rate of toxemia (25% of pregnant diabetics). Long-standing diabetes (presence of vascular or renal disease) favors occurrence of severe form of toxemia. (Eclamptogenic in over one third of the cases.)
2. Hydramnios (20%).
3. Oversized babies.
4. Edema more difficult to control.
5. Increased incidence of abortions (12%).
6. Increased incidence of premature labors.
7. More rapid aging of placenta.

### Effect of diabetes on the fetus

1. The increased size of the fetus is thought to be related to the hyperactivity of the fetal pancreas, which has been shown to contain considerably more insulin than that of the diabetic mother, due to an increase in number of islands of Langerhans.
2. Inadequate blood sugar control may contribute to damage of fetal pancreas.
3. It has been suggested that the excessive size of infants born to diabetic women is due to thiamine deficiency in the infant.[11] Others have attributed the higher birth weight to a greater amount of fat and a tendency to edema.
4. There tends to be a higher mortality rate if the fetus is left in utero until term. Degenerative changes in the placenta may lead to intrauterine asphyxia.
5. Congenital defects are five times the average. Abnormal carbohydrate metabolism during the first trimester may play a part. Insulin may act as a stressor factor contributing to teratogenesis.

structions concerning good personal hygiene. Mycotic vaginitis tends to occur in the diabetic. *Early prenatal care* may detect mild diabetes, reduce incidence of large babies, reduce perinatal mortality, and reduce maternal complications.

## Hemorrhagic complications
### Abortion

The scientific term for an unsuccessful pregnancy or termination before viability is abortion; the weight of the abortus is less than 500 grams. A fetus is believed viable at weight of 1,000 grams (usually 26 to 28 weeks' gestation). The term miscarriage and abortion differ only in the interpretation. To nonmedical people abortion brings unsavory thoughts, signifying criminal interference.

#### Classification and mechanism

*Early spontaneous.* An early spontaneous abortion occurs before the sixteenth week. Abortion before tenth week is preceded by death of the embryo.

*Late spontaneous.* A late spontaneous abortion occurs between the sixteenth and twentieth week. The embryo may be alive.

#### Etiology of early spontaneous abortion

1. Sixty-five percent of spontaneous abortions attributed to defective germ plasm
2. Faulty environment, such as abnormal development of the chorion
3. Psychic trauma

#### Etiology of late spontaneous abortions

1. Endocrine disturbance such as hypothyroidism or diabetes mellitus
2. Incompetent cervix or congenital short cervix
3. Abnormalities of the placenta (These usually occur after the twenty-fourth week, and therefore may be a premature labor.)
4. General systemic diseases

#### Clinical manifestations

*Threatened.* In a threatened abortion the bleeding appears as spotting or a trickle, and colicky pain may precede or follow the spotting. These symptoms may occur for days or extend into weeks, but there is no cervical dilatation. In a true, threatened abortion, the bloody discharge is chocolate colored (degenerated blood).

*Imminent.* If the spotting becomes actual vaginal bleeding and there is beginning cervical dilatation and effacement, the abortion is said to be imminent. The pain increases as the condition progresses.

*Inevitable.* Along with the above symptoms, in an inevitable abortion the membranes rupture, and the cord may protrude at the vaginal orifice, when spontaneous evacuation of the uterus follows.

*Incomplete.* When only part of the product of conception is expelled, it is called an incomplete abortion. The blood vessels at the site of implantation are torn by separation of parts of the chorionic villi from the decidua. The muscles cannot contract and therefore the uterus must be emptied before bleeding will stop.

*Complete.* The term complete abortion is used when the entire products of conception are expelled. Bleeding is moderate, and normal involution of the uterus takes place in a few days. This occurrence is more common before the eighth week.

*Missed.* A missed abortion is defined as the retention of the products of conception 2 months or more after death of the fetus. symptoms are few; the normal physiological changes of pregnancy cease, that is, uterus does not increase in size. The woman sometimes loses weight and may have an odorous, brownish colored vaginal discharge. Prolonged retention of the dead fetus may interfere with normal blood clotting mechanism and result in hemorrhage (hypofibrinogenemia).

If spontaneous evacuation of the uterus does not occur, the doctor may intervene with dilatation and curettage when the chorionic gonadotropic level falls to zero. There may be no symptoms, even though the fetus dies. The placenta does not detach from the uterine wall; the amniotic fluid is reabsorbed and the fetus may undergo dehydration and mummification.

*Habitual.* Habitual abortion is defined as three or more consecutive, spontaneous abortions. Etiology may be caused by (1) faulty environment such as defects in the function of the endometrium, (2) pathological ova, (3) hyperthyroid or hypothyroid, and (4) incompetent internal os of the cervix. When the patients show deficiency in endometrial function, the preconceptional treatment of diethylstilbestrol is instituted by some physicians.

*Therapeutic abortion.* Pregnancy terminated in the welfare of the mother is termed a therapeutic abortion. Just what constitutes danger to her life is left to the decision of her doctor. Since this involves his integrity and professional standing, the decision is sometimes passed on by a committee appointed by the hospital. Therapeutic abortion for probability of a defective infant has received much recognition and is now considered legal in some states. There is wide disagreement on the indications for therapeutic abortion, but some indications are (1) severe renal disease, (2) severe tuberculosis, (3) cancer of the breast, (4) heart disease, (5) psychiatric disturbances, and (6) diabetes with vascular lesions.

When termination is indicated, an effective means of inducing labor (between the twelfth and sixteenth week) is through injection of a hypertonic solution. Amniotic fluid (approximately 200 ml.) is removed by introducing a needle through the abdomen directly into the amniotic sac. This is replaced with the same amount of a 20% sodium chloride solution.

*Criminal abortion.* Sepsis associated with an abortion may be a factor in criminal interference. A criminal abortion is not only illegal but also extremely dangerous; infections of the uterine cavity are a most serious complication. Parametritis, endometritis, or general bloodstream infection may occur. It may render the woman sterile and the psychic trauma may make normal adjustment impossible.

*Psychogenic abortion.* That emotional factors play a role in abortion is purely a hypothesis. Since emotional stress can result in endocrine changes, it is believed by

some authorities that conflicts are capable of producing habitual abortions. Mention has already been made about psychogenic pregnancy (pseudocyesis) and psychogenic toxemia; the same agent may act upon the uterus to produce an abortion.

*Prognosis for abortions.* The chief danger is hemorrhage, but with modern medical treatment the prognosis is good. The mortality rate is, of course, higher with criminal abortions because of infection and hemorrhage. Abortions account for about one eighth of maternal deaths.

*Treatment and nursing responsibilities.* While the nurse is caring for the woman with the diagnosis of threatened abortion, she should observe her for extent and nature of bleeding. If the bleeding becomes increased in amount, or the pain more severe, she should notify the doctor so that treatment may be initiated promptly. The doctor may order uterine relaxants such as relaxin (Releasin and Cervilaxin) and lututrin (Lutrexin).

If the abortion becomes inevitable, the nurse should strive to show every consideration for the patient without unduly alarming her. Facing an inevitable abortion is a threat and may mean grief to the childless woman. She often feels that it is caused by some abnormality in her body. The nurse makes no false promises but does all she can to make the woman comfortable.

To reduce blood loss, the doctor may order oxytocics to hasten the abortion and antibiotics prophylactically. He may empty the uterus by curettage. Retained tissue may interfere with adequate drainage and act as a culture medium for pathogens. The nurse should keep any vaginal discharge for the doctor's examination and protect her patient from infection.

### Incompetent cervical os[2]

Incompetent cervical os, or premature dilatation and effacement of the cervix, is another cause of premature loss of the fetus. Repeated abortions of a living fetus after the first trimester (16 to 28 weeks) lead to the suspicion of incompetency of the cervical os. This may result from injury to the cervix during previous delivery or during gynecological trauma, or it may be congenital. A purse string type suture about the internal os may prevent rupture of the membranes and preserve the pregnancy until term. At term, when labor commences, the suture is encised.

V. N. Shirodkar of India was the first man to devise a method of reinforcement of the cervix by cerclage. Modifications of his procedure, such as the Würm and Lash technique, are used to correct the condition. These operative constrictions of the cervix may be done during pregnancy or be repeated in subsequent pregnancies.

### Ectopic pregnancy

Ectopic gestation is defined as one in which the fertilized ovum develops outside the uterine cavity (Gr., *ek* and *topos,* out of place).

The sites of implantation are (1) tubal, 95%, (2) cervical, (3) ovarian, and (4) abdominal or peritoneal.

#### Types of tubal ectopic pregnancies

*Interstitial.* Rare, but most serious is the interstitial type. It occurs in that part of the tube penetrating the uterine wall (cornual) in which the major blood vessels are located. Rupture results in severe intraperitoneal bleeding. Due to the greater muscularity, the pregnancy may continue longer before rupture, and it may be necessary to remove the uterus rather than repair it.

*Isthmic.* If nidation takes place in the isthmic area, intraperitoneal rupture usually follows.

*Ampullar.* The highest incidence of tubal pregnancies are in the ampullar area. Rupture occurs between the sixth and twelfth week.

*Incidence.* One in 200 pregnancies is ectopic. These pregnancies occur more often in the Negro, and this is believed to be due to the incidence of pelvic inflammatory disease that is greater among Negro women. Recurrence in subsequent pregnancies approximates 15% to 20%.

#### Etiology

1. Tubal occlusion
2. Congenital tubal development (infantile)
3. Tumors
4. Endometriosis
5. Systemic infections or toxic agents
6. Endocrine imbalance interfering with function of the tubes

#### Signs and symptoms

1. Amenorrhea of several weeks
2. Sharp, intermittent pain usually generalized over the abdomen
3. Bleeding, if present, usually scanty, brown in color (Profuse bleeding occurs in about 5% of tubal pregnancies. These symptoms usually occur 6 to 8 weeks after the last menstrual period.)

**Uterine changes.** The uterus undergoes physiological changes associated with pregnancy. The endometrium may be converted to decidua and the breasts may secrete colostrum.

**Mechanism.** The tube, not able to withstand demands of the growing fetus, thins out and finally ruptures, usually between 6 to 12 weeks. The fetus may be aborted into the abdominal cavity. If the trophoblasts implant again somewhere in the peritoneum, it may continue to grow as a secondary abdominal pregnancy. This is in contrast to a primary abdominal pregnancy where the fertilized ovum escapes through the ampulla end of the tube and attaches itself to the parietal peritoneum. If the product of conception dies, mummification may set in and when, in time, calcium salts deposit around the sac, it is then referred to as a lithopedion.

**Nursing responsibilities.** When the patient is admitted to the hospital with the diagnosis of possible ectopic (unruptured tubal) pregnancy, the nurse needs to keep in mind the signs of possible tubal rupture so that she may notify the doctor immediately, since a ruptured tubal pregnancy may be fatal without prompt treatment.

If implantation is at the ampulla end of the tube when it ruptures, blood flows into the peritoneal cavity, forming clots and a hematocele. With intraperitoneal bleeding over several days, one may note (Cullen's sign) a bluish tint around the umbilicus.

The patient may be unable to void, temperature will probably be normal or subnormal, and the pulse will be rapid. The abdomen becomes tender, rigid, and boardlike. She may express the desire to defecate and complain of shoulder pain because of increased pressure of the blood in the peritoneal cavity. External bleeding may be present but is not necessarily profuse. Nevertheless, blood transfusions are usually given before, during, and after surgery, and the nurse should see that blood is available for emergency use. Should the patient show these signs, she must be kept warm and given nothing by mouth. She may go into acute shock due to the extensive hemorrhage and the nurse must be ready (prepared) to meet such a situation. She should be able to report her observations in a clear manner and make every effort to allay fears and anxieties that are bound to overwhelm the patient.

*Prognosis.* The prognosis is good when the rupture occurs early and when the ovum is aborted. When an ectopic pregnancy becomes a secondary abdominal one, the prognosis is poor. The most frequent cause of death is lack of adequate blood replacement.

### Hydatidiform mole[6,7]

Between the third and fifth week of pregnancy, the trophoblasts proliferate and form a mass, that is, a hydatidiform mole. The abnormal embryo dies, but the mass grows large enough to fill the uterus at 7 months.

*Incidence.* Hydatidiform mole tends to occur more often among women in lower socioeconomic groups. In countries where nutrition is faulty and the intake of protein is inadequate, the occurrence is about one in 200 pregnancies. Hyperfunction of the thyroid gland exists in most all of the patients with hydatidiform mole. It is more frequent at the beginning of the reproductive age and then again toward the end. The mole may be accompanied or followed by choriocarcinoma. The cells may lie dormant for years before manifesting malignancy.

*Signs and symptoms.* About the twelfth week of pregnancy, the patient gives a history of vaginal bleeding that may be intermittent or profuse, with or without pain. This bleeding starts when part of the mole separates. The woman has edema, hypertension, and albuminuria, the symptoms of toxemia but before the twenty-fourth week of pregnancy. Hyperemesis is more frequent and severe. The uterus is larger than the expected size and the fetus is not ballottable. Persistent rise of the chorionic gonadotropic level after 100 days from last period is suggestive of hydatidiform mole because the level normally declines about this time.

The mole may be expelled spontaneously or the uterus may have to be evacuated. It is important that the chorionic gonadotropic titer is determined weekly after evacuation until results are negative, and then monthly for 1 year. If the titer is still positive 30 days after the evacuation of the mole, it may indicate continued growth of the mole or chorioepithelioma.

### Placenta previa and abruptio placentae

The most frequent causes of bleeding during the first half of pregnancy are abortions, ectopic pregnancy, and hydatidiform mole. The two most common causes of bleeding during the last half of pregnancy are placenta previa and abruptio placentae. The first is an abnormality of *implantation* and the latter an abnormality of *premature separation* of a normally implanted placenta.

*Placenta previa.* Nidation of the zygote normally takes place high on the anterior or posterior wall of the uterus. When nidation takes place in the lower uterine segment, the placenta develops close to or over the internal os; since this is the area of effacement and dilatation, hemorrhage is bound to occur.

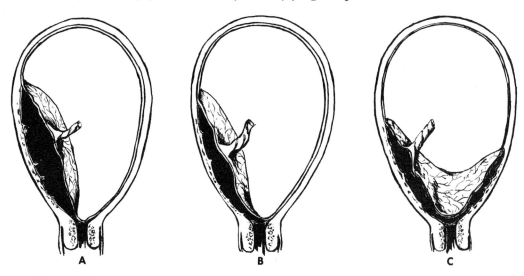

**Fig. 8-4.** Placenta previa. **A,** Low implantation of placenta. **B,** Partial placenta previa. **C,** Total placenta previa.

The classification used by the obstetrician is based on the approximate area of the internal os that would be covered by the placenta if the cervix was completely dilated. (See Fig. 8-4.)

1. Total—the placenta covers the internal os (10%)
2. Partial—the placenta partially covers the internal os (37%)
3. Marginal—the placenta is low but does not extend beyond the margin of the os

*Incidence.* Placenta previa occurs about once in 200 pregnancies. It rarely occurs in the primigravida. As parity increases, so does the frequency of this complication.

*Diagnosis.* Diagnosis is made by placentography, radioactive localization, and vaginal examination.[8]

*Etiology.* Why the zygote implants low in the uterine segment is undetermined, but predisposing factors are (1) rapid sequence of pregnancies making the upper segment of the endometrium inadequate for nidation; (2) alteration in uterine structure; (3) cesarean section scars may increase the incidence, especially if interval between pregnancies is short; and (4) fertilization late in the interval of viability of ovum. Low implantation of the placenta may cause malpresentations: engagement is usually delayed, the membranes are likely to rupture prematurely with subsequent prolapsed cord, and congenital anomalies are more frequent.

*Clinical findings and management.* Painless bleeding is the first sign of placenta previa. With partial and marginal placenta previa, the hemorrhage usually accompanies the beginning of labor. There may be several incidences of bleeding; the first is usually slight. As the lower uterine segment expands and the cervix elongates, the placental attachment is disturbed so that small gushes of blood and the passage of clots occur. Of course, if the placenta lies directly over the internal os (total), bleeding will be profuse as cervical changes take place. Management will depend on (1) amount of bleeding, (2) viability of the fetus, and (3) status of the cervix.

When the separation is marginal or partial, the fetus is viable, and labor has started, the doctor may rupture membranes to accelerate labor and allow the fetal head to descend and tamponade the bleeding.

When the fetus is not viable and the bleeding not excessive, the patient may have to remain in the hospital until term. Bleeding, in many instances, may be checked by bed rest alone. This increases fetal changes for survival. If the fetus is viable, the patient hemorrhaging, and the cervix not dilated, the doctor usually does a cesarean section.[3]

*Nursing responsibilities.* When the patient is admitted to the labor room unit, the nurse can obtain much of the pertinent information she needs concerning the bleeding while she assists the patient into bed. It is important that the nurse determine the amount of bleeding. What might be reported by the patient as a hemorrhage may be mere spotting to the nurse. How can the nurse elicit a fairly accurate estimation of blood loss from the patient? First by inquiring as to when the bleeding started and was it intermittant or continuous; how many pads she used since the bleeding started; were they saturated or heavily soiled? Was the bleeding bright or dark red, and did she pass any clots of blood? Often the nurse and patient can keep on the same level of communication by comparing how *this* bleeding compares with that experienced during a *normal* menstrual flow—same as, greater than, or less than. The doctor will also want to know if pain accompanied the bleeding. Has the fetus been active since the bleeding started and are the membranes intact? If the patient is wearing a pad on admission, the nurse estimates the amount of blood and how much bleeding has taken place since admission; she also notes tone of abdomen. If the patient has active bleeding on admission, no time should be lost in notifying the doctor. It is also the nurse's responsibility to note rate and quality of fetal heart sounds as well as the patient's pulse rate and blood pressure. She should inquire whether the patient had a fall or any severe trauma to the abdomen. With this information she can certainly give the doctor the immediate picture of the extent of bleeding. She should keep the patient quiet and give her nothing by mouth. From here on your responsibility is to function efficiently in responding to the doctor's immediate requests.

If the doctor states his intention of doing a vaginal examination, the nurse should have the room prepared for delivery, either vaginal or cesarean section. She is also responsible for having blood on hand before the vaginal is done, since hemorrhage may result from the examination. Rectal examinations are not done as they are likely to dislodge the placenta.

If the doctor states his intention of doing an amniotomy, he usually wants the patient in Fowler's position. This helps bring down the presenting part and the cord is less likely to prolapse. The nurse should check fetal heart sounds every 15 minutes and notify the doctor immediately should there be any change in rate or regularity.

When the patient is delivered vaginally, the nurse should have the doctor's choice of oxytocic at hand and packing for use as soon as the placenta is removed. The patient may bleed profusely if the lower uterine segment fails to retract, which is not unusual since the muscles in this area have poor tone.

With total placenta previa the bleeding starts earlier and cesarean section is usually performed. The woman must be treated for shock and blood loss must be replaced.

*Postpartum complications.* When implantation of the placenta is low, the placenta is usually thinner and develops over a greater area. Because of this the lower uterine segment is overstretched during pregnancy. These muscles do not have the power to compress the blood vessels and this is, of course, conducive to uterine atony.

As the placenta develops, the tissues become more friable; therefore the cervix is more likely to lacerate. Anemia is usually present and reduces the patient's resistance to infection, which is more likely to occur since pieces of placental tissue may be retained and lie close to the external os.

*Prognosis.* The prognosis depends on whether the placenta previa is marginal, partial, or total, and how quickly treatment is instituted.

*Mortality.* The mortality rate is about 1% and occurs from hemorrhage and infection.

Perinatal mortality is about 10% to 15%. The infant may be premature and suffer asphyxia or posthemorrhagic shock due to rupture of capillaries in the fetal surface of the placenta.

When the woman has vaginal bleeding, but no changes occur in her vital signs, it is likely that the bleeding is of fetal origin. When the cord attaches to the membranes "vasa praevia" occurs and may cause ruptured fetal vessels. To differentiate fetal from maternal bleeding, the Downey-Apt test is done.

*Abruptio placentae.* Abruptio placentae occurs between the twenty-eighth week of pregnancy and term. Placenta detachment before this time is an abortion. The detachment may be partial or complete; the bleeding may be revealed (50%) or concealed (20%). (See Fig. 8-5.)

Partial detachment is usually marginal and more likely to occur during labor. The hemorrhage is usually painless. The "revealed" blood escapes from the area of detachment and seeps through the cervical os.

When the hemorrhage is concealed, the condition is, of course, more hazardous to the mother and fetus, since it usually involves complete abruption. This type occurs during the last trimester and is often associated with hypertensive toxemia—"toxic abruptio." The detachment begins in the central portion of the decidua basalis (arterial bleeding) while the periphery of the placenta remains adherent to the uterus. The blood collects retroplacenta and causes outward bulging of the uterus and severe pain.

*Incidence.* Abruptio placentae occurs in about one in every 200 patients admitted to the hospital. It tends to occur more in the multipara and two thirds of the patients have toxemia. Fifty percent of the cases show albuminuria.

*Diagnosis.* Severe pain and boardlike rigidity of the uterus are classic diagnostic signs of abruption. The doctor may do a vaginal examination to rule out placenta previa or other conditions such as tumors or rupture of the uterus.

*Etiology.* The primary cause is unknown, although predisposing factors are believed to contribute to the separation, such as (1) preeclampsia, (2) chronic hypertensive disease, (3) deficiency in folic acid and vitamin C, (4) pressure on the vena cava by the enlarging uterus, (5) placental circulatory insufficiency, (6) direct trauma (but only in a very small percentage), and (7) rapid decrease in uterine volume, such as sudden release of hydramnios.

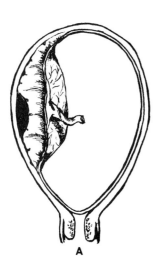 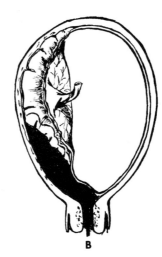 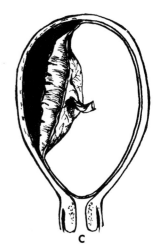

A          B          C

**Fig. 8-5.** Abruptio placentae. **A,** Partial separation (concealed bleeding). **B,** Partial separation (apparent hemorrhage). **C,** Complete separation (concealed hemorrhage).

*Clinical findings and management.* With marginal separation the woman has external bleeding in varying amounts, usually dark red (venous). The severity of the bleeding depends on the degree of separation. The uterus is relaxed, but there may be some local tenderness. When the symptoms are mild, the doctor may do an amniotomy, followed by oxytocin infusion to accelerate labor. Pressure of the head as it descends may control hemorrhage until the woman can be delivered.

With concealed bleeding the uterus becomes rigid and tender and does not relax between contractions. This makes it difficult to palpate fetal parts. The abdomen may increase in size; in some cases shock may be out of proportion to blood loss. Effective therapy includes plasma expanders until blood is obtained, and fibinogen (4 to 8 mg. as indicated by clot observation tests) in 5% glucose. Cesarean section is indicated when labor is expected to be over 6 hours, if hemorrhage continues, or if there is apparent fetal distress that is due to the hypoxia. The fetal heart rate will first show tachycardia and then slowing and irregularity. Fetal distress is indicated by hyperactivity, followed by cessation of movements. The majority of fetal deaths due to anoxia are the result of an abruptio placentae.

*Maternal complications.* Hypofibrinogenemia (decreased plasma fibrinogen), Couvelaire uterus, renal failure, and shock are the four major maternal complications. Hypofibrinogenemia occurs in approximately 10% to 12% of abruptios. During the last trimester of pregnancy the plasma fibrinogen level is 440 mg. per 100 ml. As the blood accumulates retroplacenta, the amount of circulating fibrinogen is depleted. Levels below 100 mg. per 100 ml. result in postpartum uterine bleeding. When the blood effuses into the uterine musculature and connective tissues of the broad ligaments, it is called Couvelaire uterus or uteroplacental apoplexy. As much as 1,000 to 2,000 ml. of blood may collect retroplacentally. With this extensive bleeding the uterine muscles cannot contract and hysterectomy may be necessary to prevent fatal hemorrhage.

*Maternal prognosis.* Prognosis depends on (1) whether the abruptio placentae was toxic or nontoxic abruptio, (2) extent of placental detachment, (3) extent of hemorrhage, and (4) degree of fibrinogenopenia.

*Fetal prognosis.* If the fetus suffers prolonged hypoxia, cerebral damage will result. Cerebral palsy, mental retardation, and prematurity may be the sequelae.

*Mortality.* Death of the mother is usually due to hemorrhage and renal failure and approximates 1% if separation is complete. The mortality rate approximates 50% with a mild abruptio for the fetus and 100% with a complete abruptio.

*Nursing responsibilities.* While caring for the labor patient, the nurse may notice a mild degree of bleeding. After reporting this, her responsibility is to keep an accurate, frequent check on fetal heart sounds, maternal pulse, and blood pressure so that signs of concealed bleeding may be detected early.

Patients frequently complain of constant backache in the lumbosacral region. Observe the abdomen for level of the fundus. If the uterus becomes tender and if the fetus indicates distress such as hyperactivity or tachycardia, oxygen may be given. Your prompt attention in reporting these symptoms may avoid hazards to both mother and fetus. The nurse's responsibilities are to see that fluids are at hand, that necessary blood work has been completed, and that fibrinogen is available. Blood should be placed in a water bath with a temperature of 36° C. for immediate transfusion. Guard the patient against infection and prevent heat loss. The section room should be ready for immediate response to the doctor's decision.

The danger is not over when the patient is delivered. It would be well for the nurse to remember that there is the likelihood of late postpartum hemorrhage and that both hemorrhage and trauma predispose to puerperal infection. Therefore the patient needs constant observation for at least 6 hours after delivery. Many patients with abruptio placentae tend to have oliguria during the early puerperium.

## Renal complications—urinary tract infections

Acute infections of the urinary tract frequently complicate pregnancy. The physiological changes occurring in the urinary system during pregnancy predispose to urinary stasis and infections such as cystitis and pyelonephritis. The organisms most responsible are *Escherichia coli*, *Staphylococcus aureus*, and the streptococci.

Acute pyelonephritis is the most frequent complication involving the urinary tract and occurs in 1% to 2% of all pregnancies. Pyelonephritis begins about the fifth month of pregnancy; onset is abrupt and associated with increased incidence of premature labors. The woman complains of pain in the lumbar region, which radiates to the right side, and of nausea and vomiting, malaise, dysuria, and frequency. Temperature may be elevated to 104° F.

After the urine is cultured and sensitivity tests completed, antibiotic therapy or chemotherapy is begun. Some of the drugs used are (1) nitrofurantoin (Furadantin), 100 mg., three times a day and (2) Terramycin, 250 mg., every 6 hours. The sulfa drugs are not ordered during the last 2 weeks prior to term because they enter fetal circulation and if the liver cannot detoxify these drugs, hyperbilirubinemia will result. The use of tetracyclines should also be avoided at this time, since they are believed to cause retardation of bone growth and to cause yellow staining of the teeth.

The doctor usually orders "force fluids" to 3 to 4 liters per 24 hours. It is the nurse's responsibility to encourage the patient to take fluids freely.

If catheterization is ordered, the nurse should use full surgical aseptic technique. For relief of pain the nurse may instruct the patient to lie on the side free of symptoms and elevate the foot of bed approximately 15 inches.

## Circulatory complication— heart disease[4]

In Chapter 5 you learned about the ability of the heart to withstand the stresses of pregnancy. For the woman who enjoys good health, this magnificent organ responds with competence during pregnancy, but it can be one of the great hazards to the health of the mother and fetus when injury is heaped on it, such as congenital defects or infections. Heart disease ranks fourth as a cause of maternal mortality. The various defects may first make their appearance during pregnancy as the blood vessels are making an effort to respond to the physiological changes. Rheumatic heart disease with mitral stenosis is the predominant cardiac problem.

Prevention of congestive heart failure is of prime importance. One means of accomplishing this is by reducing the heart's work. The normal physiological burden imposed on the heart cannot be reduced, but curtailment of physical activity can be. Extra periods of rest are a must in addition to 10 hours of sleep every night.

The maximum increase in cardiac output occurs between the twenty-eighth and thirty-second week of pregnancy, diminishing as term is approached to the nonpregnant levels. It is, therefore, the most dangerous period. However, with close supervision of the doctor and obstetrician and with the cooperation of the patient, women with heart trouble can go through pregnancy safely. The incidence of heart failure is observed most frequently in those who present themselves for care late in pregnancy. If the cardiac patient experiences no undue fatigue with ordinary physical activity and gives her full cooperation to the doctor, she is permitted to continue as usual with, of course, additional periods of rest. She is usually seen every 2 weeks by the obstetrician. This allows for detection of fluid retention and the development of toxemia or renal disease, for treatment of any infection, and for attention to emotional factors.

The cardiac woman in whom the disease

is moderately severe to advanced, who has marked limitations of physical activity, and who suffers from dyspnea and anginal pain is a poor risk for pregnancy. She is kept on bed rest at home and admitted to the hospital 2 weeks before the expected date of delivery.

Dietary management includes prevention of excessive weight gain and excessive fluid retention. Weight gain is limited to 15 to 18 pounds and sodium intake restricted to 1 to 1.5 grams daily. Anemia adds to demands on the heart producing dyspnea, fatigue, and an overactive heart action. Therefore an iron supplement is important. With the use of oral thiazide derivatives, fluid retention can be safely controlled in ambulatory patients. For list of diuretic drugs see reference 10. Since these drugs are administered for long periods of time, the nurse should know the side effects such as nausea and abdominal cramps, pruritus, leg cramps, and hypotensive reactions (faintness).

*Nursing responsibilities.* The nurse reinforces the doctor's instructions and stresses the importance of avoiding exertion or excitement and of reporting a cold no matter how slight it may seem to her. Intercurrent infections, even those of minor degree, may precipitate failure. The nurse can help the patient plan specific periods of rest, especially when there are small children in the home. If the woman is taking diuretics, she should encourage her to eat foods rich in potassium, such as citrus fruits, bananas, fruit juices, meats, bran products, and milk. Potassium supplement is also important for the pregnant cardiac patient on digitalis.

If the woman is an outpatient coming to the clinic, the nurse should give of her time to explain reasons for restriction of activity, avoidance of infections, and adherence to doctor's regimen. The nurse should prepare her for the possibility of admission to the hospital earlier than her expected due date, and for the probability of having to spend much of the day in bed after the thirtieth week.

Prognosis for the cardiac woman depends on functional capacity of the heart in meeting the increased demands of pregnancy as well as adequate care and full cooperation. The blood volume may increase 20% to 40% when the uterus is emptied, with consequent rise in cardiac output. (Blood that supplied the placenta now goes into general circulation.) Therefore the heart is just as likely to fail during the 24 hours after delivery as during pregnancy.

Prognosis for the fetus may depend on circulatory changes accompanying decompensation. These changes may cause intrapartum death from hypoxia.

### Infectious complication—tuberculosis

A chest x-ray film should always be included in the initial physical examination of the pregnant woman to rule out the incidence of unsuspected tuberculosis. Whether or not pregnancy aggravates tuberculosis is viewed differently by medical authorities. With modern chemotherapeutic treatment, tuberculosis by placental transmission is rare and as a rule the fetus of a tubercular mother is free from the disease. Nevertheless, there are hazards to the fetus and the infant. The fetus may aspirate infected amniotic fluid or become increasingly susceptible to the disease. Prematurity is related to the severity of the infection and cases of congenital tuberculosis are known.

Pregnant women with inactive tuberculosis are placed on modified bed rest and are more likely to cooperate if allowed to remain at home. Depending on the activity of the disease, the woman may be on required bed rest throughout the entire pregnancy, but since the advent of chemotherapy, the need for this has been debated.

The nurse can be most helpful during the prenatal period. During this time arrangements should be made for postdelivery care of the mother and infant. The woman and her family need to be educated concerning her disease if this has not been done previously. She needs explicit explanations concerning vitamin and mineral supplements as ordered by the doctor, care of the skin, elimination, and importance of adequate nutrition.

The danger of the postdelivery period should be explained to the family and arrangements should be made for the infant's care outside the home, at least until a period of postdelivery observation indicates that the mother is noninfectious. The mother may feel well and want to care for her new baby, and the thought of separation may cause anxiety and depression. The cooperation of the family is important and the rationale of the separation needs to be explained to them. With honest, simple explanations the nurse can be a source of help to the family. If the disease is inactive, the infant is not separated from the mother, but close postnatal supervision must be utilized. Breast feeding is contraindicated.

*Treatment.* Drugs prescribed are isoniazid, *p*-aminosalicylic acid (PAS), and streptomycin. These drugs have little if any known deleterious effects on the infant.

Exhausting labors and traumatic deliveries are prevented by caudal or epidural analgesia for relief of pain and by a low forceps delivery to prevent increased intrapulmonary pressure that may result from bearing down.

It is recommended that women with active tuberculosis should avoid conception until the disease has been inactive for at least 2 years.

### Hematologic complication—anemia

It is true that when a great many women become pregnant they do have a preexisting iron-deficiency anemia. A number of factors contribute to this, such as heavy menstrual periods, unsupervised weight-reducing regimens, and poor dietary planning of meals. In general when the hemoglobin level falls below 11 grams, the hematocrit falls below 35%, and reduced red cell count falls to about 4.4 million per cubic millimeter, an iron-deficiency anemia is indicated. The majority of the anemias during pregnancy are of this type.

In the healthy, nonpregnant woman the hemoglobin concentration is on an average of about 12.5 to 14 grams per 100 ml. Some women are routinely placed on oral iron preparations on their initial visit. Deficiencies are more likely to occur during the third trimester. Some women complain of weakness, dyspnea, fatigability, and nail bed pallor. Other women are asymptomatic, and the deficiency is detected only by hemoglobin determination.

During pregnancy the fetus draws on maternal reserves of iron for formation of its blood cells and for liver storage. If the woman is anemic during her pregnancy, the fetus will certainly be born with insufficient iron to carry him through the early months of life. (They have normal blood counts at birth but develop the anemia later.) It occurs more frequently in the multigravida, but with adequate prenatal care this deficiency is corrected by proper diet and oral or intramuscular iron therapy, thereby preventing hypochromic anemia. Some doctors have attributed the incidence of fetal abnormalities to iron deficiency in the mother.

Iron requirements of the pregnant woman have been estimated as 1 mg. daily during the first trimester, especially if the hemoglobin is below 13 grams; four times as much iron is needed during the second trimester, and twelve times as much during the last 3 months. Oral iron therapy may have side effects such as nausea and vomiting, diarrhea or constipation, and abdominal cramps. Medications prescribed are usually ferrous gluconate (Fergon) or ferrous sulfate (Feosol), 300 mg., three times a day after meals. If the deficiency anemia is severe, intramuscular iron therapy, iron dextran (Imferon) 2 ml. daily in each buttock, may be ordered.

Megaloblastic anemia, a form of pernicious anemia, may be caused by metabolic demands of the fetus for folic acid. It is more common among nutritionally deprived populations, in multiparas over 30, and in twin pregnancies. The woman should have foods high in folic acid, high in vitamins, high in protein, and iron supplements. Folic acid, 20 mg. daily, plus vitamin C is usually prescribed. (Vitamin C is necessary for folic-acid metabolism.)

## High-risk pregnancies associated with multiple gestations[5,9]

The added physiological burdens placed on the mother during the period of twin gestation may predispose to complications. This need not be so. If early recognition is sought, the mother may be carried through safely.

### Complications

1. Toxemia is three times as common than in a single gestation.
2. Premature termination is seven times more likely.
3. Hydramnios occurs in 5% to 7% of multiple gestations.
4. More pressure symptoms, edema, and varicosities are found.
5. Anemia and albuminuria are more likely.
6. Nausea and vomiting are more pronounced.
7. Incidence of placenta previa is higher. Surface of the placenta is greater and may reach zone of cervical dilatation.

### Management

Frequency of visits to the doctor is increased, which allows for early detection of toxemia. The patient is advised concerning the importance of adequate rest. Incidence of prematurity may be decreased by bed rest during the latter weeks of pregnancy. Adequate nutrition is stressed, since greater demands are made on the mother's reserve. Iron supplements are usually ordered. Frequent complaints of the patient are backache, hemorrhoids, and heartburn. The nurse should discuss means of relieving these minor complaints. She should also prepare the woman for the possibility of an early labor.

### STUDY QUESTIONS
*Matching*

Match the terms in the first column with their appropriate definitions in the second column.

1.
(a) Abruptio placentae — Likely to be unstable during the puerperium
(b) Placenta previa — Not unusual to have a recurrence in subsequent pregnancies
(c) Complete abruption — As parity increases so does the frequency of this complication
(d) Halo sign — Repeated abortions of living fetuses (16 to 28 weeks)
(e) Estrogen — This complication is three times as common with a multiple pregnancy
(f) Toxemia — Retention of products of conception 2 months or more after death of fetus
(g) Missed abortion — Three or more consecutive, spontaneous abortions
(h) Habitual abortion — Associated with hypertensive toxemia
(i) Early spontaneous abortion — Attributed to defective germ plasm
(j) Incompetent cervical os — Effects glucose tolerance of the liver
(k) Ectopic pregnancy — Visualization of severely edematous fetus on x-ray film
(l) Insulin requirement — Associated with toxemia

2.
(a) Hyperemesis — Antidote for respiratory depression
(b) Diuresis — Acts as a central nervous system depressant and decreases blood pressure
(c) Dextran — Diagnosis is made on presence of acetone and diacetic acid in the urine and blood
(d) Sodium Amytal — Valuable prognostic sign for the preeclamptic or eclamptic during the pueperium
(e) Edema in upper part of the body — Promotes diuresis and protects the liver
(f) Specific hypertension — Gives tone to the blood vessels
(g) Chlorothiazide — Eliminates sodium and water from tissues without causing acidosis
(h) Calcium gluconate — Possible side effect of this drug is a precipitous drop in blood pressure
(i) Magnesium sulfate — Sign of preeclampsia

(j) Dextrose, 20%  ⎯Persistant albuminuria and edema

## Multiple choice

1. Toxemia is more likely to occur in:
   (a) the very young primigravida.
   (b) the Negro.
   (c) the poorly nourished woman.
   (d) multiple gestations.
   1. b only    2. d only    3. all the above
2. Which of the following factors influence the incidence of toxemia?
   (a) age of mother.
   (b) parity of the mother.
   (c) socioeconomic.
   (d) multiple gestation.
   1. a and b    2. a and c    3. all the above
3. Complications known to predispose to preeclampsia are:
   (a) diabetes with vascular or renal involvement.
   (b) acute polyhydramnios.
   (c) hydatidiform mole.
   (d) all of these.
4. The diet recommended for the preeclamptic is usually one that is:
   (a) high in protein, high in carbohydrates, low in fat.
   (b) high in protein, low in carbohydrates, no fat.
   (c) low in protein, high in carbohydrates, low in fat.
5. Magnesium sulfate is the drug of choice for the severe preeclamptic because it:
   (a) reduces edema of the brain.
   (b) is a vasodilator, reducing blood pressure.
   (c) given intramuscularly, acts as central nervous system depressant.
   (d) all the above.
6. The signs of excessive blood levels of magnesium sulfate are:
   (a) disappearance of the knee jerk reflex.
   (b) hyperactivity of the patient.
   (c) respiratory depression.
   (d) all the above.
   1. a and c    2. b and c    3. d
7. Sodium Amytal is given to control convulsions. A possible side effect is:
   (a) damage to the vagus nerve.
   (b) hyperactivity.
   (c) precipitous fall in blood pressure.
   (d) all the above.
8. Which of the following signs should alert the nurse that the patient is about to become eclamptic?
   (a) epigastric pain.
   (b) visual disturbances.
   (c) fixed expression of the eyes.
   (d) all of these.
9. The most dangerous period of pregnancy for the cardiac patient is:
   (a) twenty-fifth to twenty-eighth week of gestation.
   (b) twenty-eighth to thirty-second week of gestation.
   (c) thirty-second to thirty-sixth week of gestation.
10. If the pregnant cardiac patient is on digitalis, you would recommend foods high in potassium. These would include:
    (a) sweet potatoes.
    (b) bananas.
    (c) oranges.
    (d) bran products.
    1. a and b    2. b, c, and d    3. a and d
11. Mrs. "D" is on oral iron preparation. The nurse knows the side effects to be expected from this drug may be:
    (a) nausea and vomiting.
    (b) diarrhea.
    (c) constipation.
    (d) abdominal cramps.
    (e) all of these.
12. Which one of the following is suggestive of diabetes?
    (a) a fasting blood sugar of 130 mg. per 100 ml. or more and a glucose tolerance of 170 mg. per 100 ml. or more.
    (b) a fasting blood sugar of 120 mg. per 100 ml. or more and a glucose tolerance of 160 mg. per 100 ml. or more.
    (c) a fasting blood sugar of 130 mg. per 100 ml. or more and a glucose tolerance of 150 mg. per 100 ml. or more.
13. Insulin requirements generally:
    (a) decrease during the first trimester, and then increase during the latter half of pregnancy.
    (b) remain constant throughout pregnancy.
    (c) decrease throughout pregnancy.
14. Diabetes affects pregnancy in that:
    (a) edema is more difficult to control.
    (b) there is an increased incidence of prolonged gestation.
    (c) there is an increased incidence of premature labors.
    1. a and b    2. a and c    3. a only
15. Which of the following are correct?
    (a) delivery is advocated at the thirtieth week for the pregnant diabetic.
    (b) the placenta ages more rapidly in the diabetic than in the nondiabetic.
    (c) infant mortality rate is higher if the fetus is left in the uterus until term.
    (d) infants tend to be large especially if the mother has transitory diabetes.
    1. a and d    2. c and d    3. b, c, and d
16. The nurse knows that:

(a) 90% of the pregnant diabetics develop toxemia.
(b) those with history of long standing diabetes favor the occurrence of severe form of toxemia.
(c) eclamptogenic toxemia is rare.
17. The chief danger of abortion is:
(a) hemorrhage.
(b) infection.
(c) hypofibrinogenemia.
18. Mrs. B had the diagnosis of partial placenta previa. Her labor was rapid and she was delivered by vaginal route. You are caring for Mrs. B in recovery room. Most likely complication to occur during this time would be:
(a) anemia.
(b) infection.
(c) uterine atony.
19. The severe pain associated with abruptio is due to:
(a) blood collects retroplacental.
(b) labor is always prolonged.
(c) labor is always rapid.
20. Complications likely to occur with an abruptio placentae are:
(a) hypofibrinogenemia.
(b) renal failure.
(c) uteroplacental apoplexy.
1. a only   2. a, b, and c   3. a and c only
21. A patient complains of constant backache in the lumbosacral region. This frequently accompanies:
(a) abruptio placentae.
(b) placenta previa.
(c) ectopic pregnancy.
22. The majority of fetal deaths due to anoxia are the result of:
(a) an abruptio placentae.
(b) a placenta previa.
(c) diabetes.

*True or false*

(T) (F) 1. A 20% dextrose solution may be ordered for the preeclamptic to promote diuresis.
(T) (F) 2. The one disadvantage of using magnesium sulfate for the mother is that it causes fetal depression.
(T) (F) 3. Toxemia tends to be more severe in the underweight woman.
(T) (F) 4. The fetus is not essential for the development of toxemia.
(T) (F) 5. A weight gain of over 1 pound a week during pregnancy is abnormal.
(T) (F) 6. It is not unusual for a patient to have a repetition of toxemia in subsequent pregnancies.
(T) (F) 7. With toxemia, edema will be noticed first in the upper extremities.

## REFERENCES

1. Adler, Frances: Textbook of ophthalmology, ed. 7, Philadelphia, 1963, W. B. Saunders Co., p. 383.
2. Babson, S. Gorham, and Benson, Ralph C.: Primer on prematurity and high-risk pregnancy, St. Louis, 1966, The C. V. Mosby Co., pp. 42-44.
3. Forbes, Donald: Application of ultrasonic scanning in obstetrics and gynecology, Hosp. Top. 46:57, Sept., 1968.
4. Gerbie, Albert: Management of heart disease complicated by pregnancy, Hosp. Med. 1:16, June, 1965.
5. Greenhill, J. P., editor: Obstetrics, ed. 13, Philadelphia, 1965, W. B. Saunders Co., chap. 39.
6. Hawkings, Pauline: Hydatidiform mole, Nurs. Times 63:721, June 2, 1967.
7. Li, Min C.: New treatment of hydatidiform mole and choriocarcinoma, Hosp. Med. 1:44, Nov., 1964.
8. Millar, K. G.: Thermography and its application to placental localization, Nurs. Mirror 127:33, Nov. 15, 1968.
9. Potter, Edith L.: Pathology of fetus and infant, Chicago, 1962, Year Book Medical Publishers, Inc., chap. 13.
10. Rodman, Morton J., and Smith, Dorothy W.: Pharmacology and drug therapy in nursing, Philadelphia, 1966, J. B. Lippincott Co., p. 301.
11. Hellman, Robert W., and Hall, J. Edward: Nutrition during pregnancy. In Wohl, Michael, and Goodhart, Robert, editors: Modern nutrition in health and disease, ed. 3, Philadelphia, 1964, Lea & Febiger, p. 1107.

## SELECTED READINGS
*Toxemia*

Barber, Hugh R. K., Graber, Edward A., and Donnenfeld, Alvin M.: Toxemia of pregnancy. In Barber, Hugh R. K., and Graber, Edward A., editors: Quick reference to ob-gyn procedures, Philadelphia, 1969, J. B. Lippincott Co., chap. 17.

Beck, A. C., and Taylor, E. Stewart, editors: Obstetrical practice, ed. 8, Baltimore, 1966, The Williams & Wilkins Co., chap. 27.

Grimm, Elaine: Psychological and social factors. In Richardson, Stephen, and Guttmacher, Alan, editors: Childbearing: its social and psychological aspects, Baltimore, 1967, The Williams & Wilkins Co., pp. 13-14.

Guyton, Arthur: Textbook of medical physiology, Philadelphia, 1966, W. B. Saunders Co., chap. 79.

Klopper, Arnold: Pre-eclamptic toxemia, Nurs. Times 64:116, Jan. 26, 1968.

Landesman, Robert: Edema of pregnancy: what to consider before giving a diuretic, Consultant 7:26, Sept., 1967.

McCartney, Charles P.: Toxemia. In Greenhill, J. P., editor: Obstetrics, ed. 13, Philadelphia, 1965, W. B. Saunders Co., chap. 31.

Montagu, M. F. Ashley: Prenatal influences, Springfield, Ill., 1962, Charles C Thomas, Publisher, pp. 241-243.

*Hyperemesis gravidarum*

Beck, A. C., and Taylor, E. Stewart, editors: Obstetrical practice, ed. 8, Baltimore, 1966, The Williams & Wilkins Co., chap. 26.

Greenhill, J. P., editor: Obstetrics, ed. 13, Philadelphia, 1965, W. B. Saunders Co., chap. 30.

Grimm, Elaine: Psychological and social factors. In Richardson, Stephen, and Guttmacher, Alan, editors: Childbearing: its social and psychological aspects, Baltimore, 1967, The Williams & Wilkins Co., pp. 11-13.

Guyton, Arthur: Textbook of medical physiology, Philadelphia, 1966, W. B. Saunders Co., chap. 79.

*Pregnancy–diabetes mellitus*

Beck, A. C., and Taylor, E. Stewart, editors: Obstetrical practice, ed. 8, Baltimore, 1966, The Williams & Wilkins Co., chap. 28.

Beckman, Harry: The nature, action and use of drugs, ed. 2, Philadelphia, 1961, W. B. Saunders Co., p. 730.

Burt, Richard L.: How to reduce the hazards of diabetes in pregnancy, Consultant 9:5, March-April, 1969.

Dolger, Henry, Bookman, John J., and Nechemias, Charles: Pregnancy in the diabetic and prediabetic. In Rovinsky, Joseph, editor: Medical, surgical and gynecologic complications of pregnancy, Baltimore, 1965, The Williams & Wilkins Co., pp. 604-612.

Garnet, James: Pregnancy in women with diabetes, Amer. J. Nurs. 69:1900, Sept., 1969.

Hagbard, Lars: Pregnancy and diabetes mellitus, Springfield, Ill., 1966, Charles C Thomas, Publisher, chap. 9.

Hellman, Robert, and Hall, J. Edward: Nutrition in pregnancy. In Wohl, Michael, and Goodhart, Robert, editors: Modern nutrition in health and disease, ed. 3, Philadelphia, 1964, Lea & Febiger, p. 1107.

Krosnick, Arthur: Counseling and managing the pregnant diabetic patient, Consultant 6:30, Oct., 1966.

Makinson, D. H.: Medical disorders of pregnancy, Nurs. Mirror 128:42, Jan. 17, 1969.

Montagu, M. F. Ashley: Prenatal influences, Springfield, Ill., 1962, Charles C Thomas, Publisher, pp. 224-231.

Shuman, Charles: The pregnant diabetic, Hosp. Med. 5:60, Sept., 1969.

Silverman, Frederick: Diabetes mellitus in pregnancy. In Barber, Hugh R. K., and Graber, Edward A., editors: Quick reference to ob-gyn procedures, Philadelphia, 1969. J. B. Lippincott Co., chap. 23.

*Abortions*

Abortion and the law, J.A.M.A. 199:211, Jan. 16, 1967.

Buxton, C. Lee: One doctors opinion of abortion laws, Amer. J. Nurs. 68:1022, May, 1968.

Carroll, Charles: Liberalized abortion—a critique, Child Family 7:157, Spring, 1968.

Copeland, William E., and Ullery, John: Therapeutic abortion, J.A.M.A. 207:713, Jan. 27, 1969.

Diamond, Eugene F.: A pediatrician views abortion, Child Family 7:47, Winter, 1968.

Fonseca, Jeanne: Induced abortion, Amer. J. Nurs. 68:1022, May, 1968.

Jakobovits, Immanuel: Jewish views on abortion, Child Family 7:142, Spring, 1968.

Klopper, Arnold: Spontaneous abortion, Nurs. Times 64:74, Jan. 19, 1968.

Knutson, Andie: When does a human life begin? View points of public health professionals, Amer. J. Public Health 57:2163, Dec., 1967.

Kummer, Jerome: Experts discuss contraception, indications for abortion, Hosp. Top. 45:92, June, 1967.

MacDonald, R. R.: Complications of abortion, Nurs. Times 63:306, March 10, 1967.

Millar, David R.: Induction of labor and abortion with intraamniotic hypertonic saline, Nurs. Mirror 124:445, Aug. 11, 1967.

Neuhaus, Richard J.: Abortions and the human community, Child Family 7:254, Summer, 1968.

Ratner, Herbert: A public health physician views abortion, Child Family 7:38, Winter, 1968.

Thurstone, P. B.: Therapeutic abortion, J.A.M.A. 209:229, July 14, 1969.

Tietze, Christopher, and Lewit, Sarah: Abortion, Sci. Amer. 220:21, Jan., 1969.

Willson, J. Robert: Abortion—a medical responsibility, Obstet. Gynec. 30:294, Aug., 1967.

*High-risk pregnancy*

Aaron, Jules, and Diamond, Bernard: Fetal and maternal hazards of surgery during pregnancy, Hosp. Med. 2:24, March, 1966.

Bowen, George L.: Pulmonary tuberculosis in pregnancy. In Barber, Hugh R. K., and Graber, Edward A., editors: Quick reference to ob-gyn procedures, Philadelphia, 1969, J. B. Lippincott Co., chap. 24.

Brainerd, Henry, Morgen, Sheldon, and Chatton, Milton J.: Current diagnosis and treatment,

Los Altos, Calif., 1966, Lange Medical Publications, chap .13.

Clinch, J.: Sydenham's chorea during pregnancy, Nurs. Times **64**:690, May 24, 1968.

Douglas, C. P.: Gestation and concurrent diseases, Nurs. Mirror **126**:25, May 24, 1968.

Gillespie, Luke: Study of high-risk patients identifies morbidity factors, Hosp. Top. **46**:79, May, 1968.

Graber, Edward A.: Heart disease in pregnancy. In Barber, Hugh R. K., and Graber, Edward A., editors: Quick reference to ob-gyn procedures, Philadelphia, 1969. J. B. Lippincott Co., chap. 22.

Greenhill, J. P., editor: Obstetrics, ed. 13, Philadelphia, 1965, W. B. Saunders Co., chaps. 37, 38, and 40.

Humphrey, Arthure: Avoidable factors in maternal deaths, Nurs. Mirror **26**:22, March 29, 1968.

Makinson, D. H.: Medical disorders of pregnancy, Nurs. Mirror **128**:15, Jan. 10, 1969.

Molyneux, Barbara C.: Rare obstetric complication, Nurs. Mirror **124**:1, July 21, 1967.

Nesbitt, Robert E. L., and Aubry, Richard H.: Recognition and care of high-risk obstetrical patients, Hosp. Med. **3**:43, Sept., 1967.

Quilligan, Edward J.: Diagnosis and management of ectopic pregnancy, Hosp. Med. **5**:27, March, 1969.

Rose, Patricia Ann: The high risk mother-infant dyad, Nurs. Forum **6**:94, 1967.

Slatin, Marion: Extra protection for high-risk mothers and babies, Amer. J. Nurs. **67**:1241, June, 1967.

Smith, G. Stewart: Clinical pathology in obstetrics, Nurs. Mirror **127**:18, July 12, 1968.

Stern, D. M.: Malignant disease and pregnancy, Nurs. Mirror **126**:19, June 14, 1968.

**For student's quick notes:**

Chapter 9

# The nurse in the prenatal clinic

If you are motivated toward maternity nursing, it will be in the prenatal clinical setting that you will have the opportunity to prove your worth and importance in counseling and teaching. The previous chapters are basic to this function. This chapter introduces you to the responsibilities of the nurse in the prenatal clinic.

Your instructor may provide an opportunity for you to visit in the homes of your patients pre- and postnatally. If you are to perform effectively in such settings, the variables in living standards and human relationships are of paramount importance so that here your knowledge of sociology and psychology will come into play.

The problem of the unwed mother is of great and increasing concern. Since you will be in contact with the unmarried mothers during your clinical experience, reference is made to the problem in this chapter. You will become aware of the girl's vital need for acceptance and of the alternative plans available to her. To further your ability in being of assistance to these girls, you should make use of the many references included in the selected readings.

## Introduction to the clinic

Now that you have acquired a basic theory covering the period of pregnancy, you are ready for observational experience, counseling, and teaching, and to give the much needed "supportive care" to women during their pregnancy. Most of this experience takes place in the prenatal clinic. It is my belief that this is a very important part of your learning experience and, therefore, this chapter is devoted to preparing you to function as a professional student in the prenatal clinic.

There is no better way to prepare you to teach pregnant women on a professional basis than to expose you to these women throughout their maternity cycle. These monthly and bimonthly visits with the pregnant woman will expand your capacity to work with people. Here you will witness, at first hand, the many facets contributing to their acceptance or rejection of pregnancy. You will acquire a knowledge of family life, gain insight into the needs of pregnant women, and become increasingly skilled in recognizing their attitudes toward motherhood. You will be rendering them a valuable service while contributing greatly to your personal and professional growth. (See Fig. 9-1.)

Most of our prenatal clinics are overcrowded and the women are reluctant to bother the doctor with questions which, if answered, might give peace of mind. Often,

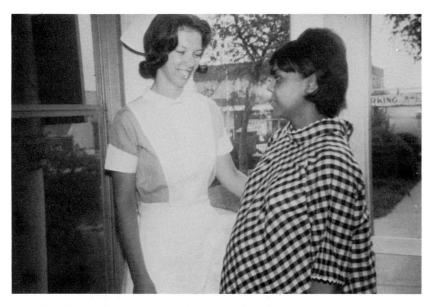

**Fig. 9-1.** Student nurse greets her assigned mother on entrance to clinic.

the line and the time of waiting is long, but the examination is all too rapid. The patient would like to tell the doctor "important" things about herself, but the atmosphere into which she is hurried makes this impossible, and she leaves with the same problems that she had when she came in.

In some of our clinics the women feel as though they are "numbers" instead of persons, that is, the personnel are rather indifferent to them. We as nurses are the guilty ones. We stand in the hall and call out a number or a "last" name, instead of approaching the "bench" and addressing the patient properly. When the clinics are overcrowded and there is a shortage of personnel, these women are mustered along a waiting line. Along with the hard benches, goes the impersonality of many of those working in these clinics. The shortage of health workers and the unusual distribution of their services are contributory factors to such conditions.

It is not my intention to criticize prenatal clinics, but rather to attempt to prepare you to face actuality. The prenatal clinic does furnish invaluable service, especially that of filtering out the high-risk mothers and admitting them to the hospital for treat-

ment. This alone has reduced fetal and maternal mortality rates considerably. (See Tables C-1 to C-4, pp. 323 to 325.)

It gives the mother-to-be a great deal of satisfaction during the "waiting months" to know that someone really cares. Traveling a long distance to get to the clinic is less tiring when she knows that a nurse will be at the door to greet her. Sitting on a bench for an hour or more is also less tiring if someone talks with her, shares her experiences, and cares whether or not she comes to the clinic. Here is where you become a supportive person. If the woman understands something about the physiological and psychological changes, she is more likely to accept them without complaint, and she can more easily turn a deaf ear to advice of well-meaning acquaintances.

It is with relative ease that the nurse discusses the physiological changes accompanying pregnancy, but it is with more difficulty that she acquires some understanding of the psychological factors because they are so much more complex. However, we are not being fair if we consider only the woman's physical well-being. We place so much emphasis on adequate prenatal care, yet ignore the emotional as-

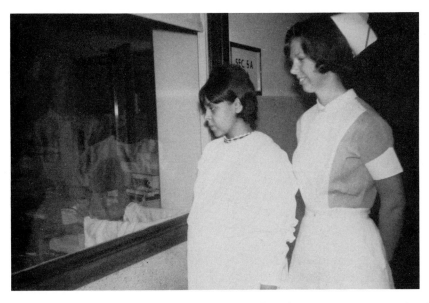

**Fig. 9-2.** Student takes her assigned mother on a tour through maternity unit. Here they both enjoy viewing newborn infants.

pects which predominate during the maternity cycle. What are dismissed as unimportant side effects of pregnancy often weigh heavily on the emotions of the woman. You neglect an important phase of maternity nursing when you ignore her emotional needs. It is not within the realm of the student nurse to get to the root of the psychological problems. The nurse should nevertheless be aware of the propelling factors, develop skills in recognizing how variable these emotional responses may be, and recognize when the problem is no longer within her scope and needs the attention of the doctor.

One of the students' problems is learning how much to discuss with the patient. She starts by listening and observing so that she may sense her emotional needs and her expected behavior in labor. In this way the nurse improves her own understanding of social and cultural variations. It is important that you realize that your teaching and counseling levels are those of a student nurse, not an authoritative person.

The greatest contribution the nurse can make is to be genuinely sincere in displaying concern for the patient's interests. In no

other field of nursing does the student have more opportunity to show this interest in human needs than in maternity nursing. (See Fig. 9-2.)

### Preparation for and assistance with the initial examination

While the nurse is assisting the woman in preparation for the examination, she should notice whether she appears nervous or apprehensive, especially if she is a primigravida. Often this can be minimized if the nurse explains the procedure of the examination and assures the woman that she will be in attendance.

Prior to the examination, the nurse takes the blood pressure, weighs the patient, and charts her findings for the doctor. Remember that this first blood pressure reading may not be a reliable one because of the emotional trauma involved during this first visit. Her blood pressure reflects the condition of her heart and blood vessels; a sudden rise is a danger signal of poor kidney function and developing toxemia.

During the examination the doctor asks the patient about her previous pregnancies, labors, and deliveries; he inquires about her present pregnancy, such as date of her last period and the regularity of her menses. This is important, since it evaluates her glandular status. He examines her chest and breasts and palpates the abdominal organs. He examines her for varicosities or edema and questions her about past illnesses, since it is important that he know whether she had any diseases, for example, rheumatic fever that might have affected her heart or the kidneys, since these two organs have an especially important function during pregnancy. All of this is highly valuable in helping the doctor detect any organic pathology.

The nurse then prepares the patient for the pelvic examination. Some doctors do pelvic measurements, since this allows for accurate planning by revealing any structural abnormality, or inadequate measurements for labor and prepares the woman for the possibility of a cesarean section.

The vaginal examination is important because (1) it establishes the diagnosis of pregnancy by the presence of such signs as von Fernwald's, Chadwick's, or Ladin's; (2) it estimates the probable duration of the pregnancy; (3) it allows for the opportunity of taking smears for a cyto-logical examination to detect early cellular changes, that is, possibility of future development of carcinoma (cultures may be taken if there are any vaginal discharges); and (4) it detects abnormalities such as cysts and infections.

The incidence of *Trichomonas* and *Candida albicans* varies with the socioeconomic level of women and is found to be higher among clinic than private patients. The discharge in trichomoniasis is greenish white in color, malodorous, and usually purulent. It causes the vulva to become tender, reddened, and edematous. The discharge in candidiasis causes flaky, white particles to adhere to the vagina.

On completion of the examination, the doctor notates his findings on the woman's chart, while the nurse assists the patient in dressing. The examination gives the doctor the opportunity to estimate the woman's health status and her fitness for pregnancy. He evaluates her weight in comparison with the average curve and plans for her total gain or loss during her pregnancy. If she has a weight problem, he or the nurse discusses this with her. Her weight will be a guide to her well-being throughout her pregnancy. He may prescribe a vitamin-

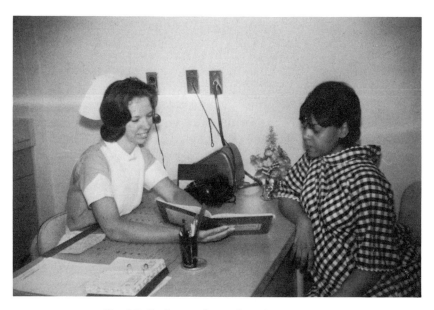

**Fig. 9-3.** Student reinforces doctor's instructions.

mineral supplement. If her initial visit is after the twentieth week, the doctor auscultates fetal heart beat and estimates presentation, position, and engagement of presenting part.

The woman should be allotted time for a personal interview with the doctor so that she may have her questions answered. When others are waiting, unfortunately, this interview may be in a hurried instead of in a relaxed, casual atmosphere. She may sense this and yet feel the need to discuss her problems. Then, too, some women feel their discomforts are too trivial to tell the doctor. Therefore the nurse should be ready to assume responsibility for the interview, and this is not an unimportant responsibility. Simply by giving her of your time and showing that you are interested and care, you may contribute a great deal toward putting her at ease. In talking with her you may learn something about her educational background and suggest suitable booklets, of which there are many, for her to read. If there is a weight problem during this time, the nurse reviews thoroughly, with the patient, whatever diet the doctor may desire that she follow. This must be done with tact since too much emphasis on weight gain may predispose to anxiety in the patient. (See Fig. 9-3.)

Before she leaves she may be sent to the laboratory to have blood drawn from her veins. The nurse should explain to the patient that this is done (1) to determine presence of anemia, (2) for a Wassermann test, and (3) for blood type in case of blood discrepancies.

## Teaching and counseling during the period of pregnancy

The nurse also instructs the patient to bring a specimen of her urine at each visit. Routine examination of the urine permits detection of unusual contents such as plasma proteins, increased amounts of sugar (glycosuria frequently occurs as a functional disturbance), and pus, indicating pyelitis.

She explains the importance of keeping her clinic appointments; usually once a month until the thirty-second week; every 2 weeks until the thirty-sixth week; then weekly until delivery.

Some of the topics you might discuss with the patient during the visits to the clinic are given below.

*Rest, relaxation, and sleep.* If we consider the extra energy the body requires for maternal and fetal physiology, we can easily understand why the expectant mother requires more rest and sleep. Some women are normally filled with energy and keep going throughout the day; others are less active and accustomed to frequent rest periods. A code of rest and sleep should be planned according to each individual's needs, taking into consideration her age and her usual habits and stressing especially that she should avoid fatigue. (See Fig. 9-4.)

*Care of the breasts.* The nurse should discuss the changes the woman may expect in her breasts during the first trimester, such as the feeling of fullness and noticing that they may be a little more tense, turgid, with perhaps a broadening and dark-

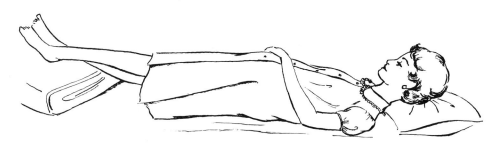

**Fig. 9-4.** A code of rest should be planned for each individual according to her needs.

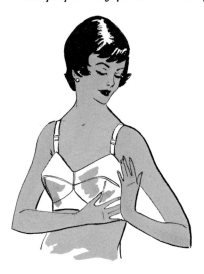

**Fig. 9-5.** Nurse instructs mother-to-be how to properly support breasts.

ening of the areola. Instruct the woman to wear a well-fitted brassiere and as she adjusts it, to bring her breasts to the center of the cups instead of compressing them tightly. As the breasts increase in size this proper support helps retain their normal contour. (See Fig. 9-5.) One of the little worries of the young primigravida is that she will lose the lovely contour of her breasts. Actually these instructions concerning the wearing of a support should be given to any girl when she reaches puberty.

At a later visit the nurse may also mention the secretion of colostrum from the breasts. She can also learn whether the woman has any feelings about bottle or breast feeding. This gives the patient time to think about what method of feeding she would like to use; then it can be discussed again during the second trimester.

*Care of the teeth.* If the woman has regular examinations of her teeth, little need be said. If not, she should be encouraged to see a dentist or referred to the dental clinic. Changes in pH or bacterial flora may enhance occurrence of dental caries. Decaying teeth are a source of infection. Some women do experience irritation of the gingivae, but this regresses after parturition.

*Personal hygiene.* During the first trimester the woman should be encouraged to take daily tub baths, although she may prefer to shower. It has been proved that there is no validity to the statement that tub baths should be avoided because water enters the vaginal canal. A warm bath can be a means of relaxation, but if she does not have access to the tub or shower, then you should instruct her to take a daily sponge bath.

*Body mechanics.* The pregnant woman must make adjustments in her posture to balance the weight of her protruding abdomen. There is bound to be added strain on the spinal column and muscles of the back. Instruct the woman to balance her weight on both feet, to train her buttock muscles by tucking them under (contracting them), and to stand erect with head held high. This will keep her pelvis level while walking, permit full chest expansion, free diaphragmatic action, and minimize strain on muscles in lumbar area. If she advances one foot forward before squatting, this will act as a prop to transfer her weight.

*Intestinal elimination.* You will recall that intestinal motility is apt to be reduced during pregnancy, which is believed to be due, in part, to the relaxin hormone and to the displacement of the intestines by the enlarging uterus. To forestall increasing difficulty, you might discuss dietary readjustment by increasing intake of fluids, especially fruit juices. If this does not help, then the doctor should be informed of this condition.

*Abdominal support.* The value of an abdominal support during the first trimester is questionable. If she is accustomed to wearing one, she should, of course, continue. If she has been wearing round garters, the nurse should caution her about this by explaining that they do constrict the flow of blood. You might suggest the advisability of a garter belt. (See Fig. 9-6.)

*Exercise.* Exercise needs to be defined for each individual. The woman who tends to be athletic would not consider walking as exercising, yet for the woman who is sedentary, you would recommend walking. Women who participate in the so-called

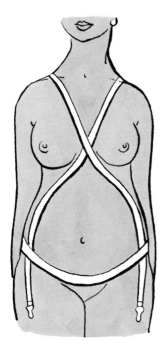

**Fig. 9-6.** Form of stocking support to avoid use of round garters.

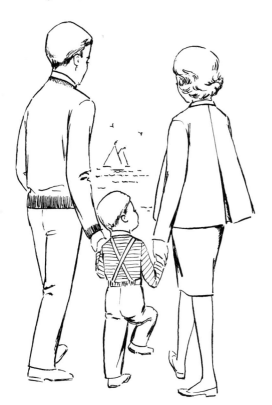

**Fig. 9-7.** Walking—a form of exercise for the family to enjoy together.

"strenuous" exercises should discuss the continuation of these with the doctor. Some doctors do restrict horseback riding, or participation in any new type of exercise. If the patient questions exercising, you should see that she is given an opportunity to discuss this with the doctor. (See Fig. 9-7.)

*Traveling.* Most doctors advise women to avoid long and arduous traveling. It may produce fatigue and overexertion. Air travel is not restricted, except during the last 2 months.

*Employment.* Many pregnant women are employed outside the home and have no choice but to continue, even into the last trimester. Some women work away from home all day, then cook and care for their family during the evening hours. If it is imperative that she work during the last trimester, all that we can do is caution her about undue fatigue and about the danger involved in lifting or any type work involving physical trauma.

Studies done on factors influencing a woman's health during pregnancy show that hard work during the last months increases the rate of prematurity and low birth weight infants. When the woman attending clinic is employed outside the home, it is primarily for economic reasons.

*Teaching during the second trimester*

It is during the second trimester when the patient begins to "show" that she is often concerned about her changing figure. She should be encouraged to walk with pride—to be proud of her ability to fulfill her greatest function in life. She may be assured that if she obeys the doctor's pattern of weight gain, she can have just as lovely a figure after delivery and that the process of pregnancy, labor, and delivery need not cause her to become shapeless.

As the abdomen protrudes, the center of gravity changes and the nurse should explain to the woman that it would be far better if she wore shoes with low heels, since high heels cause added strain on back muscles and tend to throw the pelvis forward. This is the time when she might find that a girdle gives added support to the protruding abdomen and relieves her backache.

The woman coming to the clinic may not be able to afford to purchase a maternity girdle, but a stretch girdle serves the same purpose. The nurse must be certain that the woman understands that it should not be so tight as to constrict circulation. She might also mention Braxton Hicks's contractions and inquire whether she has felt the fetus "quicken." Her recognition of quickening may aid the doctor in pinpointing the period of gestation.

If the woman continues to show excessive gain in weight (due to overeating) after adequate counseling, the nurse needs to learn why she is overeating. This may be her way of responding to inner anxieties. We cannot expect women to change deep-rooted food patterns, but if we display genuine concern, we can often motivate their interest in trying to follow instructions.

If at any visit the patient shows a sudden gain in weight and edema, the doctor may restrict her sodium intake. It is then the nurse's duty to review (with the woman) the foods containing considerable salt such as most frozen and canned vegetables, all seafoods, meats, processed cheese, butter, peanut butter, margarine, pickles, catsup, and soft drinks. Low-sodium milk (Lonalac) and salt-free butter or margarine are available.

At one of the visits during the second trimester, the nurse should again discuss methods of feeding the infant. If she has no preference for either method, she needs encouragement toward breast feeding. The emotional value of the infant at the breast should be explained to her rather than ignored. Breast feeding meets the infant's and mother's emotional needs. Parturition interrupts the symbiotic relationship between these two—lactation reestablishes this relationship. It certainly contributes toward the mother's feeling of adequacy and relieves her of the emptiness many women experience after the infant is delivered. *There is no finer way for her to experience complete mothering.*[1]

Explain the great emotional satisfaction her baby will derive from this warm, close skin to skin contact. Explain also how the infant's sucking stimulates the uterine muscles to contract and helps her uterus return more naturally to its prepregnant size and position. If the woman has inverted nipples, you may instruct her to put *gentle* traction on the nipples. This mild stimulation promotes erection of the nipple due to contraction of muscle fibers. If she does this nipple exercise twice a day, every day, by the time she delivers she will find the infant will be able to get a better grasp of the nipple.

With tact the nurse should instruct the prospective mother regarding danger signals that tell us all is not well. Severe headaches or swelling of the extremities is a sign of preeclampsia; escape of fluid from the vaginal canal could mean the membranes have ruptured; and vaginal bleeding could mean the possibility of a slight abruption of the placenta.

You might suggest she write to the LaLeche League for information about their organization and activities. The LaLeche League was formed by a group of young parents interested in the *natural* way of feeding their infant. LaLeche (lay-chay) is the Spanish title of Mother of Christ and means "the milk."

Mothers who are members of the league always show a friendly interest in the new mother and sincerely try to give her a happy introduction into the natural way of mothering. When she has problems or questions concerning breast feeding, they respond with "time," "patience," and "kind words," all so essential to the new mother who may be unduly concerned about her ability to nurse her infant. Their slogan, "Good mothering through breastfeeding the world over," well describes their main function of promoting the natural way of mothering.

### Teaching in preparation for the onset of labor

During the third trimester, the nurse instructs the woman in preparation for the onset of labor. All women fear for their safety during labor and delivery. In discussing labor with them, especially primigravidas, you will learn that they have vague concepts of this process. The primigravida's fears about labor are usually associated with the unknown. By listening to her comments, the nurse can acquire insight into how much explanation the patient needs.

We know that preparation for labor influences attitudes toward and progress made during parturition, and to a certain degree the extent of discomfort. For some women the impact of early life experiences have a tremendous effect on them. The nurse must develop a sensitivity to the inner conflicts the woman is trying to master. Her questions may never have been answered or what information she has received is often distorted and superstitious. Multigravidas recall unfortunate distressing situations during previous labors and may be relieved by having someone with whom they may discuss these experiences.

More commonly today women fear developmental imperfections in their babies. If you help her understand that labor is safe, then she will be more likely to want to participate in the birth instead of requesting the "black-out" method that so many of our American women request. Women who receive adequate instructions and are properly prepared enjoy the experience of giving birth. If the woman understands the forces of uterine contractions, she will be ready to assist nature—not resist the normal powers. A little of the nurse's time during this trimester can remove much of the emotional trauma and physical discomfort.

It is during this time that she will instruct the patient about the signs of approaching labor. Nature has ways of signaling women that the "time to be born" has arrived: (1) the primigravida experiences lightening about 2 weeks before true labor starts (this provides relief in the upper abdomen, eases breathing, and decreases epigastric pressure; however, it increases pressure in the pelvis, causes difficulty in walking, and increases urinary frequency); (2) vaginal secretions increase in amount and the oper-

culum that corked the cervical canal may escape from the vaginal canal (this is usually tinged with blood and mucus from changes occurring in the cervix and is referred to as the show); (3) a loss of weight, as much as 2 to 3 pounds, may be caused by excretion of body water; (4) a backache may persist; and (5) rupture of the membranes may occur. These prodromal symptoms usher in the climax to the period of waiting.

The nurse may invite the woman on a tour of the maternity department. This clears many misconceptions; the hands are merely fitted into the cuffs—the patient is *not* strapped to a table! The nurse may also direct her to the entrance used for admissions during the night.

Some of the women like to discuss the layette they have prepared; others prefer to wait until after the infant is born. Either way, the nurse may be of assistance in discussing her plans for the care of the infant.

The early signs and symptoms of impending labor may confuse the woman and she may come to the hospital when she could have remained at home with her family. It is the nurse's responsibility to explain prodromal labor to the patient.

When should the woman come to the hospital? This depends on various factors. If on admission the woman is assigned to the room that she will occupy after delivery and allowed to remain there with her husband until her labor becomes active or until she needs sedation, then coming to the hospital early may have its advantages. Not all hospitals are equipped with such an environment; they do not even have a room where the woman can read, relax, or walk around. Upon admission she is put to bed, and there she stays until her baby is ready to be born.

Women in false labor, or the early phase of the first stage, should *never* be placed in a room with patients in active labor. One must feel sorry for the primigravida who comes to the hospital "early" because she was told to do so and then is placed in a bed along side an active patient. This can be a frightening experience for her. All that the nurse might have tried to teach the woman in preparation for labor is defeated when she is in such an environment. Great pity that not one room can be spared or set aside for these women, where they could read, rest, or just relax in a quiet environment. The woman in false labor is discouraged, is disappointed, and wonders just what is going to happen to her. Her need for emotional support is greatly neglected through our thoughtlessness. Women in "false" labor are *not* safer in the hospital when subjected to such an environment. There is no need for the primigravida to come to the hospital as soon as labor starts. She can remain at home with her loved ones and continue with her usual activities. The woman should be instructed how labor may start, such as low back discomfort radiating to the front or definite, distinct uterine contractions, and how to time contractions. She has ample time to come to the hospital when the contractions are 8 to 5 minutes apart and regular, unless she has a great distance to travel. If the membranes rupture or there is any vaginal bleeding, the woman should come to the hospital and not wait for contractions to start.

Valuables should be left at home. This simplifies admission procedures and avoids loss of personal effects. Instruct the woman to pack a suitcase with her personal articles. Her husband can bring this to her after delivery and she is transferred to her room. If she did buy a layette, she might also like to pack the clothes she wants to use for the baby when discharged. This makes it more convenient for her husband or member of the family than if they have to gather the articles. Invariably they forget the essentials, the diaper or safety pins!

*Evaluation of experiences*

After each visit to the clinic you should evaluate your teaching and learning experience. Your instructor may arrange for a conference at which time each student has the opportunity to relate her experiences so that all may benefit. The following might be considered in preparation for your conference report: (1) What trimester of pregnancy was the patient in when you met with her? Review the physiological changes occurring during this trimester. (2) If you met the woman on a previous occasion, did you observe any response to what you may have taught her? If so, discuss. (3) How did this visit contribute toward your knowledge of maternity nursing? (4) What do you plan to discuss with her on the next meeting?

## The nurse and the unwed mother-to-be

It is known that the number of unmarried mothers is increasing and that the average age is decreasing. There is no "average" unmarried mother. These girls come from every social and economic level of society, but you are more likely to come in contact with those girls from the lower income level; the others have the financial support from their families and can be secluded in a maternity home.

What can the unmarried girl do when she becomes pregnant? In despair she may terminate the pregnancy, yet very few unmarried mothers consider this possibility. She may not know who the father is, and if she does, she may not wish to marry him. Whatever is the case, her predicament is the result of complicated environmental factors, not necessarily lack of morals. Our complex society condones extramarital sex, yet condemns the result.

The stigma placed on the unwed mother and her child is centuries old. Society's view was to *prevent by punishment*. The laws of the Puritans in the 1600s is an example of this. The girl was displayed in the public square and then imprisoned. It was not until the middle of the nineteenth century that the maternity home movement got underway. The church was influential in founding and operating many such homes. Although those interested worked for humane treatment, the victims were still labeled "fallen" and were viewed as moral problems of society.

In 1898 the nationwide Florence Crittenton organization was granted a national charter by act of Congress. Today there are over 200 such homes. The Salvation Army, out of their mission work for women, opened their first home in 1887 in Brooklyn. Fortunately, today most of those responsible for these homes recognize social conditions contributing to the girl's dilemma and do more than give her physical shelter. The philosophy today is one of tolerance and understanding, but the stigma established by society is still with us.

The unwed girl that you meet in the clinic is facing motherhood before adulthood and lacks the basis on which to develop her motherliness. She is confronted with an overwhelming situation and is bound to react in various ways. She will display her defense mechanism with hostility, suspicion, or the pose of adequacy. You will meet girls with attitudes of rigidity and those with laxity with regard to moral standards.

We need to offer these girls more than our physical facilities of prenatal care and delivery, but it is your function neither to pry nor to prod into the wherefore of her predicament. She has come to the clinic, and that in itself is good, for here she is assured of prenatal care. Some clinics turn away the unmarried girl if she is a minor. Others will not accept her if she has not lived in the locality for a period of time, or they may refer her to another clinic. Some girls have no choice but to do without prenatal care and present themselves as emergency patients when labor starts. This, of course, contributes to our high infant mortality rates.

The unwed girl expects to be poorly received and to be condemned. She may be reluctant to talk with you; you may feel insecure in knowing just how to respond to her, but you can start by offering warmth and respect for her and by being noncritical and nonjudgmental. You are not to disapprove her behavior but to understand behavior. If the girl wishes to talk, then encourage her by being an interested, uncensorious listener. Whatever information she volunteers must be accepted matter-of-factly. Guard against reflecting your own personal attitudes or allowing personal emotions to influence you. You need to encourage her to continue prenatal visits and this she will do when she learns that your interest is genuine. You also need to explain about the doctor's procedures, especially the internal examination. Then discuss the physiological and psychological changes she may expect during her pregnancy and prepare her for the labor and birth process.

It is not within the realm of the student nurse to try to deal with the many deep psychological problems that beset this individual. She needs professional counseling of a caseworker. If there is no social service worker available in the hospital, then it is the function of the nurse to direct the girl to an agency in her vicinity. It is the trained social service worker who counsels the girl during her pregnancy, and when the time comes for her to decide what is best for the baby, the caseworker will guide her with the plan that seems most feasible for her. The social service worker can direct her and see that the infant is adopted through a reputable agency.

She needs help in rehabilitating herself in society after the ordeal is over. This takes stamina, more than is needed to tread through pregnancy without a husband, more than to make the decision to place the infant. The caseworker makes every effort to place her in a noncensuring environment.

The greatest contribution you can make is helping to promote a warm environment for these bewildered girls.

Physiologically these young mothers-to-be react favorably to their pregnancy. The incidence of miscarriage and nausea is rare, although toxemia is relatively common. They deliver their babies with fewer than the average complications, but many of them show a postpartum anemia. The infants tend to be classified as low birth weight.

**REFERENCE**

1. Rawlins, Carolyn M.: The expectant mother. Should you nurse your baby, Redbook **131**:44, July, 1968.

**SELECTED READINGS**

*Maternity clinics*

Anderson, Edith, and Lesser, Arthur: Maternity care in the United States: gains and gaps, Amer. J. Nurs. **66**:1539, July, 1966.

Barnard, Jan: Your part in helping to reduce infant mortality, RN **30**:43, Nov., 1967.

Beebe, Joyce, Pendleton, E. M., and King, E.: Bench conferences in a large obstetric clinic, Amer. J. Nurs. **68**:85, Jan., 1968.

Ely, Carol, Diulio, R. J., and Koster, E. C.: Are maternity clinic dropouts necessary, Nurs. Outlook **15**:41, July, 1967.

Freeman, Ruth: The criterion of relevance, Amer. J. Public Health **57**:522, Sept., 1967.

Hilliard, Mary E.: New horizons in maternity nursing, Nurs. Outlook **15**:33, July, 1967.

Kovner, Anthony R., and Seacat, Milvoy: Continuity of care maintained in family-centered outpatient unit, Hospitals **43**:89, July, 1969.

Lake, Alice: Why do so many babies die? Good Housekeeping **167**:63, Aug. 1968.

Melber, Ruth: The maternity nurse specialist in a hospital clinic setting, Nurs. Res. **16**:69, Winter, 1967.

Reid, Duncan: To everything there is a season, Obstet. Gynec. **30**:269, Aug., 1967.

Schlesinger, Richard, Davis, Clarence, and Milliken, Sewall: Out-patient care—the influence of interrelated needs. In Lytle, Nancy A., editor: Maternal health nursing, Dubuque, Iowa, 1967, William C. Brown Co., sect. 2, pp. 50-61.

Seacat, Melvoy, and Schlachter, Louise: Expanding nursing role in prenatal and infant care, Amer. J. Nurs. **68**:822, April, 1968.

Wagenheim, Helen: Reactions of women to gynecologic examination, Obstet. Gynec. **30**:152, July, 1967.

Williams, Sue Rodwell: Nutrition and diet therapy, St. Louis, 1969, The C. V. Mosby Co., chap. 14.

Yeaworth, Rosalee: Identification and maternity nursing, Nurs. Forum **7**:249, 1968.

*Exercises during pregnancy*

Bruser, Michael: Sporting activities during pregnancy, Obstet. Gynec. **32**:721, Nov., 1968.

Chabon, Irwin: Awake and aware, New York, 1966, The Delacrote Press, chap. 9.

Juzwiak, Marijo: Exercises for the expectant mother, RN **29**:52, Dec., 1966.

Liley, H. M. I.: Modern motherhood, New York, 1966, Random House, Inc., pp. 216-221.

Smith, Christine: Maternal-child nursing, Philadelphia, 1963, W. B. Saunders Co., pp. 96-108.

Wiedenbach, Ernestine: Family-centered maternity nursing, New York, 1968, G. P. Putnam's Sons, pp. 144-161.

*The unwed couple*

Adams, Hannah M., and Gallagher, Ursula: Some facts and observations about illegitimacy. In Lytle, Nancy, editor: Maternal health nursing, Dubuque, Iowa, 1967, William C. Brown Co., pp. 177-187.

Anderson, Ursula, Jenss, R., Mosher, W. E., and Richter, Virginia: The medical, social, and educational implications of the increase in out-of-wedlock births, Amer. J. Public Health **56**:1866, Nov., 1966.

Auerbach, A., and Rabinow, M.: Parent education groups for unmarried mothers, Nurs. Outlook **14**:38, March, 1966.

Bolby, John: Child care, and the growth of love, ed. 2, Baltimore, 1965, Penguin Books, Inc., chap. 10.

Burgess, Linda C.: The unmarried father in adoption planning, Children **15**:71, March-April, 1968.

Burton, M., and Holter, I.: Health education classes for unwed mothers, Nurs. Outlook **14**:35, March, 1966.

Calderone, Mary: Young men and their influence on the girls who love them, Child Family **6**:69, Winter, 1967.

Daigel, C.: Unwed pregnant adolescents, Clin. Pediat. **6**:281, May, 1967.

Daniels, Ada M.: Reaching unwed adolescent mothers, Amer. J. Nurs. **69**:332, Feb., 1969.

Duvall, Evelyn Millis: Why wait till marriage, New York, 1965, Association Press, chap. 7.

Gregory, Diana J.: Problems connected with illegitimacy, Nurs. Mirror **127**:19, July 19, 1968.

Howard, Marion: Comprehensive service program for school age pregnant girls, Children **15**:193, Sept.-Oct., 1968.

Iungerich, Zoe: High school for unwed mothers, Amer. J. Nurs. **67**:92, Jan., 1967.

Kotaska, J. G.: Prenatal classes for unmarried expectant parents, Canad. Nurse **64**:35, Jan., 1968.

LaBarre, Maurice: Pregnancy in adolescence, Amer. J. Orthopsychiat. **37**:265, March, 1967.

LaBarre, Maurice: Pregnancy experiences among married adolescents, Amer. J. Orthopsychiat. **38**:47, Jan., 1968.

Markovits, Andrew S.: How I counsel pregnant, unwed girls, Consultant **6**:42, Nov.-Dec., 1966.

McGregor, Angus: Teen-age aspects of illegitimacy, Nurs. Mirror **128**:13, March, 28, 1969.

Murdock, C.: The unmarried mother, Amer. J. Public Health **58**:2217, Dec., 1968.

Pollack, Jack Harrison: New help for pregnant teen-agers, Good Housekeeping **164**:84, May, 1967.

Roberts, Robert W.: The unwed mother, New York, 1966, Harper & Row, Publishers.

Russell, J. K.: Pregnancy in the young teen-ager, Nurs. Mirror **127**:30, June 28, 1968.

Sarrel, Philip M.: Teen-age pregnancy, Pediat. Clin. N. Amer. 16:347, 1969.

Sarrel, Philip, Holley, M. and Anderson, G.: The young unwed mother: the role of the obstetrician in a comprehensive care program, Obstet. Gynec. 32:741, Dec., 1968.

Semmens, J. P.: Fourteen thousand teen-age pregnancies, Amer. J. Nurs. 66:308, Feb., 1966.

Visotsky, Harold M., Barglow, Peter, Bornstein, Dolores B. Exum, and Wright, Mattie K.: Some psychiatric aspects of illegitimate pregnancy during early adolescence, Amer. J. Orthopsychiat. 37:266, March, 1967.

Von Der Ahe, Clyde V.: The unwed teen-age mother, Amer. J. Obstet. Gynec. 104:279, May, 1969.

Wright, M. K.: Comprehensive services for adolescent unwed mothers, Children 13:170, Sept.-Oct., 1966.

**Student's quick notes:**

# Chapter 10

# Preparation for cooperative childbirth

There are women who wish to participate with nature in the process of labor and delivery; they desire to cooperate in bringing forth their infant. This chapter discusses preparation for active participation in the miracle of birth.

Cooperative childbirth means actively participating in the process of labor and birth of the infant. The objective of a training program for active participation is to help make childbirth a *satisfying, emotionally rewarding experience* and *to replace culturally instilled fears with understanding and confidence.*

Cooperative childbirth is a challenging experience, but not all women can be conditioned to participate. Some women experience labor and delivery with relative ease without any prenatal training; other women intend to cooperate, receive prenatal instructions, but are unable to overcome the firmly rooted misconceptions; and then there are the women who do benefit.

The first step in preparation for cooperative childbirth is the woman's own interest. Her contribution must be voluntary. Those who show doubt or reluctance should never be "sold" or forced into participating.

Cooperative childbirth does not mean that the woman receives no medication, nor does it mean noninterference in the birth process. It is important that the mother-to-be is never misled to believe that labor and birth are painless and that there is any guarantee of complete analgesia and amnesia for the entire labor and delivery.

Instructions in preparation for cooperative childbirth during the period of pregnancy include simple, clear explanations concerning the process of labor and birth. This will eliminate those anxieties resulting from misunderstanding or lack of knowledge. The mother-to-be is taught exercises that will help her contract certain muscles and relax others. Ideally the exercises are started early in the second trimester. She learns to change her breathing technique to conform to the contraction. She is trained to cooperate with nature during the labor and birth process, that is, to work with the uterine contractions. As she practices, she will master slow, deep intercostal breathing, the pattern used during the early part of the first stage. Powerful muscular pull of the uterine contractions need not be interpreted as pain if she conditions herself to react to the contractions with concentration on patterns of breathing. Learning to establish these breathing patterns conserves energy and prevents fatigue. She will learn the Kegel exercise of alternately contracting and relaxing the perineal muscles. But effective bearing down is accomplished by learning to contract the abdominal muscles, not by bearing down on perineal muscles. As she approaches the second stage, she will have (to some extent) the ability to control her expulsive efforts by panting, thus preventing lacerations.

Panting exercises, if not practiced correctly, may result in muscle spasms that can be extremely painful.[1] This hyperventilation further reduces the flow of blood through the placenta and causes fetal metabolic acidosis. Therefore panting exercises should be done under direct supervision of trained personnel. For detailed explanation of these various exercises see reference 2. Practicing relaxation of muscles does help her maintain control during labor and is beneficial to the woman even though she does not wish to be awake for the birth nor actively participate. It gives her the opportunity to develop confidence in the doctors, in the nurses and in herself. Women participating tend to develop wholesome attitudes toward giving birth. Their labor tends to be shorter and certainly less traumatic. They require less sedation, and consequently there is little delay in initiating respirations in the infant.

When the expectant mother enters the hospital and has had prenatal preparation for cooperative childbirth, the first prerequisite to routine admission procedures is the assurance that someone will be with her to support the confidence she has in her ability to cooperate throughout labor and delivery. She should be permitted to labor in a private room. All the months of preparation during the period-of-waiting can be destroyed in a few minutes, if we usher her into a noisy environment. If it is agreeable with the obstetrician, the husband, of course, will furnish the support she needs and deserves. If her husband is not with her, then the nurse coaches her in carrying out the various breathing technics she has practiced during her period of waiting.

Patterns of breathing and effleurage are reinforced. Physical fitness during the period of pregnancy through good nutrition, adequate rest, and exercise pays off as she approaches the transitional phase, for she is likely to become weary and anxious.

Should complications arise the husband will be requested to leave. Since he had been prepared during pregnancy, he understands and complies with the request, knowing that this is being done in his wife's best interest.

To some women childbirth is revered with a spiritual significance and they want to experience the consciousness of birth. A feeling of pride and accomplishment fills the new mother's heart when she first sees her infant. This is intensified when they both share in the unfolding miracle before them.

Interestingly enough, studies show that these women are also interested in breast feeding; that is, they have positive feelings toward their biological destiny and show delight in putting the infant to their breast immediately after birth.

## REFERENCES

1. Battaglia, Frederick C.: Dangers of maternal hyperventilation, J. Pediat. 70:313, Feb., 1967.
2. Hytten, Frank E., and Leitsch, Isabella: The physiology of human pregnancy, Oxford, 1964, Blackwell Scientific Publications, Ltd., p. 102.

## SELECTED READINGS
*Cooperative childbirth*

Bradley, Robert: Husband-coached childbirth, New York, 1965, Harper & Row, Publishers.

Buxton, C. Lee: Psychophysical training in preparation for childbirth. In Lytle, Nancy A., editor: Maternal health nursing, Dubuque, Iowa, 1967, William C. Brown Co., sect. 3, chap. 3.

Chabon, Irwin: Awake and aware, New York, 1966, The Delacrote Press, chaps. 10 and 11.

Estey, Gretta: Word from a mother, Amer. J. Nurs. 69:1453, July, 1969.

Hazell, Lester: Commonsense childbirth, New York, 1969, G. P. Putnam's Sons.

Hazlett, Wm.: The male factor in obstetrics, Child Family 6:3, Fall, 1967.

Hoff, Florence E.: Natural childbirth. How any nurse can help, Amer. J. Nurs. 69:1451, July, 1969.

Juzwiak, Marijo: Intimate look at husband-coached childbirth, RN 29:45, Dec., 1966.

Liley, H. M. I.: Modern motherhood, New York, 1966, Random House, Inc., pp. 216-223.

Meerloo, Joost A. M.: Mental first aid in pregnancy and childbirth, Child Family 5:11, Fall, 1966.

Newton, Niles: New methods for easing childbirth, Child Family 5:17, Fall, 1966.

Sinsibar, Judith L.: Why we choose natural childbirth, Redbook 132:22, Jan., 1969.

Ulin, P. R.: Changing techniques in psychoprophylactic preparation for childbirth, Amer. J. Nurs. 68:2587, Dec., 1968.

Wessel, Helen S.: Natural childbirth and the Christian family, New York, 1963, Harper & Row, Publishers.

Young, E. W.: Prepared childbirth: its impact on nursing, Canad. Nurse 64:39, Jan., 1968.

**For student's quick notes:**

# UNIT II

# The period of parturition

Even though the event of birth occurs somewhere throughout every minute of the day and night, it still remains miraculous. Hidden forces of nature have been at work throughout pregnancy, and now after ten lunar months of preparation, nature unfolds the handiwork of her mysterious performance by initiating labor. Only after this mechanism is completed will the miracle of birth be revealed.

# Chapter 11

# The female pelvis and fetomaternal anatomical relationships

This chapter deals with the structure of the female pelvis and explains how it functions during the process of labor and delivery. You will learn about the anatomical relationship of the mother's pelvis to the various presentations and positions the fetus may assume.

## Bony pelvis (the passageway)
### Important pelvic landmarks

The bony pelvis is the starting point for the fetus to make its entrance into the world, and the normal female pelvis is so constructed that it facilitates its passage. The pelvis is made up of the two innominate bones, which form the front and sides, and the sacrum and coccyx, which form the back. To facilitate understanding, the pelvis is divided into an upper (false pelvis) and a lower (true pelvis). The upper, or false, pelvis is that portion above the linea terminalis (pelvic brim). It supports the enlarging uterus during pregnancy, but has no function in the mechanism of labor. (See Fig. 11-1.)

The true pelvis lies below the pelvic brim. It is further divided into the *inlet* (superior strait), or upper boundary, a *cavity*, and an *outlet* (inferior strait).

On p. 151 you will read about the mechanism whereby the fetus rotates and adapts to the inlet, cavity, and outlet. When pelvic measurements are inadequate, this mechanism is interfered with, and labor may then be protracted or vaginal delivery impossible.

There is no need for the nurse to know pelvic measurements, but she should have an understanding of the importance of their adequacy. If she familiarizes herself with the obstetric pelvic landmarks, she will have a better understanding of the

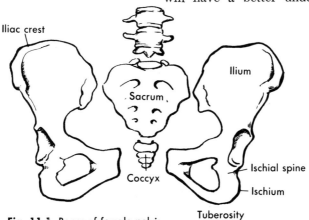

**Fig. 11-1.** Bones of female pelvis.

mechanism of labor. Pelvic capacity is more accurately determined by x-ray examination, but since most deliveries are uneventful, it is used specifically late in pregnancy or during labor when progress is delayed. Pelvic measurements are no longer a ritual with the obstetrician, but many doctors include clinical evaluations as part of the initial examination.

### Pelvic inlet (Fig. 11-2)

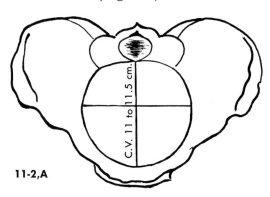

**11-2,A**

One of the anteroposterior measurements of the pelvic inlet is the *conjugate vera* (C.V.), or *true conjugate*. This measurement extends from the middle of the promontory of the sacrum to the upper margin of the symphysis pubis *(A)*.

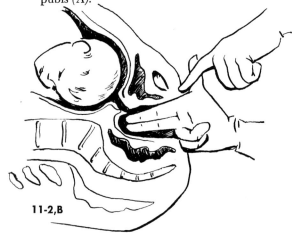

**11-2,B**

Another anteroposterior measurement of the pelvic inlet is the *diagonal conjugate*. This is the distance from the promontory of the sacrum to the lower margin of the symphysis pubis. This measurement can be determined by vaginal examination, and it is from this measurement that the conjugate vera can be estimated by subtracting 1.5 cm. *(B)*.

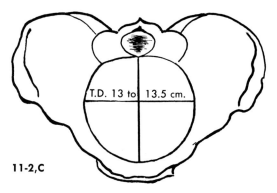

**11-2,C**

The transverse diameter (T.D.) of the inlet is the widest distance between the iliopectineal lines. This diameter can be determined only by x-ray examination *(C)*.

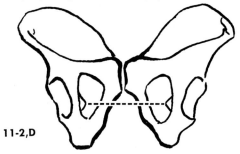

**11-2,D**

Extending from the middle of each ischium are the *ischial spines*. The distance between the ischial spines represents the shortest diameter of the pelvic cavity. When the biparietal diameter of the fetal skull has just passed the inlet, or superior strait, it is said to be engaged *(D)*.

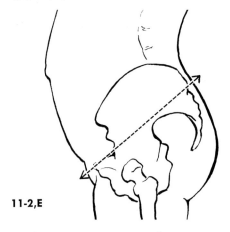

**11-2,E**

The important external measurement is Baudelocque's diameter. This measurement extends from the depression below the last lumbar spine to the anterior surface of the symphysis pubis *(E)*.

*Pelvic outlet* (Fig. 11-3)

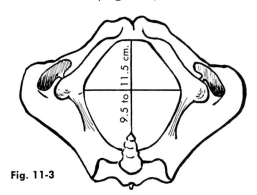

**Fig. 11-3**

The anteroposterior diameter extends from the lower margin of the symphysis pubis to the tip of the sacrococcygeal joint. Because of the motility of the sacrococcygeal joint, the distance spreads from 9.5 to 11.5 cm. as the presenting part advances during labor.

*Transverse diameter* (Fig. 11-4)

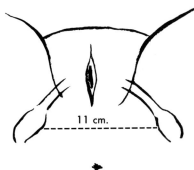

**Fig. 11-4**

The transverse diameter is the distance between the inner surfaces of the tuberosities of the ischium.

|  | Female pelvis | Male pelvis |
|---|---|---|
| **Bones:** | Smaller and lighter | Larger and heavier |
| **Pelvic cavity:** | Round and shallow | Funnel shaped |
| **True pelvis:** | Roomier | More narrow at the outlet |
| **Pubic arch:** | Wider | Angle of arch more narrow |

*Varieties of pelves* (Fig. 11-5)

The Caldwell-Moloy-D'Esopo classification of the four major types of pelves is given below.

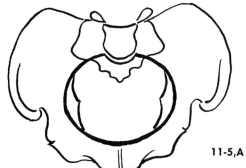

11-5,A

*Gynecoid pelvis.* The gynecoid pelvis, also referred to as the female type pelvis, has a well-rounded inlet (*A*).

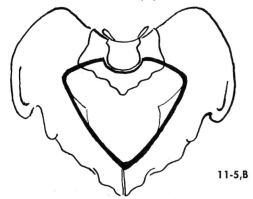

11-5,B

*Android pelvis.* Also referred to as the male type pelvis, the android pelvis has a wedge-shaped inlet (*B*).

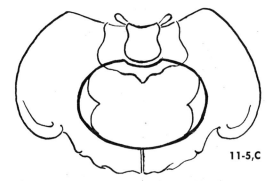

11-5,C

*Platypelloid pelvis.* Also referred to as the flat pelvis, the platypelloid pelvis has a short inlet anteroposteriorly, with the long diameter transverse (*C*).  **Continued.**

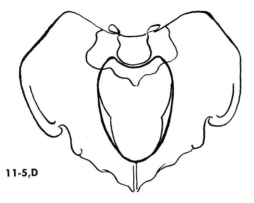

**11-5,D**

*Anthropoid pelvis.* The anthropoid pelvis is oval shaped, causing the transverse diameter to be narrow *(D)*.

### Motility of pelvis

During pregnancy the pelvic joints and ligaments are capable of expansion. It is believed by some doctors that the relaxin hormone, along with estrogen, contributes toward this motility and elasticity.

## Fetomaternal anatomical relationships
### Fetal skull

Just as the mother's pelvis is constructed to facilitate birth, so the fetal cranium with its incomplete ossification makes it possible to adapt more easily to the birth passage. Indeed, from the obstetrician's viewpoint the head is the most important part of the fetus. (See Fig. 11-6.)

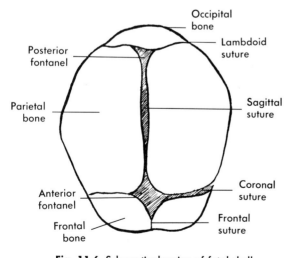

**Fig. 11-6.** Schematic drawing of fetal skull.

The important bones of the cranium are (1) the two parietal bones, on the side, (2) the temporal and frontal, anteriorly, and (3) the occipital bone, posteriorly. At birth these bones are poorly ossified and joined only by membranes (suture lines). At points of intersections, these membranes form areas called *fontanels.*

As the head adjusts its position to adapt to the passageway, it is compressed and the soft tissues overlap; this is termed *molding.* Molding may be quite extensive and the resulting shape of the newborn's skull may cause anxiety to the mother. It is the nurse's responsibility to explain to the mother that in a few days the head will assume the normal contour.

**Suture lines**

1. Sagittal: lies between the parietal bones.
2. Lambdoidal: extends transversely to separate occipital bone from the two parietals.
3. Coronal: extends transversely to separate frontal from parietal bones.
4. Frontal: a continuation of the sagittal suture; separates the two frontal bones.

**The fontanels**

1. Anterior: The intersection of the sagittal, frontal, and coronal sutures forms the bregma (anterior fontanel), or the "soft spot." It is diamond shaped and becomes ossified between 12 and 18 months of age.
2. Posterior: The intersection of the sagittal and lambdoidal sutures forms the posterior fontanel (lambda). It is triangular, smaller than the anterior, and closes between 6 and 8 weeks of age.

### Presentations and positions

The term "lie" of the fetus refers to the relation of the long axis of the fetus to the long axis of the mother and is either *longitudinal* or *transverse.* The lie of the fetus at term is longitudinal in 99% of all labors. For a vaginal delivery the body of the fetus must always be vertical, either head upward toward her chest, in which case the presenting part will either be *feet* or *sacrum,* or the head downward toward the cervix; the latter is the best possible position for the fetus to make its entrance into the world. This means, then, that in general there are two "lies"—vertical or longitudinal.

That part of the fetus presenting over the inlet is called the *presenting part.* It may be (1) cephalic (head), (2) breech, buttocks, or footling, or (3) shoulder.

To indicate *position,* the pelvis is divided into four quadrants; anterior, left or right, and posterior, left or right. The way the presenting part lies in relation to these quadrants determines its position. For example, if the presentation is vertex, the occiput may be to the left or to the right;

it may be direct, anterior, transverse, or posterior. There are, then, two positions, left or right, with eight varieties for each presentation, except in the transverse lie, where there are only four varieties.

### Points of designation for presentations and positions

**Presentations** (Fig. 11-7)

| | |
|---|---|
| Longitudinal | |
|   1. Cephalic | |
|     a. Vertex (occiput) | O. |
|     b. Mentum (face) | M. |
|     c. Brow | Br. |
|   2. Breech | |
|     a. Buttocks (sacrum) | S. |
| Transverse | |
|   1. Shoulder (scapula) | Sc. |

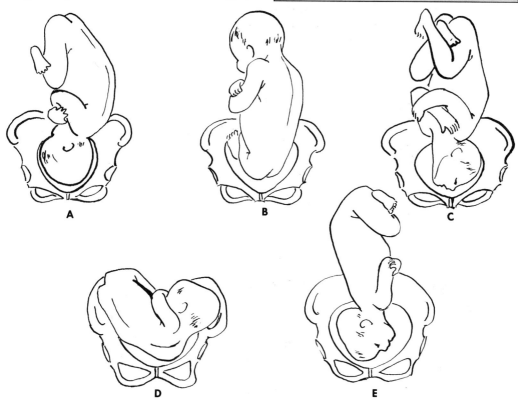

**Fig. 11-7.** Presentations and positions. **A,** Longitudinal presentation, with left occiput anterior position (L.O.A.). **B,** Longitudinal presentation, with left sacrum anterior position (L.S.A.). **C,** Longitudinal presentation, position right mentum anterior (R.M.A.). **D,** Transverse presentation, position left scapula anterior (L.Sc.A.). **E,** Brow presentation.

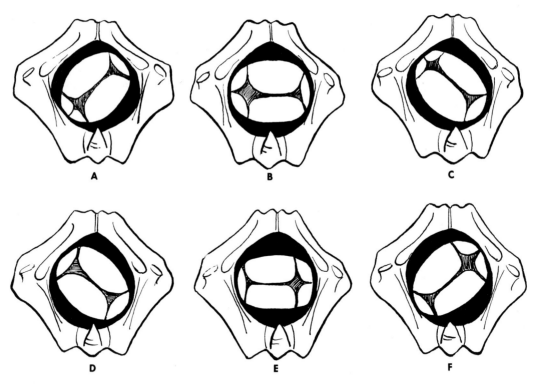

**Fig. 11-8.** Varieties of positions with occipital presentation. **A,** Left occiput anterior (L.O.A.). **B,** Left occiput transverse (L.O.T.). **C,** Left occiput posterior (L.O.P.). **D,** Right occiput anterior (R.O.A.). **E,** Right occiput transverse (R.O.T.). **F,** Right occiput posterior (R.O.P.).

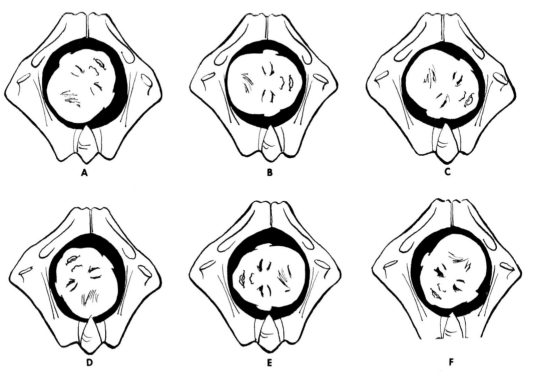

**Fig. 11-9.** Varieties of positions with face presentation. **A,** Left mentum anterior (L.M.A.). **B,** Left mentum transverse (L.M.T.). **C,** Left mentum posterior (L.M.P.). **D,** Right mentum anterior (R.M.A.). **E,** Right mentum transverse (R.M.T.). **F,** Right mentum posterior (R.M.P.).

**Variety of positions with occipital presentation**
**(Fig. 11-8)**

| | |
|---|---|
| Anterior direct | O.A. |
| Left occiput anterior | L.O.A. |
| Left occiput transverse | L.O.T. |
| Left occiput posterior | L.O.P. |
| | |
| Posterior direct | O.P. |
| Right occiput anterior | R.O.A. |
| Right occiput transverse | R.O.T. |
| Right occiput posterior | R.O.P. |

**Variety of positions with transverse presentation**

| | |
|---|---|
| Left scapula anterior | L.Sc.A. |
| Right scapula anterior | R.Sc.A. |
| Left scapula posterior | L.Sc.P. |
| Right scapula posterior | R.Sc.P. |

Approximately 96% of presentations are vertex, 3% are breech, and 0.5% are face and transverse. When the head enters the pelvis first, it accommodates itself to the shape of the inlet, most often in the transverse position, and as a result the back of the fetus will be either to the left or right of the mother's pelvis.

One of the reasons why the position of the vertex is more frequently to the left (L.O.A.) and anterior is because the bladder is frequently displaced toward the right, allowing more room for the head on the left side. Also the flexed fetus accommodates more readily to the soft *anterior* wall of the abdomen than to the back.

A factor of interest is that when the breech is the presenting part, the placenta is usually found to be implanted high, reducing the amount of room for the buttocks in the upper portion of the uterine cavity.

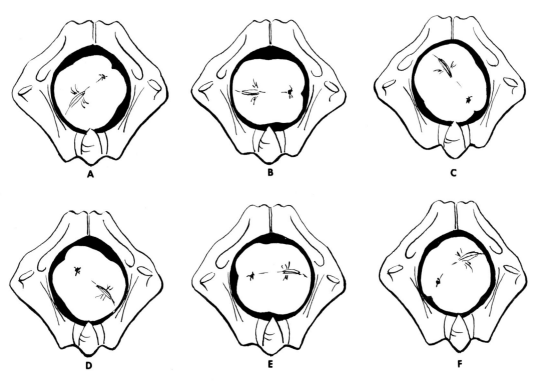

**Fig. 11-10.** Varieties of positions with breech presentation. **A,** Left sacrum anterior (L.S.A.). **B,** Left sacrum transverse (L.S.T.). **C,** Left sacrum posterior (L.S.P.). **D,** Right sacrum anterior (R.S.A.). **E,** Right sacrum transverse (R.S.T.). **F,** Right sacrum posterior (R.S.P.).

## Attitudes

Attitude refers to the relation of fetal extremities to its trunk; the normal attitude is one of flexion of the head (chin in contact with the sternum), legs flexed and

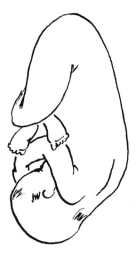

**Fig. 11-11.** Normal attitude—complete flexion.

knees bent with thighs on the abdomen and the feet on the anterior surfaces of the legs, and arms folded against the chest. (See Fig. 11-11.)

With complete flexion of the head the suboccipitobregmatic diameter enters the pelvis. This is important because it is the smallest diameter of the head (9.5 cm.). In this attitude the fetus conforms (more readily) to the shape of the uterine cavity.

## Engagement

The presenting part is said to be *engaged* when it reaches the level of the ischial spines. The fetal head engages most frequently with the sagittal suture in the transverse diameter of the pelvis. Engagement in the primigravida generally takes place late in pregnancy or at the onset of labor; it is not synonymous with *lightening*. If the head is not engaged (in primigravida) at the onset of labor, the nurse may expect

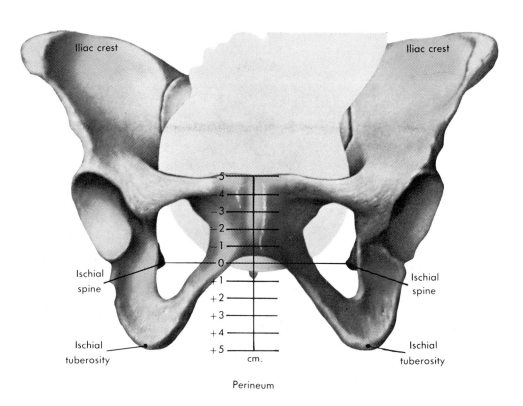

**Fig. 11-12.** Stations of presenting part (degree of engagement). (From Ross Nursing Education Service No. 7, Ross Laboratories, Columbus, Ohio.)

careful evaluation of the patient's progress by the obstetrician. The nurse, too, needs to be alert to delay in her progress. Fetopelvic disproportion, abnormal presentation or position, or abnormalities in the fetus may prevent engagement. In such cases the abdomen becomes quite pendulous. It is also true that a relaxed abdominal wall contributes to delay in engagement. (See Fig. 11-12.) Engagement in the multigravida at the onset of labor is unusual.

### Stations

The relation of the presenting part to the level of the ischial spines is called the station. When the presenting part has reached the level of the ischial spines, it is said to be at *zero station;* if it is above the spines, the distances are designated in minus figures (−1 cm., −2 cm.); if the presenting part is below the ischial spines, the distances are designated in the plus figures (+1 cm., +2 cm.). At +4 cm. the presenting part is on the perineum and can be seen easily if one separates the vulva. (See Fig. 11-12.)

*Floating.* Floating designates that the presenting part is freely movable above the inlet (Fig. 11-13, *A*).

*Dipping.* When the presenting part has passed partially through the plane of the inlet, but is not engaged, it is called dipping (Fig. 11-13, *B*).

*Fixation.* Fixation means that the head has partially entered the true pelvis, cannot be moved from side to side, but is not engaged.

• • •

To determine fetomaternal anatomical relationships one may use (1) a roentgenogram, (2) vaginal examinations, (3) rectal examinations, (4) auscultations, and (5) abdominal examinations. When the fetomaternal anatomical relationship is determined by abdominal palpation, it is called maneuver(s) of Leopold.

The nurse may become proficient in determining presentations and positions by abdominal palpations and rectal or vaginal examinations, but this requires practice over a period of time.

### STUDY QUESTIONS
### Matching

Match the terms in the first column with their appropriate definitions in the second column.

1. (a) Anthropoid   ___Bony protuberance where the sacrum joins the last lumbar vertebra

  (b) Superior strait   ___Widest diameter across the pelvic inlet

  (c) Gynecoid   ___Abnormally flat inlet

  (d) Distance between ischial spines   ___Has a heart-shaped inlet

  (e) Platypelloid   ___Transverse diameter of the outlet

  (f) Inferior strait   ___Represents shortest diameter of the pelvic cavity

  (g) Sacral promontory   ___Pelvis contracted transversely

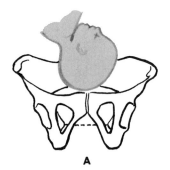 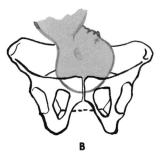

**Fig. 11-13.** Schematic drawing showing, **A,** presenting part above inlet of pelvis, and **B,** head "dipping" into pelvic cavity.

2. (a) Dipping     —Forms posterior fontanel
   (b) Ischial     —Smallest diameter through
   spines       which the fetus's head
           must pass
   (c) Floating     —Relation of presenting
           part of fetus to level of
           ischial spines
   (d) Conjugate     —Presenting part has
   vera       passed through the inlet
           but is not engaged
   (e) Intersection     —When fetal head passes
   of sagittal       this level of the pelvis,
   and lamb-       it is said to be engaged
   doidal su-
   tures
   (f) Position     —Presenting part is freely
           movable above inlet
   (g) Station     —Forms the bregma
   (h) Intersection     —Relation of presenting
   of sagittal,       part of fetus to quadrants
   frontal, and       of mother's pelvis
   coronal su-
   tures

**SELECTED READINGS**

Beck, A. C., and Taylor, E. Stewart, editors: Obstetrical practice, ed. 8, Baltimore, 1966, The Williams & Wilkins Co., chaps. 9 to 11.

Brantigan, Otto C.: Clinical anatomy, New York, 1963, McGraw-Hill Book Co., chap. 13.

Oxorn, Harry, and Foote, Wm. R.: Human labor and birth, New York, 1964, Appleton-Century-Crofts, chaps. 5, 6, and 7.

Reith, Edward J., and Breidenbach, Bertha: Textbook of anatomy and physiology, New York, 1966, The Williams & Wilkins Co., pp. 53-55.

Ross, Janet S., and Wilson, Kathleen J.: Foundations of anatomy and physiology. ed. 2, Baltimore, 1966, The Williams & Wilkins Co., pp. 61-64.

**For student's quick notes:**

# Chapter 12

# Course of labor and delivery—I

The period of waiting is over! Physiological changes now occur that will set into motion the forces necessary to direct the fetus through the birth canal. Nature does this (1) by preparing the birth canal (beginning with cervical effacement), (2) by bringing about preparatory changes so that intermittent, irregular contractions of muscle cells become more efficient and forceful, propelling, directing, and guiding the fetus into a new existence, (3) by severing the infant's life line (placenta) from the mother's body, and finally, (4) by, without ado, bringing about preparatory changes in the muscle cells, thereby returning her physiology to the pregravid state within 6 weeks.

## Onset of labor

Hippocrates attributed the onset of labor to insufficient nutrition for the fetus, but the modern obstetrician recognizes the interaction of several factors: (1) physical aging of the placenta may lend support to Hippocrate's contention, but there are other hypotheses; (2) the uterus reaches a crucial point of distention, causing tension on muscle fibers and stimulating their activity; (3) nerve impulses from the uterus to postpituitary gland may bring about release of oxytocin; and (4) changes in level of hormones may render the myometrium irritable. Whatever factors are involved, the onset of labor finds both mother and fetus in readiness for the event.

Intermittent contractions of the uterus (Braxton Hicks's contractions) become more pronounced as pregnancy nears term. Some women interpret these as beginning labor and may be admitted to the hospital prematurely, only to be discharged as a case of false labor. The nurse can lessen the woman's disappointment and embar-

rassment by explaining how the contractions differ. There are various ways in which true labor may be distinguished from false labor, and the nurse should be familiar with them.

The intensity of the contractions force the presenting part in the direction of the cervix. The upper segment is thicker, stronger, and more powerful and exerts pressure downward, while the less muscular lower segment becomes greatly distended as contents descend. In addition to uterine contractions, pressure of the presenting part, especially when the membranes are intact, also assists nature.

Discomfort experienced during contractions is caused by (1) stretching of the ligaments, (2) pressure or stretching of the nerve endings, (3) distention of soft tissues, and (4) emotional factors.

## Duration of labor

The duration of labor depends on the force produced by uterine contractions and on the resistance offered by soft tissues as

**True labor**

1. Contractions occur at regular intervals and increase in frequency, duration, and intensity as labor progresses.
2. The cervix is soft and admits the finger easily.
3. Discomfort is not relieved by mild sedation.
4. Descent of the presenting part occurs.
5. There is backache due to stretching of the cervix.

**False labor**

1. Contractions occur at irregular intervals and tend to disappear when the patient lies down. Contractions do not increase in frequency or intensity.
2. The cervix does not change.
3. Discomfort may be relieved by mild sedation.
4. Presenting part does not descend.
5. Discomfort is mainly in the anterior region of the abdomen and pelvis.

the fetus passes through the birth canal. These may be affected by (1) parity of the patient, (2) presentation and position of the fetus, (3) fetopelvic diameters, (4) sedation, (5) hormone levels, and (6) emotional factors such as anxiety and tension.

The contractions are initiated at the pacemakers, one situated at each end of the cornu of the uterus, and travel downward from this area. As labor progresses, uterine contractions cause the muscle fibers in the upper segment of the uterus to shorten. This retraction of muscle fibers marks a division of the uterus into (1) an *upper segment*—thick, muscular, and retractile; and (2) a *lower segment*—thin, muscular, and passive. The transition area is called Braun's retraction ring, or physiological retraction ring. When labor or passage of the fetus is obstructed, this stretching is increased and the retraction ring of muscle fibers may reach the area of the umbilicus; it is then known as Bandl's ring. This is a warning of impending rupture and labor must be terminated. See discussion on the rupture of the uterus, p. 195.

Nature's way of starting the new life on its journey into existence is a progressive pattern of uterine activity occurring in three stages.

## First stage of labor

This stage is said to start when musculature of the uterus starts true, pronounced contractions and brings about *progressive cervical effacement* and *dilatation of the cervix*. To simplify understanding of the mechanism of this stage, it is further divided into three phases—a latent phase, an active phase, and a transitional phase.

### Latent phase

The contractions start slowly with rhythmicity and occur about every 15 to 20 minutes. They are described by some women as "cramplike" pains, radiating from the lumbar region to anterior part of the abdomen. The contractions are usually of *short* duration (20 to 30 seconds) and of *mild* intensity. The cervix dilates to approximately 4 cm. Two thirds of the first stage is completed when the cervix reaches 5 cm. dilatation.

### Active phase

During this phase the contractions occur at shorter intervals (2 to 5 minutes) and are of greater intensity and duration (40 to 45 seconds). The cervix dilates to approximately 8 cm. during this phase.

### Transitional phase

This phase represents transition from first to second (expulsive) stage. The contractions occur at about 2-minute intervals and bring about the final stretching of the cervix as it retracts over the fetal head. These contractions of the first stage are under the control of the autonomic nervous system; therefore the patient has no control over them. The cervix dilates from 8 to 10 cm.

Nature's pace is slow in completing this first stage. For the primigravida the usual length of this stage of labor is about 12 hours; for the multipara it is about 6 hours. All physical and anatomical factors being normal, today's young mothers have shorter first stage labors than did their elder sisters and mothers. This is attributed to prenatal education and a better understanding of the psychological aspects of labor. The end result, however, is cervical effacement and complete dilatation.

*Cervical effacement and dilatation.* Toward the end of pregnancy the cervix has been undergoing progressive changes that favor effacement (thinning) whereby the cervical canal blends in with the lower uterine segment. This is brought about by (1) pressure of the presenting part and (2) traction as the upper segment becomes thicker and shorter, and the lower segment becomes thinner and longer. (See Fig. 12-1.)

In the primigravida effacement precedes dilatation and is expressed in percent. As the first stage of labor progresses, the cervix shortens and the external os dilates. *Dilatation* is expressed in centimeters, indicating diameter of the opening of the cervical os. When the os dilates to approximately 10 cm., dilatation is said to be complete and the head is able to pass through. These two processes may occur simultaneously. However, multigravidas often are fully effaced and 2 to 4 cm. dilated before labor

even begins. When these two phases are complete, the first stage is ended and the second stage starts and continues on until the fetus is born.

*Rupture of membranes.* When do the membranes rupture? Ideally, they rupture at the end of the first stage of labor, after they have performed their functions of protecting the fetus and of forming a wedge to help dilate the cervix. The nurse may note that the contractions slow down after the membranes rupture, but this is only temporary because very soon they become stronger and of more expulsive force.

Rupture of the membranes may herald the beginning of labor, or if the pregnancy is at or near term when this occurs, labor usually starts within 24 hours. Eastman cites that ordinarily labor is shorter following premature rupture of the membranes.[1] See discussion on premature rupture of the membranes, p. 183.

*The amniotomy.* If the force of the uterine contractions is not sufficiently strong enough to cause rupture of the membranes by the end of the first stage, the doctor may do an amniotomy (artificial rupture of the membranes), allowing the fluid to drain from the vaginal canal. If the head is allowed to egress in the unruptured sac, there is a greater possibility that the fetus will aspirate quantities of the amniotic fluid, which may result in a possible pneumonia. Some obstetricians prefer an amniotomy because in their opinion descent

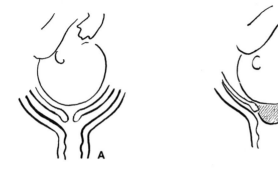 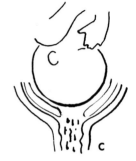

**Fig. 12-1.** Cervical effacement and dilatation. **A,** Starting dilatation and effacement. **B,** Membranes bulging through partially dilated cervix. **C,** Rupture of the membranes with almost complete dilatation.

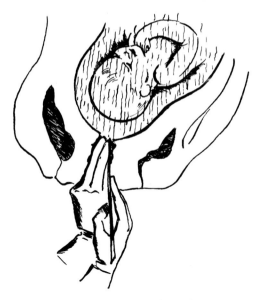

**Fig. 12-2.** Artificial rupture of membranes (amniotomy).

of the hard fetal head brings about reflex stimuli of the myometrium. (See Fig. 12-2.)

*Mechanism of fetal adaptation to pelvis and birth canal.* During the time that the cervix is dilating and effacing, the fetus is being moved toward the cervix by force of uterine contractions. Because of the various shapes and sizes of the pelvic bones, the presenting part must adjust its position as it passes through the pelvis and down through the birth canal.

You are now ready to learn about these intricate movements of the fetus as it adapts to the passageway. There are seven movements; they are *gradual* and *interrelated* and a continuum from the first stage on through the second. These movements are (1) *descent,* (2) *flexion,* (3) *internal rotation,* (4) *extension,* (5) *restitution,* (6) *external rotation,* and (7) *expulsion.* As the

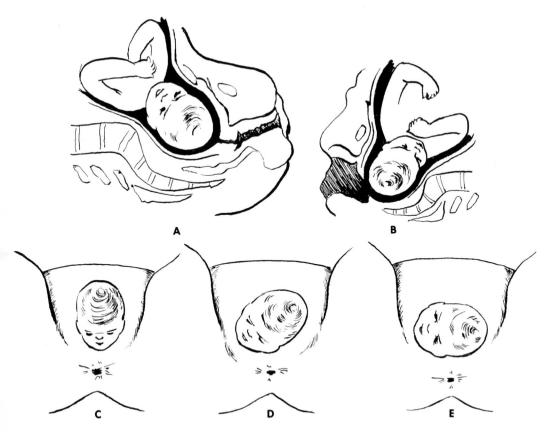

**Fig. 12-3.** Schematic drawing showing mechanisms of fetal adaptation to the birth canal. **A,** Descent with flexion. **B,** Internal rotation. **C,** Extension. **D,** Restitution. **E,** Restitution complete (external rotation).

head *descends*, it *flexes;* as it *flexes,* it *rotates,* etc.; *descent* is the common denominator.

The position of the head of the fetus is so directed that it can be flexed to fit the heart-shaped pelvic inlet. Using the L.O.A. as an example, the head as it *descends* also *flexes* and *rotates* to the right and anteriorly toward the midline. Thus it descends beneath the symphysis pubis with the sagittal suture in line with the anteroposterior diameter of the pelvic outlet (L.O.A. to O.A.). (See Fig. 12-3.)

## Second stage of labor

The second stage of labor is said to start with complete *dilatation* and *effacement* of the cervix and end with the actual birth of the infant.

As stated on p. 148 the upper segment of the uterus is the contractile portion, which is now very active; contracting about every 2 minutes, the contractions are strong and last approximately 50 seconds. The lower segment is rather passive and the external os completely dilated. The central nervous system now comes into play and the auxilliary forces of voluntary efforts of abdominal and diaphragmatic muscles contribute to completion of labor.

As the presenting part approaches the perineal floor, it produces a reflex which initiates involuntary bearing down effort, and even though the patient may be under sedation, she cannot resist this force of nature. The levator ani muscles may aid as the head extends, but their action is largely passive.

As the head is ready to emerge, one will observe a bulging of the perineum with each contraction (Fig. 12-4). If the membranes have not ruptured, they will appear in front of the head. As each contraction subsides, the head recedes. This process continues, but the head emerges farther each time, that is, it is said to be "crowning" with each contraction until finally a larger segment (the biparietal diameter) becomes visible and the perineum becomes thin. A Ritgen maneuver is performed be-

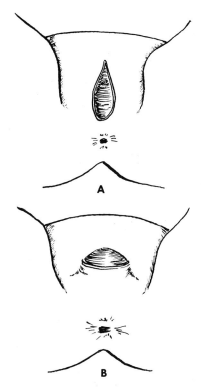

**Fig. 12-4. A,** Schematic drawing to illustrate "bulging of the perineum" and visible caput. **B,** Further bulging of labia and perineum with visible rectal pressure as anus dilates.

tween contractions when the doctor has control, and the head can be delivered slowly. As the head crowns, the doctor places a towel over the rectum and exerts pressure on the infant's chin through the perineum. With the other hand he exerts pressure on the occiput. This controls egress of the head and helps prevent tissue damage. (See Fig. 12-5.) As the head approaches the pelvic floor, to overcome resistance of the perineum, the doctor does an episiotomy at the height of a contraction.

Meanwhile the mechanism of fetal adaptation continues on. The head is born by *extension* and then *restitutes* back 45 degrees (O.A. to L.O.A.). By this maneuver the head resumes its original position in the pelvis. One can observe nature at work because her powers will restitute the head, although the doctor may aid this maneuver

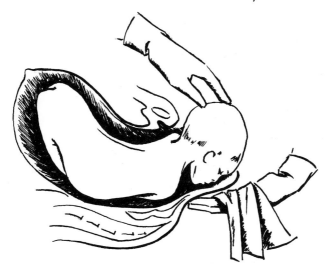

**Fig. 12-5.** Ritgen maneuver to control egress of head and prevent tissue damage.

manually. As this occurs, the shoulders are approaching the perineum and rotating to the anteroposterior position; the posterior delivers over the perineum and the anterior beneath the pubic arch. During this maneuver there is additional *external rotation* of the head by another 45 degrees (L.O.A. to L.O.T.), with *expulsion* of the body.

The duration of this stage is approximately 1 hour in the primigravida and 30 minutes in the multipara. The discomfort of this stage is caused by (1) uterine contractions and (2) distension of perineal muscles. The second stage of labor is said to be the most dangerous for the fetus because this journey is tedious.

After the birth of the head, the doctor removes secretions from the nose and mouth and then aspirates the nasopharynx with a bulb syringe. After delivery of the infant, the obstetrician suspends it by its feet so the head is the most dependent portion, and he again aspirates mucus from the nose and throat. (See Fig. 12-6.) He may also "milk" the trachea.* The first contraction of the third stage forces blood through

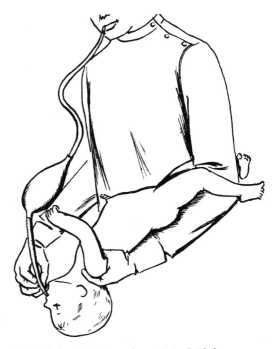

**Fig. 12-6.** Aspiration of amniotic fluid from nose and throat.

the placenta and cord to the infant. Some obstetricians place the infant at a slightly lower level than the placenta. Approximately 60 to 100 ml. of blood will drain from the placenta through the cord into the newborn. For this reason some doctors do not sever the cord until they have

*The value of milking the trachea to help the infant eject mucus is questionable. It is believed by some doctors that the manipulation may be traumatic.

milked this blood into the infant. The advantage of this is questionable. See discussion on physiology of newborn, pp. 261 and 282.

### Third stage of labor

This is termed the placental stage or stage of expulsion. The third stage is divided into two phases: (1) the phase of separation and (2) the phase of extrusion. Normally within 3 to 5 minutes after delivery of the infant, nature will complete the third stage of labor. The mechanism of this separation and expulsion is brought about by contractions and retractions of uterine musculature, moving the placenta away from the uterine wall, to the midline, and then into the lower uterine segment. The bulky consistency of the placenta forces the fundus upward and toward the right. If the patient is anesthetized, the doctor may place his hand on the abdomen and press between the fundus and the symphysis, elevating the fundus. With the other hand he puts gentle traction on the cord and the placenta will be expelled (Fig. 12-7). This is known as the Brandt-Andrews' maneuver. If the mother is awake, voluntary bearing-down efforts of the mother may force the placenta from the vagina. Contractions of the levator ani muscles may also assist in the expulsion. See p. 165 for a discussion of the nurse's function.

There is very little, if any, bleeding during the birth process itself. If excessive bleeding does occur, it is usually due to cervical lacerations or premature separation of the placenta; both can cause the death of the mother and fetus if immediate action is not taken.

In some instances the placental margin separates first. In others the central portion is freed first, in which case bleeding will occur retroplacental. When the placenta detaches completely, blood is released and gushes from the vagina. The blood loss accompanying the third stage averages 200 to 250 ml.

The uterus cannot contract and retract sufficiently to close off the bleeding vessels unless all of the products of conception are expelled. It is extremely important that all the placenta and tissues (chorion and amnion) are expelled. Sometimes pieces of cotyledon remain attached to the wall of the uterus; the patient will continue to bleed because the uterine muscles are unable to contract and retract sufficiently.

When the central portion of the placenta is forced into the vagina first, that is, the fetal surface is expelled first, it is called the Schultze mechanism. When the placenta folds on itself as separation occurs, the maternal surface will be expelled first and this is called Duncan's mechanism.

When the placenta does not separate

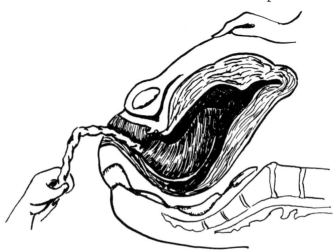

**Fig. 12-7.** Brandt-Andrews method of expressing placenta.

## DRUGS USED TO CONTRACT THE UTERUS

**Generic name:**    Ergonovine maleate, U.S.P.
**Trade name:**      Ergotrate*

| Action | Dosage |
|---|---|
| Acts slowly; produces sustained tetanic contractions of uterine musculature. | |
| **Second stage of labor** | |
| Given intravenously as head is born; causes uterus to contract within 1 minute. This helps to separate the placenta and keep uterus firm, thus keeping bleeding to minimum. It is important that the nurse give the drug precisely when ordered to do so by the doctor. Prematurely induced contractions may trap the placenta in the uterus. | 1 ml. (0.2 mg.) |
| May be given intramuscularly as the infant is being born. Uterus will contract within 2 to 5 minutes during placenta separation. | |
| **Third stage of labor** | |
| May be given intravenously or intramuscularly directly after placenta has been expelled. | 1 ml. (0.2 mg.) |
| **Fourth stage of labor** | |
| May be given intramuscularly if fundus feels boggy or has tendency to relax. | 1 ml. (0.2 mg.) |
| **Postpartum period** | |
| Produces long-lasting uterine contractions. Believed by some to hasten involution. | 0.18 mg. orally 3 or 4 times daily |

*Since Ergotrate has a long-lasting action on the myometrium, it is never used to induce labor. The effect of ergot is largely limited to myometrical smooth muscle, but may cause abnormal rise in blood pressure. Chlorpromazine given intravenously will counteract such a reaction. Ergotrate is not used for patients with peripheral vascular disease.

**Generic name:**    Oxytocin injection, U.S.P.
**Trade names:**     Pitocin, Syntocinon, Uteracon

| Action | Dosage |
|---|---|
| Acts quickly but contractions are not sustained. | |
| **Second stage of labor** | |
| May be given intramuscularly as shoulder is being born. | 3 to 10 units |
| **Third stage of labor** | |
| May be given intravenously after placenta is expelled. | 10 units in 1 ml. of water |
| May be given intramuscularly after placenta is expelled. | 10 units |

**Generic name:**    Methylergonovine maleate, U.S.P.
**Trade name:**      Methergine (a semisynthetic derivative of Ergotrate)

| Third stage of labor | Dosage |
|---|---|
| Is usually given intramuscularly after placenta is expelled. It is said to have less tendency to raise blood pressure than ergonovine. | 0.2 mg. intravenously or intramuscularly |

within 30 minutes after the birth of the baby or if the patient bleeds excessively as separation takes place, the doctor will do a manual removal of the placenta. (See pp. 194 and 195 and Fig. 12-8.)

This stage is the shortest, but nature is methodical in completing the birth process and should not be hurried by forceful manual removal of the placenta from the uterine wall, nor should the uterus be massaged before the placenta separates. This may result in complete relaxation of the uterus with subsequent fatal hemorrhage. This is why the third stage of labor is the most dangerous stage for the mother.

After the placenta has been expelled, hemorrhage from the placenta site is prevented by contractions and retractions of the uterine muscles. The contractions compress the blood vessels, but it is the retractions (shortening of muscle fibers) that accomplish the permanent arrest of hemorrhage. To prevent too much blood loss, oxytocic drugs are administered as prophylaxis against postpartum hemorrhage.

Some obstetricians order Ergotrate intravenously with delivery of anterior shoulder to produce immediate placenta separation. The buttocks, not having been born,

keep the cervix open while contractions separate the placenta and prevent considerable blood loss.

Oxytocin (Pitocin, Syntocinon, Uteracon), ergonovine (Ergotrate), and methylergonovine (Methergine), when administered intravenously, sometimes initiate hypertension and nausea. Where there is evidence of hypertension, Ergotrate or Methergine should not be given. In such instances, intravenous Pitocin, 2 units in 1,000 ml. glucose solution, at 15 drops per minute is usually ordered. (See "Drugs used to contract the uterus," p. 155.)

## Fourth stage of labor

Our continued nursing care following the third stage of labor is most important, for, as stated above, if the uterine muscles are unable to contract and retract sufficiently to close off the bleeding vessels, the mother will suffer a postpartum hemorrhage. Referring to this recovery period as the *fourth stage of labor* may help the student keep in mind that the labor and delivery room nurse's responsibilities are not over with completion of the third stage, but that her constant vigilance is needed during this crucial period. For her detailed responsibilities see pp. 166 and 167.

### STUDY QUESTIONS
*Matching*

Match the terms in the first column with their appropriate definitions in the second column:

(a) Change of hormone level — Indicates opening of cervical os
(b) Amniotomy — Most dangerous stage of labor for fetus
(c) Latent phase — Physiological cervical dilator
(d) Braun's ring — Placenta and membranes
(e) Transient phase — Factor in onset of labor
(f) Effacement — Contractile portion of the uterus
(g) Third stage — Transitional area dividing uterus into upper and lower segment
(h) Crowning — Artificial rupture of membranes
(i) Second stage — Doctor may use Brandt-Andrews maneuver during this stage

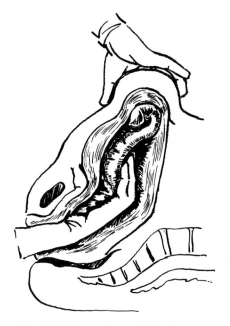
Fig. 12-8. Manual removal of placenta.

(j) Dilatation ___Patient is quite cooperative during this phase of
labor

(k) The "bag of ___Thinning of cervix
waters"

(l) Upper segment ___Contractions are force-
of the uterus ful and expulsive in nature during this phase

(m) Secundines ___Biparietal diameter of
fetus's head is visible on
the perineum

*Multiple choice*

1. Posture of the fetus in utero is referred to as:
   (a) presentation.
   (b) position.
   (c) attitude.
2. The most reliable means of differentiating true from false labor is that with true labor:
   (a) there is descent of the presenting part.
   (b) contractions are regular with short intervals between.
   (c) the cervix is soft and dilatable.
3. During the transitional phase of labor the cervix dilates from:
   (a) 5 to 9 cm.
   (b) 2.5 to 5 cm.
   (c) 9 to 10 cm.
4. The primigravida has completed two thirds of her first stage of labor when the cervix reaches dilatation of:
   (a) 5 cm.
   (b) 8 to 9 cm.
   (c) 2.5 to 4 cm.
5. The ideal time for membranes to rupture is:
   (a) at the end of the first stage of labor.
   (b) at the beginning of the active phase of labor.
   (c) at the beginning of labor.
   (d) when contractions occur every two minutes.
6. The second stage of labor starts:
   (a) with involuntary bearing down.
   (b) when caput is visible.
   (c) when cervical dilatation and effacement are complete.
   (d) with the transitional phase.
7. As the presenting part approaches the perineum, the nurse may observe:
   (a) bulging of the perineum.

(b) involuntary micturition during bearing down.
(c) increase in bloody show.
(d) all of these.

*True or false*

(T) (F) 1. Emotional factors contribute to discomfort experienced during labor.
(T) (F) 2. The patient will have the desire to "bear down" with contractions when she starts the active phase of labor.
(T) (F) 3. If a woman is at term and her membranes rupture, labor most always starts spontaneously within 24 hours.
(T) (F) 4. Contractions may slow down temporarily after rupture of the membranes.
(T) (F) 5. Flexion aids engagement and descent.
(T) (F) 6. The second stage of labor is the most dangerous stage for the mother.
(T) (F) 7. During normal labor the interval between contractions is always longer than the contractions themselves.

**REFERENCE**

1. Eastman, Nicholson J., and Hellman, Louis M., editors: Williams' obstetrics. ed. 13, New York, 1966, Appleton-Century-Crofts, p. 407.

**SELECTED READINGS**

Beck, A. C., and Taylor, E. Stewart, editors: Obstetrical practice, ed. 8, Baltimore, 1966, The Williams & Wilkins Co., pp. 175-188.
Bradford, Wm. D.: The case for careful examination of the placenta, Clin. Pediat. 7:716, Dec., 1968.
Freedman, Emanuel: The use of labor pattern as a management guide, Hosp. Top. 46:57, Aug., 1968.
Guyton, Arthur: Textbook of medical physiology, Philadelphia, 1966, W. B. Saunders Co., pp. 1163-1166.
Oxorn, Harry, and Foote, Wm. R.: Human labor and birth, New York, 1964, Appleton-Century-Crofts, chap. 11.

**For student's quick notes:**

# Chapter 13

# Course of labor and delivery—II

This chapter deals with the nursing responsibilities from admission of the patient until completion of her fourth stage of labor. You will learn the importance of psychological support during labor and of the value in reducing the need for drugs to alleviate pain. The end of the chapter discusses your responsibilities in caring for the newborn during the period immediately after birth.

## Nursing responsibilities during first stages

### Admission of the patient

Admission procedures and management of the patient in the labor room vary from hospital to hospital, but the objective should be the same—to provide environment conducive to the best welfare of the mother and infant. Whether the admission clerk directs the patient to the labor room suite or the nurse goes to the admission office to escort the woman makes little difference. It is the dignified, pleasant manner in which she is greeted that leaves its impact. It is the personnel who helps put the woman at ease and dispels the frightening strangeness of hospital environment. The good labor room nurse uses this first contact with the mother-to-be to establish good rapport by showing her sincere interest in the woman's welfare.

Every consideration should be shown to the husband, especially when he is forced to leave his wife in the lobby and turn her welfare over to the hospital staff.

When admitting a patient, the nurse first ascertains the status of her labor and then notifies the obstetrician. If delivery is imminent, the physician is notified immediately, and the patient prepared for delivery without any delay.

Whenever possible the student nurse should be assigned to the primigravida for admission procedures to become familiar with routines. The following is a general plan of admission for a woman whose labor is in the latent phase of the first stage: (1) parity of the patient, (2) estimated date of delivery if prenatal record is not immediately available, (3) when labor contractions started, (4) status of membranes, (5) presence of the "show," and (6) whether or not the doctor has been notified.

As the nurse proceeds with her work, she should inquire whether this patient has been previously exposed to a hospital environment. If not, this experience is likely to be more traumatic for her and it will ease her fears if the nurse informs her of the necessary, preliminary procedures such as the perineal preparation, midstream urine specimen, enema, and methods of examination. During this preliminary admission, it is important for the nurse to take into consideration her emotional status. Labor heralds in thoughts of parting and disrupts symbiosis. The emotional aspects of labor are as real and significant as the physical. Every woman has fears concerning the outcome of the delivery and the condition of her baby. When reporting the status of labor to the physician, remember to report her emotional response. A mild sedative at this time may prove of value.

### Clinical preparation

*Perineal shaves.*[2] The perineal shave has been dispensed with in many hospitals. The pubic hair is merely clipped with a scissors. However, some doctors feel that shaving the vulva is a good means of cleansing and disinfecting the area and that it facilitates inspection of the episiotomy during the early puerperium.

*Vital signs and blood pressure.* Any variation in vital signs should certainly be reported to the doctor. Blood pressure increases slightly during labor. Most women show a rise of about 10 to 20 mm. Hg during the latter part of the first stage. The nurse should check the blood pressure after a contraction has completely subsided.

*Fetal heart rate.*[3] Auscultation of the fetal heart rate gives the doctor valuable information concerning condition of the fetus. The normal rate is between 100 and 160 per minute and should be checked every hour during the first stage and every 30 minutes during the second stage. The nurse should listen to the fetal heart sounds after a contraction, after allowing time for restoration of the normal rate, because they are indistinct and become slower at the height of a contraction. The doctor may take them during a contraction to tell him how the fetus is withstanding the labor.

The student nurse may have difficulty hearing fetal heart sounds in obese patients, polyhydramnios, or posterior position of the occiput (back of fetus is away from anterior abdominal wall). She should not hesitate asking for assistance in checking the rate and quality.

*The enema.* The enema or suppository is almost routine, unless delivery is imminent. The enema serves many purposes: (1) cleans out the lower bowel making more space for passage of the fetus, (2) facilitates rectal examination, (3) prevents contamination of the delivery field during the second stage when expulsive forces initiate bearing-down efforts, and (4) has the effect of stimulating contractions. Enemas are withheld if the patient has vaginal bleeding or is in premature labor.

After the admission procedures have been completed, the doctor, intern, or head nurse examines the patient abdominally, vaginally, or rectally. The rectal or vaginal examination determines the extent of dilatation, effacement, station, presentation, position, and status of the membranes. A vaginal examination, with proper vulvar preparation and adherence to aseptic technique, is a safe method and furnishes more accurate information than does the rectal examination.[5] When performed by trained personnel, the examinations can be limited to one or two during the course of normal labor.

### Evaluating uterine contractions

Labor contractions are measured in terms of (1) frequency, (2) duration, and (3) intensity.

*Frequency* of contractions is defined as the number of contractions per 10 minutes and for accuracy the nurse should time them for this period before recording her findings. The uterus starts contracting before, and subsides after, the patient feels the discomfort. To time contractions accurately the nurse places her hand over the fundal area to feel the oncoming contraction. The contraction may be at its height before the woman complains of discomfort; therefore the nurse should not depend on when the patient says she feels the contraction. The *duration* of the contraction is measured in seconds and is timed from the time the contraction starts until the fundus relaxes and the contraction fades.

The *intensity* is measured by degree of

firmness during the height of the contractions. They are recorded as *mild, moderate, or severe*. The student learns to measure these by practice and should not rely on patient's subjective symptoms.

The patient may come to the hospital when she thinks her membranes have ruptured. It may have been involuntary escape of urine. If the state of the membranes cannot be determined accurately, the nurse may do the Nitrazine test. Normally the pH of vaginal secretions is 4.5 to 5.5; the pH of amniotic fluid is 7 to 7.5. The nurse inserts sterile cotton applicator gently into the vaginal canal, withdraws it, and applies it to Nitrazine paper. If the membranes are intact, the color change will be yellow to olive green (pH 5 to 6); if ruptured, blue-green to deep blue (pH 6.5 to 7.5).

If the membranes ruptured previous to admission and the patient seems concerned because labor has not started, the nurse can assure the woman that this does not necessarily mean her labor will be longer. This phenomenon is sometimes called *dry labor*. The amniotic fluid usually seeps slowly from the vaginal canal between pains because the presenting part recedes slightly from the external os. This allows a small amount of amniotic fluid to flow past the presenting part.

### Phases and progress

It is in part the nurse's responsibility to maintain the patient's strength. Solid foods should be withheld during labor to avoid the possibility of vomiting and aspiration during delivery. The patient must be maintained in a state of good hydration during labor and should be encouraged to take fluids during *early* labor; ginger ale and fruit juices are usually welcome. If the patient cannot take enough fluids orally, intravenous infusions of glucose-water are given. When labor is prolonged, these infusions are especially important. The nurse needs to explain why fluids are not taken orally after labor has advanced or is prolonged.

If the mother-to-be is not too uncomfortable with the contractions and the membranes are intact, she is usually allowed to ambulate until analgesia is administered or the membranes rupture. Walking stimulates the cervix and reflexly intensifies uterine contractions.

As stated on p. 149 the contractions begin with rhythmicity, and the duration and intensity increase as labor progresses. This results in cervical effacement and dilatation.

The nurse urges the woman to pass her urine every few hours to prevent overdistention of the bladder; a full bladder contributes toward discomfort, impedes the progress of labor, and is conducive to urinary tract infection. If the mother has no desire to void, palpate the abdomen frequently to detect bladder fullness because contractions and pressure felt by the patient may make her unaware that her bladder is full. It is also wise to have the patient empty her bladder before the administration of sedation.

During the latent phase of the first stage of labor the nurse impresses on the woman the importance of relaxing *with* contractions. If she breathes slowly and deeply *during* the contractions, she is likely to experience less discomfort. Effective relaxation enhances cervical dilatation.

During this time she is usually cooperative and pleased that the "time" has finally arrived. Bearing down during this stage should be discouraged; it delays cervical dilatation and is exhausting. Instruct her that when the cervix is fully dilated, the urge to bear down will come into its own and she will bear down involuntarily.

When the mother-to-be reaches the *active phase,* she may require sedation. Much of this depends on (1) the individual's threshold to the discomfort, (2) prenatal education, and (3) how the doctor feels about sedation for his patients. As labor progresses, she may begin to feel that she is unable to cope with the contractions, become anxious about her progress, and show less concern as to what is going on about her. Here the nurse must learn to use tact in answering questions. Honesty is important, but the nurse must guard against expressing her estimate of the hour at which labor will be completed, since she does not know. Diaphragmatic breathing (deep breathing) with contractions is helpful. When the mother is given medication to dry secretions, such as scopolamine, frequent mouth care or *small* amounts of cracked ice are appreciated. Fetal heart rate should be auscultated every 15 minutes during this phase and after rupture of the membranes.

The nurse should assist the patient in assuming the position most comfortable to her and suggests that she change her position at intervals. A change of position may often affect a change in the pattern of uterine contractions. The doctor may request that the woman be in Sims' position on the side opposite the infant's back. This prevents pressure of the uterus on the inferior vena cava and favors anterior rotation of the fetal head. Hand pressure on the sacral region brings relief, especially when the presenting part is in a posterior position. Much of the backache that the patient complains of is due to stretching of the cervix.[9]

### Maternal danger signals

One of the important functions of the nurse while caring for the patient in labor is her observation of any deviation from normal progress. The doctor depends on her early recognition of signs indicating all is not well and reporting them promptly.

*Elevated temperature.* It is normal to find a slight elevation of temperature during labor, that is, about 1° F. above normal. This may be due to dehydration, but should be reported.

*Elevated pulse.* During normal labor the pulse rate averages between 70 and 80 per minute. There is a slight increase during a contraction and bearing-down efforts. A pronounced increase may be a sign of internal hemorrhage or dehydration.

*Respirations.* There should be no change

in respirations except during the second stage, when there may be a slight increase.

*Blood pressure.* A blood pressure higher than 140 systolic and 90 diastolic should be reported, as should a sudden drop.

*Tone and contour of the uterus.* A uterus that does not relax becomes exhausted. This means danger to mother and fetus.

*Vomiting.* Nausea and retching are experienced by some women during the transitional phase of their labor. The nurse should assist the patient to turn on her side and avoid aspiration of any emesis. Excessive vomiting leads to dehydration.

### Fetal danger signals

*Fetal heart rate.* Changes in fetal heart rate may be due to a neural stimuli and are not necessarily a sign of fetal distress. Fetal heart rate tends to be more rapid at the first sign of distress, but persistence of a *slow* rate has a greater significance than a rapid or irregular rate. However, a rate out of normal range should always be reported promptly.

*Meconium.* Passage of meconium is not *always* a sign of distress. This can be attributed to a vagal reflex that will produce increased bowel motility or it may be due to pressure on the fetus if it is presenting in breech. This, too, should be reported. Either change in fetal heart rate or passage of meconium may be the first sign of fetal anoxia.

With use of the amnioscope the doctor can detect presence of meconium through the intact fetal sac. Changes in blood and urine levels of chorionic gonadotropins and estriol determinations may also be of value in detecting fetal distress prior to the onset of labor.

After rupture of the membranes changes in composition of blood can be determined by microanalysis of minute samples taken from the fetal scalp.

*Hyperactivity.* Hyperactivity also indicates that the oxygen supply is being interfered with. The nurse's observation and prompt action in reporting this might give the obstetrician time to intervene and prevent the possibility of a stillbirth. There are a number of reasons why the oxygen supply might not be adequate: (1) premature separation of the placenta, (2) rupture of the membranes when the presenting part is above the inlet of the pelvis allows for prolapse of the cord, and (3) pressure on the cord as the fetus rotates through the birth canal.

*Prolapse of the cord.*[1,6] Prolapse of the cord is likely to occur when the presenting part does not fill the inlet of the pelvis, such as a footling breech or transverse, and the membranes rupture prematurely. When the nurse knows the presenting part is high and the membranes have ruptured, she should notify the doctor and take the fetal heart sounds more frequently, immediately reporting any change in rate or irregularity. If the cord protrudes from the vulva, the nurse should observe whether it is pulsating and carefully place the patient in an elevated Sims' or Trendelenburg position (with hips elevated). The patient should be instructed not to bear down and is given oxygen by mask until the doctor arrives. (See Fig. 13-1.)

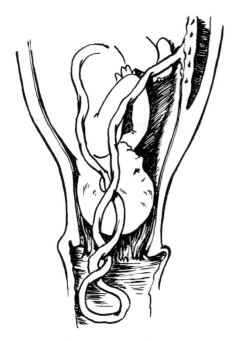

**Fig. 13-1.** Cord prolapse.

## Psychological support

All women need someone to be with them during labor. This is especially true of the primigravida. She usually comes to the hospital in the latent phase of the first stage. Loneliness can be threatening, especially in strange surroundings, and time seems endless. These mothers-to-be need psychological support to maintain self-restraint.

Ideally, the patient should be admitted to a quiet environment, and her husband should be permitted to be by her side if they so desire. Numerous pros and cons are voiced by the personnel as to the value of psychological support of the husband during labor. Those fathers who are not interested or who feel they cannot give of their time use the adjectives "sentimental" or "nonsense" to express their disapproval. It has been stated many times by both doctors and nurses that the mother-to-be needed little if any sedation while her husband was by her side during labor. The husband's own need to help is being met when he recognizes that he can comfort and support his wife and, therefore, share in the experience. His need to feel adequate is met only if he may function in his role of support to his wife.

During your early months of training you were taught and you practiced the basic skills for administering physical care to ill patients. Physical skills are relatively unimportant to the woman in *active* labor. She needs a nurse with warmth, understanding, and genuine concern. Reassurance and frequent encouragement will help the woman relax; this itself accelerates the progress of labor. The woman wants to feel accepted regardless of her behavior, but when she is placed in a cubicle with curtains drawn around her, she feels stripped of her defenses. This fosters fear and loss of self-control. When the patient is said to be "out of control," it is usually true of the nurse also. This further frightens the patient and the situation seems hopeless. Vocal response may be the only means the patient has of coping with stress. She may tell you that it makes her feel better if she screams—it reduces her tension. We need to help the patient before she reaches this point of "loss of control." Encouragement and measures of comfort by the husband or nurse will prevent this unfortunate state.

During your clinical experience in the labor rooms you need to develop skills for giving supportive care. This you will do by observing attitudes of women toward motherhood and how it affects their reactions toward labor. It has been cited that the feelings that women have toward giving birth may influence the nature of their labors.[4] Highly emotional women tend to have irregular labor patterns. These women have increased epinephrine circulating in their blood. They require medication early and tend to develop uterine inertia. You will observe how variable their pain threshold can be and recall that their attitudes toward pain is often conditioned by society. You will observe various reactions to stress and learn to accept the patient's behavior without showing personal signs of disapproval.

*The greatest and most important need in our labor rooms is for nurses willing to function in emotionally supporting roles.*[8]

### Nursing responsibilities during second stage

The transitional phase represents the end of the first stage and the beginning of the second stage. There may be (1) an increased bloody show, (2) nausea and retching, (3) irritability and uncooperativeness, (4) desire to defecate, and (5) anxiety to have it over with.

During this phase the bearing-down efforts of the mother are the result of reflex phenomenon. This reflex is initiated with full cervical dilatation as the head approaches the pelvic floor and stretches the perineum, thus stimulating receptors of sensory nerves. It is the responsibility of the nurse to coach the mother in the proper technique of using her abdominal muscles, since they are under her control.

As the contraction begins the nurse instructs the mother to take a deep breath and hold it; with knees flexed, heels tight against the mattress, she exerts downward pressure exactly as though she were straining to have a bowel movement. Here "labor" is truly defined. The woman is anxious and eager to participate and she can truly labor on when coached and encouraged. Here, too, is where the labor room nurse uses her skills. Because only during the contractions is force exerted, she encourages the patient to relax between times; this is important, since the patient needs to resupply her muscle tissues with oxygen and conserve her strength. (Oxygen and glucose are a *must* for the fetus during labor.) To be effective these bearing-down efforts must be sustained for the duration of the contraction, for grunts and short endeavors merely tire and discourage the mother.

Patients who practice deep breathing exercises during pregnancy can, of course, hold their breath longer, usually for the duration of the contraction. The nurse will soon observe as the result of the patient's efforts an increased bulging of the perineum from further descent of the presenting part. For needed encouragement the nurse should share this sign of progress with the patient. During this phase of bearing down, check the maternal pulse frequently as the mother must not be allowed to become exhausted. If the nurse coaches the mother, the birth process, then, will be more gentle; this is an important factor for both mother and infant.

Women are subject to muscle cramps in the legs, especially during this stage, because of pressure. The nurse should not ignore the woman's complaint because these cramps are most painful. She should change the position of the leg or straighten the leg and apply pressure on the ball of the foot, forcing the ankle toward the anterior aspects of the leg. (See Fig. 7-3.)

When the caput is visible on a primigravida, the woman is moved to the delivery room. The doctor or nurse in charge determines the time when the multigravida should be transferred. The multigravida is moved to the delivery room long before the caput is visible because she delivers more quickly. The time to move her depends on various factors. Do not expect the woman to move during a contraction. She should be assisted onto the table *between* contractions. If the patient is to be delivered in lithotomy position, the wrists are restrained and the legs placed in stirrups. Most of the mothers object to this, but if the nurse explains that it is done only to prevent injury, they are less likely to resist. Flannel or muslin leggings are placed on the patient. These should extend well above the knees. Both legs should be elevated at the same time and placed gently and properly into the stirrups. No area of the skin should be against the metal extension of the stirrups, since this pressure predisposes to thrombophlebitis.

If the mother is to be delivered in a recumbent position, she is assisted to turn on her side and assume Sims' position. A pillow or quilted padding is placed between the knees. In this position the patient has freedom of movement of the legs and is not subjected to the rigidity of the stirrups. Another advantage of this position is that there is no pressure by the uterus upon the inferior vena cava, and if vomiting occurs, the vomitus is readily ejected with less danger of aspiration. After the patient is positioned, the circulating nurse proceeds with whatever method is used for cleansing the delivery area. As the head crowns, the woman is told to cease bearing down. She can do this by panting through her mouth during the contractions. This, of course, should not be done over a period of time because hyperventilation causes dizziness and vomiting and reduces blood flow through the placenta, which results in fetal metabolic acidosis.

The doctor applies gentle pressure against the infant's head to prevent too rapid delivery and avoid lacerations. See p. 152 for a discussion of the Ritgen maneuver and p. 200 for a discussion on episiotomy.

When the doctor has completed aspirating the infant, the nurse places him in a warm blanket and takes him to the mother's side. It is her just reward that she so truly deserves—to see and hold her newborn infant, if only for a few minutes. The infant is then placed in a heated crib under constant observation of a nurse.

If the nurse is functioning in an emergency situation where the doctor is not present, she should remember to rupture the bag as it is forced ahead through the vaginal canal, thereby preventing the fetus from aspirating the fluid. When only the chorion ruptures, the head may be born with the amnion enveloping it; the infant is then said to be born with a caul, or veil. As the head advances she controls its progress by pressure applied laterally beneath the symphysis and over the perineum to steady the egress of the head and prevent lacerations. (See p. 152.)

### Ophthalmic prophylaxis

The newborn is protected against gonorrheal conjunctivitis by instillation of silver nitrate drops. Two drops of a 1% silver nitrate solution are dropped on the inner aspects of the lower eyelid. This was introduced in 1884 by Carl Credé and is known as Credé's prophylaxis. One minute after instillation of the drops, the eyes should be irrigated by isotonic saline solution or sterile distilled water. This reduces the incidence of chemical conjunctivitis. (See p. 249.)

### Nursing responsibilities during third stage

The mechanism of placental separation and expulsion was discussed on p. 154. The nurse can detect this separation if she will place her hand on the uterus immediately after delivery of the infant. She will feel a change in the form of the uterus from the flattened to globular mass (Calkins' sign). As the placenta is forced into the lower segment, she can feel a bulging above the

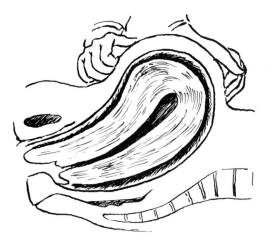

**Fig. 13-2.** Guarding fundus immediately after delivery.

symphysis pubis; this is the fundus becoming firm and rising. The placenta is then expressed from the vaginal canal by the Brandt-Andrews method or bearing-down efforts of the mother.

After completion of the third stage of labor, the doctor inspects the cervix, vagina, and perineum for lacerations. See p. 194 for degrees of lacerations.

Immediately after expulsion of the placenta, the nurse should *guard* the fundus, massaging it gently if it does not maintain its contractile tone (Fig. 13-2). You will observe the doctor examining the placenta and membranes. He is doing this to see if all the cotyledons are intact and the membranes expelled. If not he must remove them manually. See p. 194 for manual removal of the placenta.

### Nursing responsibilities during fourth stage

The immediate hours after birth are crucial for the mother. The nurse is an indispensable member of a team administering to her care. The importance of this time leads some doctors to refer to this period as the fourth stage of labor.

The mother should be transfered to the postpartum recovery room or remain in the delivery room until the postpartum condition is stabilized. Normally this takes 1 to 2 hours. This allows for (1) close observation as the mother recovers from the anesthesia, (2) observation of the condition of the uterus and amount of vaginal bleeding, and (3) a check on the vital signs. She may expect a slowing of the pulse rate and a slight rise in temperature. The blood pressure usually shows a rise of 10 to 20 mm. Hg. This is because at least 300 ml. of blood is restored to the maternal circulation after expulsion of the placenta. Also, oxytocins such a Gynergen elevate the blood pressure. A constant trickle of blood can progressively lower the pressure and atonia also aggravate hypotension. A *sustained* rise in blood pressure may indicate intrapartal toxemia.

If the uterus relaxes during this time, the nurse massages it until firm, but avoids overstimulation since this predisposes to fatigue of the muscles and later relaxation. Should this occur frequently, it should be reported to the supervisor.

It is important that the nurse in the recovery room and on the postpartum unit know whether the patient had an overdistended uterus during pregnancy, such as with hydramnios or a multiple pregnancy. "Late hemorrhage" is more likely to occur in such women and in those heavily sedated.

### Transition to extrauterine environment
*Establishment of respirations*[7]

Birth is a traumatic transition from a parasitic to an independent existence, and this is the infant's first crisis, rapid and complex. For some the transition is delayed, but it is achieved successfully by the majority of newborns.

During fetal life, nature has been busy developing the mechanism that will have to function adequately to meet this transition—the respiratory system. Just as in postnatal life, this system is controlled largely by carbon dioxide and oxygen levels in the blood. Hyperventilation of the mother leads to apnea in the fetus also.

It has been hypothesized that contraction and expansion of the lungs is not newly inaugurated at birth but is a continuation of intrauterine respiratory movements that occur from the end of the first trimester until the latter months when they are inhibited. You may ask why then does the fetus not drown if he inspires while in the bag of fluid? The answer is that because respirations are very shallow and that although amniotic fluid moves continually in and out of the lungs, little fluid is aspirated and it is rapidly absorbed through the capillary bed of the alveoli. If anoxia occurs, stimulation will cause more fluid to be inspired and the alveolar ducts become distended, a state that can seriously interfere with extrauterine respirations.

The reasons the infant gasps and begins to breathe on delivery are still unknown. There may be several, for example: (1) the immediate decrease in arterial oxygen tension with the accompanying rise in carbon dioxide tension and the lowering of the pH of the blood, (2) thermal stimuli from the temperature change, (3) transient rise in blood pressure on occlusion of the cord, and (4) as respirations are established, the steady increase of oxygen saturation of blood and tissues initiates rhythmical activity in the respiratory center.

The normal healthy infant will breathe within 30 seconds to 1 minute after birth. With the first inspiration, circulation of blood takes a different course, and the infant is independent of his intrauterine environment.* His initial responses are intense muscular activity and a lusty cry. His peak respirations are 80 and the heart rate is 180 per minute. Within the hour he settles down, relaxes, and falls asleep. His heart rate then averages 130 to 140 and his respirations 40 to 60 per minute.

It is the responsibility of the delivery room nurse to assist the newborn in this transition. She gently clears his airway, positions him in head-down posture on his right side, stimulates crying gently, and keeps him warm. Constant observation is of extreme importance.

### Anoxia

Anoxia may be defined as insufficient oxygen saturation in the tissues. The fetus and newborn possess some immunity to anoxia. However, the degree that can be tolerated is variable and questionable and depends to a great extent on the degree of maturity and development of the central nervous system. There are also other protective mechanisms that see him safely through the early period of adjustment to extrauterine respirations; for example, the fetal red blood cells are larger, contain more hemoglobin, and can take up oxygen more readily than do the mother's red cells, and there is a decline in the newborn's temperature at birth. Thus the lowered metabolism in turn lessens the infant's oxygen requirement. Nevertheless, anoxia is the leading cause of death during the perinatal period.

During labor the doctor and nurses assess the status of the fetus by monitoring the heart rate. The first sign of intrauterine anoxia is the slowing of the fetal heart rate between uterine contractions. A temporary increase plus fetal hyperactivity may precede the slowing. When anoxia is severe, peristalsis in the fetal intestines is increased and the nurse will note meconium-stained amniotic fluid coming from the vagina. See p. 162 for a discussion on fetal danger signs with complications. The nurse, in such instances, should administer oxygen to the mother.

Asphyxia of the newborn (asphyxia neonatorum) is a syndrome in which apnea (absence of respirations) is the outstanding clinical symptom that all is not well. If this occurs it is spoken of as *initial apnea;* late apnea is cessation of respirations for more than 60 seconds after spontaneous breathing has been established and sustained.[7] Oxygen deprivation is not the only cause of asphyxia. The degree of acidosis is most important. (See Fig. 13-3.)

---

*The student is referred to Chapter 4, p. 43, for review of changes in circulation.

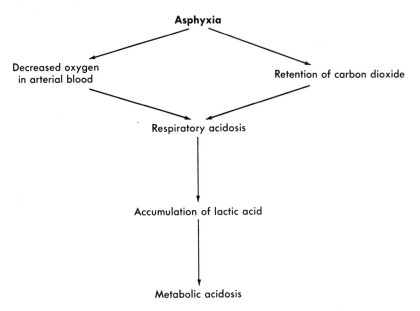

**Fig. 13-3.** Oxygen deprivation and retention of carbon dioxide results in respiratory and metabolic acidosis.

There are infants born showing no evidence of intrauterine anoxia and yet they fail to breathe. This may be caused by intracranial hemorrhage, debris in the alveoli preventing exchange of gases, or excessive doses of analgesics or anesthetics. In the premature infant it may be due to immaturity of the lungs.

The infant in distress will attempt to meet his oxygen need by using his intercostal muscles to elevate his ribs, thereby increasing the size of the intrathoracic cavity. Deep sternal retraction is then observed.

**Conditions during prenatal period that predispose to asphyxia neonatorum**

1. Anemia
2. Multiple pregnancies
3. Bleeding during the third trimester
4. Toxemia
5. Diabetes
6. Excess pressure on vena cava
7. Placenta insufficiency
8. Postmaturity
9. Age of the mother (over 40 years)

**Conditions during parturition that predispose to asphyxia neonatorum**

1. Compression or prolapse of the umbilical cord
2. Precipitate delivery
3. Dystocia
4. Premature delivery
5. Uterine tetany usually as the result of inductions with oxytocics
6. Hypotension from spinal anesthesia and injudicious use of analgesics and anesthetics
7. Difficult delivery resulting in cerebral hemorrhage or damage to the central nervous system
8. Narcosis from excessive analgesia or anesthetics; loss of laryngeal reflex necessary to produce cough response

**Conditions in the infant that predispose to asphyxia**

1. Obstruction of respiratory passage by mucus
2. Immaturity of the lungs
3. Tumors or stenosis of respiratory passage
4. Diaphragmatic hernia

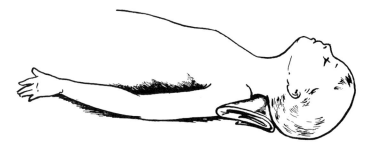

**Fig. 13-4.** Position of infant for laryngeal intubation and aspiration.

Table 13-1. Apgar scoring system

|  | 0 | 1 | 2 |
|---|---|---|---|
| Heart rate | Absent | Slow, below 100 per minute | Above 100 per minute |
| Respiratory effort | Absent | Slow, gasping, irregular | Good, strong cry |
| Muscle tone | Flaccid | Flexion of extremities poor | Good flexion, active motion |
| Reflex response | No response | Grimace, some motion | Active, crying |
| Color | Body pale or blue | Body pink, extremities blue | Completely pink |

### Management of the infant in respiratory distress

The infant should be placed in a prewarmed incubator and positioned in head-down posture. This position is contraindicated in premature infants or where intracranial hemorrhage is suspected.

When in a head-down posture, extend the neck gently to clear the upper airway of mucus. This position may easily be maintained by placing a folded pad or blanket at nape of infant's neck. (See Fig. 13-4.) A small bulb syringe is used to aspirate the *throat first* and then the nostrils, or gentle suction with soft rubber catheter may be used. *After* the airway has been cleared, oxygen is administered to relieve cyanosis. If these simple measures do not relieve the distress, then oxygen should be administered under controlled intermittent pressure by an anesthesiologist, or a skilled, experienced delivery room personnel.

Coramine or alpha-lobeline should not be used, since the dosage necessary to act as a respiratory stimulant may predispose to convulsive seizures. Nalorphine hydrochloride (Nalline) can be given to counteract effect of narcosis caused by administration of morphine or Demerol to the mother during labor, but not if narcosis is caused by anesthetic gases or barbiturates. Caffeine sodium benzoate in doses of 30 to 50 mg. intramuscularly is also used. As soon as condition of infant permits, the stomach should be aspirated to remove fluid, especially in those delivered by cesarean section.

*Since an infant in respiratory distress is in a state of shock, or close to shock, warmth and extreme gentleness in handling are of utmost importance.*

In 1953, Dr. Virginia Apgar presented a means of evaluating the newborn by a scoring system. This method appraises the newborn within 1 minute after birth is completed. This score also furnishes an excellent clinical evaluation for use during the immediate neonatal period. Every delivery room and nursery nurse should be familiar with the method of scoring, since many doctors depend on her to furnish the evaluation. The evaluation for scoring is based on the following five clinical signs:

> **Heart rate:** should be between 100 to 140 per minute.
> **Respiratory effort:** cry should be clear and lusty.
> **Muscle tone:** should flex muscles on external stimuli.
> **Reflex irritability:** should respond to gentle stimulation.
> **Color:** entire body should be pink.

The Apgar sheet should be kept at hand to evaluate the infant at 1, 5, and 10 minutes. After identification and ophthalmic prophylaxis, the infant should be transferred to the "recovery nursery" where he can be observed during the precarious first hours of life. (See Table 13-1.)

The nurse should keep the following in mind as she cares for the immediate newborn:

> 1. Cyanosis is not as grave a sign as pallor.
> 2. Flaccidity indicates a greater degree of asphyxia than does hypertonicity.
> 3. Tachycardia (heart rate above 140) does not indicate severe asphyxia, but bradycardia (heart rate below 100 per minute) does.

### Baptism

Every person has the right to be baptized. This applies to embryos and fetuses as well as newborn infants. For those of the Catholic faith, it is a sacrament of significance. There are numerous circumstances where the nurse may be called on to administer the rites of baptism. Without hesitance she should know how and when to baptize. She needs to know the essential words and whether to pour or sprinkle the water or to immerse the baby.

Every aborted embryo or fetus should be baptized. If in doubt about "life," con-

fer the baptism conditionally, saying "If you can be baptized." When the embryo or fetus is expelled in the sac, it must be ruptured and then baptism conferred. When baptizing an infant of Catholic parents, the water should be poured on the forehead while pronouncing the words, "I baptize you in the name of the Father, and of the Son, and of the Holy Ghost." The water is sprinkled on the forehead when the infant is born to Protestant parents. Holy water should be kept in the delivery room, but in an emergency, other water may be used.

### The stillborn infant

An intrauterine fetal death may occur as a complication of placenta insufficiency, maternal diabetes, or accidents to the fetoplacental circulation, such as separation or a compressed cord. Confirmation of the doctor's suspicion of an intrauterine fetal death can be made by palpating the macerated skull bones. When death is due to hydrops fetalis, the mother's weight will increase rapidly due to the developing hydramnios. When the fetus dies due to other causes, the mother loses weight and the chorionic gonadotropic hormone level decreases. After the fetus has been dead for approximately 10 days, an x-ray film may show an overlapping of the skull bones (Spalding-Horner sign) and curvature of the fetal spine.

Labor usually starts spontaneously. Carrying a dead fetus produces anxiety for the patient and her family and the danger of hypofibrinogenemia. If labor does not start within 30 days after fetal death, the doctor usually starts an induction of labor by intravenous oxytocin or intraamniotic hypertonic saline solution. (See p. 101.)

**STUDY QUESTIONS**

*Multiple choice*

1. A full bladder:
   (a) impedes progress of labor.
   (b) is conducive to urinary tract infection.
   (c) contributes to patient's discomfort.
   (d) all of these.
2. To prevent pressure of the uterus on the inferior vena cava the nurse would assist the

patient in assuming the following position:
(a) Sims' on side opposite the fetus's back.
(b) Sims' on the side same as fetus's back.
(c) on back in Fowler's position.

3. Nausea and retching is a sign of approaching:
(a) toxemia.
(b) transitional phase of labor.
(c) active phase of labor.
(d) internal hemorrhage.

4. The enema may serve many purposes but the main reason for administering one during labor is that:
(a) it prevents contamination of delivery field.
(b) it makes more space available for passage of the fetus.
(c) it stimulates contractions.
(d) it facilitates rectal examinations.

5. During labor the blood pressure should be checked:
(a) during contractions.
(b) as the contraction starts.
(c) after the contraction completely subsides.

6. The nurse knows that the fetal heart rate is:
(a) more rapid at the height of a contraction.
(b) slower at the height of a contraction.
(c) more distinct at the height of a contraction.

7. On admission to the labor room a patient tells you she is "leaking" fluid but she is not certain that her membranes have ruptured. To be certain about this the nurse may do the Nitrazine paper test. She knows that with ruptured membranes the color change will be:
(a) orange to brown.
(b) blue green to deep blue.
(c) yellow to yellow green.

8. Women tend to suffer from muscle cramps in their legs during the transitional phase of labor. This is primarily due to:
(a) pressure.
(b) decrease in phosphorus content of the blood.
(c) anxiety and fear.

9. Hyperventilation (if not practiced properly) during the transitional phase of labor can be dangerous because it may:
(a) reduce blood flow through the placenta.
(b) prolong labor.
(c) reduce blood flow to the perineum.

10. Change in form of the uterus during the third stage of labor is called:
(a) Ritgen's sign.
(b) Calkin's sign.
(c) Brandt-Andrews' sign.

11. The placenta may be expressed from the vaginal canal by the following maneuver:
(a) Ritgen.
(b) Calkin.
(c) Brandt-Andrews.

12. The nurse knows that a prolapsed cord will cause death of the fetus unless pressure is relieved. Her immediate duty is to inform her supervisor. She also knows that chances for fetal survival are less favorable if the presentation is:
(a) vertex.
(b) breech.
(c) transverse.

13. The clinical signs whereby the nurse can tell that the placenta has separated from the uterine wall are:
(a) change in the form of uterus from discoid to globular mass.
(b) fundus is in the midline.
(c) cord protrudes further from the vaginal canal.
(d) all of these.

14. After delivery the nurse should:
(a) massage the uterus vigorously.
(b) apply pressure over fundal area.
(c) guard fundus and massage gently if contractile tone is poor.

15. Overlapping of cranial bones occurs in fetal death. This is referred to as:
(a) halo sign.
(b) Spalding's sign.
(c) Homan's sign.

16. In assisting an infant in respiratory distress due to mucus the first thing you will do is:
(a) give oxygen.
(b) clear air passages.
(c) stimulate infant to cry.

17. If you see the need to baptize an infant in an emergency and holy water is not available, you would:
(a) send someone for holy water.
(b) contact a minister or priest.
(c) use ordinary water.

18. A prolapsed cord is more likely to accompany premature rupture of the membranes when the fetus presents as:
(a) footling breech.
(b) shoulder.
(c) vertex.
(d) mentum.
1. a and b    2. b and d    3. c and d

19. A *pronounced* increase in pulse may indicate:
(a) dehydration.
(b) hemorrhage.
(c) transitional phase.
1. a and b    2. b only    3. all of these

20. During the fourth stage of labor, the nurse may normally expect:
(a) a loss of approximately 200 ml. of blood.

(b) a temporary rise in blood pressure of 10 to 20 mm. Hg.

(c) a slowing of the pulse.

   1. b only    2. b and c    3. a and c

21. The nurse would be alert for a postpartum hemorrhage if the patient had the following:

(a) hydramnios.

(b) multiple pregnancy.

(c) premature delivery.

(d) deep, prolonged anesthesia

   1. a, b, and c   2. a, b, and d   3. all of these

22. The following conditions may predispose to asphyxia of the fetus during labor and delivery:

(a) dystocia.

(b) excessive analgesics or anesthetics.

(c) blood pressure 140/90.

(d) precipitate labor and delivery.

   1. b and c   2. a, b, and c   3. a, b, and d

## True or false

(T)  (F)  1. For accuracy in checking pulse rate it should not be taken during a contraction.

(T)  (F)  2. It is normal for the patient to have a slight elevation of temperature during labor.

(T)  (F)  3. No woman should be left alone during labor, especially the primigravida.

(T)  (F)  4. Much of the backache experienced during labor is due to stretching of the cervix.

(T)  (F)  5. Changing position of a patient may effect a change in pattern of contractions.

(T)  (F)  6. A sustained rise in blood pressure during the fourth stage of labor may indicate intrapartal toxemia.

(T)  (F)  7. Persistence of a slow fetal heart rate has a greater significance of distress than a rapid or irregular rate.

(T)  (F)  8. Fetal red blood cells are larger and contain more hemoglobin than the mother's.

(T)  (F)  9. Both fetus and the immediate newborn possess some immunity to anoxia.

(T)  (F)  10. Anoxia is the leading cause of death during the perinatal period.

(T)  (F)  11. The first evaluation on the Apgar score is respiratory effort.

(T)  (F)  12. If you are baptizing an infant and you know the parents are of Protestant faith, you would *pour* the water on the infant's forehead.

## REFERENCES

1. Goldthorp, W. O.: Umbilical cord prolapse, Nurs. Mirror **127**:19, Dec. 13, 1968.

2. Long, A. E.: The unshaved perineum at parturition, Amer. J. Obstet. Gynec. **99**:333, 1967.

3. Matousek, Irene: Fetal nursing during labor, Nurs. Clin. N. Amer. **3**:307, 1968.

4. Newton, Niles: Maternal emotions, New York, 1955, Paul E. Hoeber, Inc., p. 30.

5. Ottoway, John P.: Vaginal vs. rectal examination in evaluation of labor status, Hosp. Top. **45**:101, March, 1967.

6. Oxorn, Harry, and Foote, Wm. R.: Human labor and birth, New York, 1964, Appleton-Century-Crofts, chap. 21.

7. Schaffer, Alexander: Diseases of the newborn, Philadelphia, 1965, W. B. Saunders Co., p. 54.

8. Tryon, Phyllis: Assessing the progress of labor through observation of patients' behavior, Nurs. Clin. N. Amer. **3**:315, 1968.

9. Ueland, Kent, and Hansen, John M.: Maternal cardiovascular dynamics: posture and uterine contractions, Amer. J. Obstet. Gynec. **103**:1, 1969.

## SELECTED READINGS

*Transition to extrauterine environment*

Broadribb, Violet: Foundations of pediatric nursing, Philadelphia, 1967, J. B. Lippincott Co., pp. 64-69.

Du, Joseph N. H., and Oliver, Thomas K., Jr.: The baby in the delivery room, J.A.M.A. **208**:1502, Feb. 24, 1969.

Hurlock, Elizabeth: Child development, ed. 4, New York, 1964, McGraw-Hill Book Co., chap. 3.

James, L. Stanley: Onset of breathing and resuscitation, Pediat. Clin. N. Amer. **13**:621, Aug., 1966.

Latham, Helen, and Heckel, Robert V.: Pediatric nursing, St. Louis, 1967, The C. V. Mosby Co., p. 14.

Montagu, M. F. Ashley: Prenatal influences, Springfield, Ill., 1962, Charles C Thomas, Publisher, pp. 472-481.

Towell, Molly: The influence of labor on the fetus and the newborn, Pediat. Clin. N. Amer. **13**: 575-595, Aug., 1966.

*Management of infant in respiratory distress*

Apgar, Virginia: Resuscitation of the newborn—when and how to do it, Hosp. Top. **44**:105, Nov., 1966.

Avery, Mary Ellen: The lung and its disorders in the newborn infant, Philadelphia, 1964, W. B. Saunders Co., chap. 17.

Drage, J. S., and Berendes, H.: Apgar scores and outcome of the newborn, Pediat. Clin. N. Amer. **13**:635, Aug., 1966.

Heller, M. L.: Resuscitation procedures in neonatal crises, Hosp. Top. **44**:105, April, 1966.

James, L. Stanley: Resuscitation of the newborn. In Gellis, Sydney, and Kagan, Benjamin, editors: Current pediatric therapy, Philadelphia, 1966, W. B. Saunders Co., sect. 23, p. 844.

*Detection of fetal distress*

Bergen, Margaret A.: Monitoring the fetal heart, Nurs. Clin. N. Amer. 1:559, 1966.

Cunningham, T. M.: Detection of fetal distress, Nurs. Mirror 126:37, Feb. 9, 1968.

Lefebrve, Yves: Urinary estriol levels indicative of insidious fetal distress, Hosp. Top. 47:63, Jan., 1969.

Milic, Ann, and Adamson, Karlis: Fetal blood sampling, Amer. J. Nurs. 68:2149, Oct., 1968.

*Psychological support during labor*

Grimm, Elaine: Relationship of personality variables to psychological and physiological reactions during labor and delivery. In Richardson, Stephen A., and Guttmacher, Alan F., editors: Childbearing: its social and psychological aspect, Baltimore, 1967, The Williams & Wilkins Co., pp. 24-29.

Hazlett, Wm. H.: The male factor in obstetrics, Child Family 6:3, Fall, 1967.

Kelman, Norman: The father, Child Family 6:55, Fall, 1967.

Liley, H. M. I.: Modern motherhood, New York, 1966, Random House, Inc., pp. 57-72.

Miller, J. S.: Return to joy of home delivery with fathers in the delivery room, Hosp. Top. 44:105, Jan., 1966.

Morton, J. H.: Fathers in the delivery room—an opposition standpoint, Hosp. Top. 44:103, Jan., 1966.

Roberts, John A.: I watched my baby being born, Parents' Magazine 64:60, Jan., 1969.

*Miscellaneous selected readings*

Claman, A. D.: Evaluation of some obstetrical traditions, Canad. Nurse 64:44, Feb., 1968.

Du, Joseph, and Oliver, Thomas K.: The baby in the delivery room, J.A.M.A. 207:1502, Feb. 24, 1969.

Klopper, Arnold: Intra-uterine fetal death—diagnosis of hormone excretion, Nurs. Times 65:146, Feb. 2, 1968.

Russell, J. K.: Ligation of the umbilical cord, Nurs. Times 65:747, June 12, 1969.

Shanklin, D. R., and Wolfson, S. L.: Oxygen as a cause of pulmonary hemorrhage in infants, New Eng. J. Med. 277:833, Oct. 19, 1967.

Towell, Molly: The influence of labor on the fetus and the newborn, Pediat. Clin. N. Amer. 13:575, Aug., 1966.

Tryon, Phyllis: Use of comfort measures as support during labor, Nurs. Res. 15:109, Spring, 1966.

**For student's quick notes:**

# Chapter 14

# Alleviation of pain

Hlow much pain will I have to endure? This is the question that each
woman asks as she faces the inescapable fact that she is about to give birth.
The first part of this chapter reviews our forefathers' views about relieving
pain accompanying childbirth. The methods of pain relief used in today's
obstetrics and the clinical aspects of various drugs are then discussed.

## Historical background

Hippocrates said, "Divine is the work to
subdue pain." The deadening of pain by
potions was practiced among primitive persons. Wine made from European mandrake
plants was the popular anesthetic substitute during the Middle Ages. Potions of
honey and niter were among some of the
drinks prepared by herbal doctors, along
with their music of drums and chanting.

The use of anesthesia to alleviate pains
of childbirth was not introduced until the
middle of the nineteenth century. Even
during the Renaissance of Western Civilization when progress was being made, to
be sure, relief of any pain during childbirth
was not considered progress. Even as late
as the sixteenth century, men were burned
at the stake for attempting to assuage the
pains of labor. The feeling of this era was
that pains associated with childbirth were
meant to be; this was woman's ordained
function to be endured with fortitude. The
absence of pain might alter her love for
her child and lessen her fear of God. When
there were no "pangs of childbirth," there
would be no maternal instinct.

Credit goes to Sir James Simpson (1811-
1870) for having contributed much toward
the acceptance of anesthesia for labor and

delivery. He was among the first to use
ether and chloroform. In 1847 he introduced anesthesia into obstetrics. From the
pulpits came the cry that man must not
interfere with God's plan and the popular
text of their sermons was taken from Genesis 3:16: ". . . in sorrow thou shalt bring
forth children." To prevent pains of childbirth was a sacrilege.

What these preachers did not understand
was that translators are often influenced
by their culture. This was so true in Bible
times; thus the experience of childbirth
was related according to the phrasing given
it by the culture. The word "sorrow" translated from the Greek word *lupe* refers to
anxiety or exertion. The words "sorrow"
and "pain" translated from the Hebrew
language mean toil.

Dr. John Snow, English anesthetist, administered anesthesia to Queen Victoria at
the birth of her son Prince Leopold in 1853.
This may have helped pave the way for
others who previously objected so strenu-
ously to its use for childbirth.

Although tremendous strides have been
accomplished, there is still much to be
learned and improved upon to control pain
accompanying childbirth; never for a moment can we forget that there are always

two lives involved, the mother's and her baby's. One of the goals in obstetrics today is to provide comparable freedom from pain for the mother without endangering the fetus. Such an ideal drug has yet to be discovered.

Most drugs given to control pain during labor and delivery do pass to the fetus. As long as there is adequate oxygen, the fetus suffers no damage. The blood of the fetus normally has a low oxygen tension, and a degree of hypoxia that appears insignificant to the mother may prove lethal to the fetus. Maternal hypotension, the result of so many tranquilizing drugs, is also responsible for fetal hypoxia. It is often after birth that serious problems arise; the infant's respiratory center may be so severely depressed that it is unable to breathe for itself. See discussion on fetal anoxia, p. 167.

The obstetrician does not guarantee a completely painless labor and delivery. The type of analgesia and anesthesia the patient is to have and the optimal time for starting sedation is left to the discretion of the obstetrician. If he gives the woman intelligent, satisfying answers to her questions she is likely to understand that in relieving her discomfort, he must consider her welfare and the safety of her baby. She is also more likely to cooperate if she understands something about the techniques of administration.

The nurse needs to know (1) how the drug affects the physiology of the fetus, (2) physiology of labor, (3) routes of administration, (4) maximum dosage, (5) reactions to expect from the patient, and (6) advantages and disadvantages of the drug.

## The analgesics

*Meperidine (Demerol).* Demerol produces satisfactory analgesia for patients during labor. It is a synthetic preparation with mild atropine-like action. It relaxes smooth muscles of the uterus; it has a relaxing effect on the cervix and may therefore shorten labor in the primipara.

The patient experiences pain relief in about 20 minutes after the injection. The nurse will observe peripheral vascular flush, especially of the face. She will also note restlessness during contractions, evidencing discomfort, but the patient has no recollection of what has transpired. Since Demerol dries secretions, the patient experiences dryness of tongue and mouth. To relieve this, the nurse may swab the mouth with antiseptic mouth wash or apply cracked ice to her lips. The frequency and intensity of contractions are not affected unless the drug is given early in the first stage of labor.

If Demerol is given intravenously, it should be administered *slowly* and the nurse should have oxygen ventilation and airways at hand. Demerol may produce profound depression of vital centers when administered by this route.

The effect of Demerol on the fetus is related to the dosage, not to the time at which it is given.

*Alphaprodine hydrochloride (Nisentil hydrochloride).* The desired analgesic effect is obtained by the mother with alphaprodine much more rapidly than is the case with Demerol. Onset of noticeable relief is often seen within 10 minutes. Thus it is excellent in multigravidas who are first seen when close to the time of delivery. Effects wear off more rapidly both in the mother and in the infant.

*Scopolamine hydrobromide (hyoscine hydrobromide).* Scopolamine is a cerebral depressant used as an amnesic agent for the first stage of labor in combination with other drugs. Scopolamine produces drowsiness and affects structures concerned with the emotions. It passes over the placenta but has no significant effect on the fetus. Scopolamine raises the basal metabolism, produces peripheral vascular flush, reduces secretions of the respiratory tract, and prevents laryngospasms. The action of scopolamine is variable. It may cause delirium in the presence of pain unless administered with analgesic drugs. Scopolamine may counteract respiratory depression after the administration of morphine. Since scopolamine causes hypotension, it should not be given when the infant is premature.

## Tranquilizers and ataractics

The phenothiazine derivatives have little analgesic effect themselves, but they enhance the effect of analgesics, sedatives, and anesthetics. This allows for the dosage reduction of narcotics. These drugs reduce anxiety, suppress nausea and vomiting, potentiate hypotensive drugs, and counteract hyperactivity sometimes seen with scopolamine.

A few of the phenothiazine derivatives used for obstetrical patients are (1) promazine hydrochloride (Sparine), (2) chlorpromazine (Thorazine), (3) promethazine (Phenergan), and (4) propiomazine (Largon). Phenergan and Largon are primarily antihistamines, but they produce drowsiness and have sedative effect on patients in labor.

Since these drugs tend to cause hypotension, they are not given when the doctor expects to use spinal anesthesia. They are contraindicated when the patient has eclampsia or severe hypertension or when a sudden drop in blood pressure is undesirable. The nurse should remember to keep the patient recumbent to prevent a sudden drop in blood pressure after any of these drugs is given.

With the administration of these tranquilizers, little or no scopolamine is needed, and the patient may participate in the delivery if she so desires. Pudendal block is often the choice for delivery when the phenothiazine derivatives have been used during labor.

Nalorphine (Nalline) or levallorphan (Lorfan) is given as an antagonistic to morphinelike drugs. They relieve respiratory depression (asphyxia neonatorum) due to the action of narcotics. They should never be used when inhalation anesthetics are given, since they then cause further depression of the infant. The drug may be given to the mother (10 mg. intravenously, 15 minutes prior to delivery) or into the umbilical vein of the newborn (0.25 mg.) immediately after delivery.

## General anesthesia

*Nitrous oxide.* Usually limited to the second stage of labor, a nitrous oxide oxygen mixture is given *during* the contractions, with 100% oxygen as the contraction ceases. The anesthetist gives 100% oxygen after birth of the baby until the cord stops pulsating. There is little danger of asphyxia neonatorum if given correctly.

*Cyclopropane.* Cyclopropane acts quickly and is eliminated rapidly. It is good to use where the doctor desires rapid induction. It is not given intermittently because of its explosive properties. The gas does not depress the fetus unless given over a period of more than 8 to 10 minutes.

*Trilene.* The gas Trilene is used during the latter part of the first stage and during the second. The mother may apply the mask herself and inhale during contractions. She needs coaching and the constant attention of the nurse. It should be used during delivery only under the surveillance of an anesthetist. Trilene causes asphyxia of the infant only if administered over a prolonged time.

When labor begins without warning, the patient most likely has food in her stomach. Vomiting with possible aspiration of gastric contents can be fatal to mother and fetus. Therefore these gases should not be administered unless the stomach is empty and then only by a trained anesthetist.

## Intravenous anesthesia

Thiopental sodium (Pentothal sodium) is more prompt than nitrous oxide. It is used for quick induction; recovery is prompt and without vomiting. It takes about 5 minutes before enough of the drug crosses the placenta to narcotize the fetus. It is used for the eclamptic patient when convulsions are anticipated and for manual removal of the placenta.

## Conduction or regional anesthesia

Spinal anesthesia is used for control of pain during the latter part of the first stage of labor and during the second stage, or it may be used for delivery only. The anesthetic agent is injected into the subarachnoid space.

In preparation for spinal anesthesia the nurse assists the patient to turn on her side and flex her spine. The nurse should have a pillow available and place it under the patient's head immediately after the anesthetic agent is injected. Blood pressure and respirations are checked every 10 minutes. If the blood pressure drops, encourage the patient to breathe deeply and have oxygen available. Approximately half of the patients receiving spinal anesthesia reveal a lowering of blood pressure, on an average of 10 mm. systolic. It is the nurse's responsibility to have vasopressor drugs, such as ephedrine, at hand should the doctor order an immediate dose to counteract marked fall in blood pressure. The nurse should also remember that nausea and vomiting frequently occur with spinal anesthesia. A marked hypotension would be the only means by which spinal anesthesia would affect the fetus.

Postspinal headaches are experienced in 5% to 10% of the patients receiving spinal anesthesia. Headaches are attributed to use of incorrect type needle, to leakage of spinal fluid, or to too rapid injection of the drug.

### Saddle block

Saddle block anesthesia is spinal anesthesia confined to the perineal area. When the cervix is dilated 8 to 10 cm., the patient is moved to the delivery room. The nurse assists the woman in sitting with legs over the side of the delivery room table with her feet resting on a chair. Her arms are folded across her chest and she leans forward as the nurse supports her shoulders. This makes the vertebrae more prominent and facilitates location of posterior spines. The anesthetic agent is injected into the subarachnoid space between the third and fourth lumbar interspace. The patient remains in sitting position for *30 seconds* after the drug is administered and is then

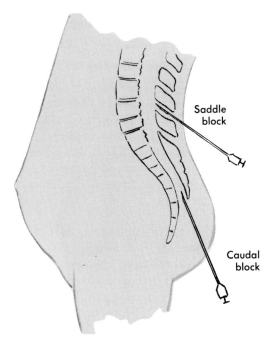

**Fig. 14-1.** Regional anesthesia to control pain of parturition.

assisted in resuming the supine position with pillow under her head to keep the neck flexed. A saddle block is not used when the perineum is bulging, since injury to the head of the fetus may occur with the mother in upright position for its administration. (See Fig. 14-1.)

### Caudal analgesia and anesthesia

Caudal analgesia and anesthesia control pain impulses by nerve block. The drug is injected through the caudal canal into the extradural space and does not mix with the spinal fluid. It may be given continuously from the latter part of the first stage all through the second stage, or it may be given terminally at time of delivery. Therefore it provides analgesia for labor and anesthesia for delivery. The nurse assists the patient in assuming the left lateral Sims' position for administration of the drug. (See Fig. 14-1.)

The drug does not disturb fetal oxygenation unless maternal blood pressure falls below 100 mm. Hg, decreasing blood flow to the uterus. This hypotension, if reported promptly, can be controlled by vasopressor drugs or by elevating the patient's legs.

Caudal anesthesia is recommended for patients with heart disease, severe toxemia, nephritis, and diabetes and for women in premature labor. Women delivering premature infants tend to have forceful labors. With caudal anesthesia the obstetrician can control the delivery and prevent intracranial pressure. Caudal analgesia can impair frequency and strength of uterine contractions, especially if started early in labor, and the second stage tends to be prolonged. With continuous caudal analgesia during labor the patient loses the normal sensation of a full bladder so that the nurse should check frequently and report this immediately. Both spinal and caudal anesthesia provide the same effect but from a different anatomical approach.

For hypotension, the nurse may be instructed to start an intravenous infusion of 500 ml. of dextrose solution with 10 mg. of Neo-Synephrine. The doctor may also order the patient's legs to be elevated to a 90-degree angle. This is usually done when the blood pressure falls below 80 mm. (a critical level).

### Peripheral or pudendal nerve block

This method blocks pudendal nerves at the ischial spine level and anesthetizes nerve supply to lower birth canal. It is administered to the primigravida when the cervix is fully dilated and the station is +2 and to the multigravida when the cervix is dilated 7 to 8 cm.

Pudendal block anesthesia is the choice in many instances for premature deliveries; asphyxia occurs less often than with general anesthesia.

Pudendal block, saddle block, and caudal block will eliminate the reflex urge, but when properly executed none of these procedures will significantly affect the power of the auxiliary forces because the patient still retains the muscle power to bear down, and, if coached by the nurse, she can use her expulsive forces for a spontaneous delivery.

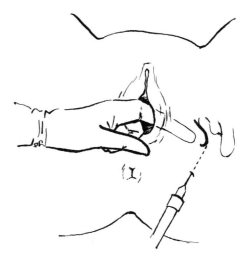

**Fig. 14-2.** Local infiltration anesthesia.

### Regional or local perineal anesthesia

The anesthesia producing drug is injected locally into the vulva and perineal body to desensitize the delivery area. Drugs such as Metycaine, Xylocaine, and procaine are used. They are preferred when delivery is imminent and episiotomy must be performed. (See Fig. 14-2.)

The advantages of regional anesthesia are (1) the mother is awake, (2) the infant's respiratory center is not depressed, (3) the cough reflex is not depressed and therefore there is less danger of aspiration if the patient does vomit, and (4) it is also preferred for premature births to avoid increasing the depression of vital centers so characteristic of these infants.

### Hypnosis

The word hypnosis means sleep and is derived from the Greek word *hypnos.* This "state of sleep" is quite different from sleep as we experience it. It is a state of sleep in which the subject's attention is fixed on the hypnotist, with an awareness of her surroundings and concentration on his suggestions.

During one of the visits with the obstetrician, he may discuss the subject of what type anesthesias are available. Hypnoanesthesia was practiced long before the introduction of chemical anesthesia. An ob-

## 180    *The period of parturition*

stetrician well-trained in the basic principles of hypnotherapy may suggest that she consider hypnosis, explaining to the woman that it involves a period of physical training and mental conditioning. The decision to use it is, of course, based on sound medical opinion. Its use is considered when chemical analgesics and anesthesias are contraindicated.

The initial induction to the hypnotic state does not usually begin before the seventh month of pregnancy, which provides time for the doctor to educate the woman in all the aspects of hypnosis that he advocates. The doctor may recommend that she practice exercises in relaxation. This therapy seems to be more effective when done with a group of mothers-to-be, and for this reason she may wish to attend group training classes. Here she will become familiar with techniques of breathing and relaxation used during labor and gradually learn to relax *all* her muscles, thereby making her labor and delivery a healthier, happier event.

The doctor explains that hypnosis is a means whereby she can help herself during labor and delivery. Reassurance that she will approach labor with confidence is continuously given throughout her pregnancy. Such understanding and confidence between patient and doctor during pregnancy heightens the patient's susceptibility to his suggestions during parturition, such as when to breathe deeply and when to bear down. (She is reassured that analgesic drugs will be available should she need them.)

In some women a diminished sensitivity to pain is produced, whereas in others a marked degree of anesthesia may be obtained. With "light hypnosis" the woman remembers, that is, she recalls her labor and delivery. This is ideal for women who wish to participate in the delivery and remember the climax to her ultimate goal —giving birth.

Posthypnotic suggestion means the subject will carry out acts suggested by the doctor after awakening from the trance.

This is used sometimes for puerperal women. With posthypnotic suggestion she is less likely to experience the depression that sometimes follows labor.

In giving nursing care to the woman under hypnotic suggestion, the nurse should remember that these women are in a "suggestive state," that conversation must be chosen with care, and that whispering should not be engaged in at the bedside.

### STUDY QUESTIONS
### Matching
Match the terms in the first column with their appropriate definition in the second column.

(a) Demerol —Tends to cause hypotension

(b) Nausea and vomiting —Although this drug passes over the placenta, it has no ill effects on the fetus

(c) Nisentil —Can be self-administered
(d) Scopolamine —May be injected into the umbilical vein to counteract respiratory depression caused by oversedation with Demerol or morphinelike substances

(e) Phenothiazines —Safe anesthetic for delivery of premature infants

(f) Levallorphan —Synthetic preparation with mild atropine-like action

(g) Pudendal nerve block —Has more rapid effect than Demerol but of shorter duration

(h) Chlorpromazine —Occurs with spinal anesthesia

(i) Trichoroethylene —Incidence of nausea and vomiting is reduced significantly with this drug

### Multiple choice
1. With continuous caudal analgesia the nurse would check the patient frequently for signs of:
   (a) full bladder.
   (b) cold extremities.
   (c) dyspnea.
2. The doctor orders 25 mg. of chlorpromazine and 0.4 mg. of scopolamine. In preparing the medication, the nurse knows:
   (a) chlorpromazine may be mixed with the scopolamine.
   (b) chlorpromazine should be given separately.

(c) the chlorpromazine should be given subcutaneously.

3. Before saddle block is given, the cervix must be dilated:
   (a) 8 to 10 cm.
   (b) 2 to 4 cm.
   (c) 5 to 7 cm.

4. Within 15 to 30 minutes after administration of Demerol, the nurse may expect the following:
   (a) peripheral vascular flush to the patient's face.
   (b) restlessness between contractions.
   (c) dryness of tongue and mouth.
   (d) pronounced nausea.
   1. b and c    2. a and c    3. all the above

5. The effects of chlorpromazine are:
   (a) the patient assumes a quiet, phlegmatic acceptance of pain.
   (b) it lessens the amount of inhalation anesthesia required.
   (c) it produces amnesia in all patients.
   1. a and b    2. c only    3. all the above

*True or false*

(T)  (F)  1. With epidural anesthesia the patient must always be delivered with forceps.

(T)  (F)  2. When oxygen to uterine muscles is inadequate, the severity of the pain is increased.

(T)  (F)  3. Chlorpromazine potentiates analgesics and sedatives.

(T)  (F)  4. Emotional distress increases parturient's demand for oxygen.

(T)  (F)  5. Patients must be kept flat with peridural and caudal block anesthesia.

(T)  (F)  6. The parturient patient with an android pelvis must always be delivered by cesarean section.

(T)  (F)  7. Chlorpromazine controls psychomotor hyperactivity sometimes encountered with scopolamine.

(T)  (F)  8. Demerol administered intravenously may produce profound depression of vital centers.

(T)  (F)  9. Scopolamine does not effect the pain threshold.

## SELECTED READINGS

Beck, A. C., and Taylor, E. Stewart, editors: Obstetrical practice, ed. 8, Baltimore, 1966, The Williams & Wilkins Co., chap. 46.

Gordon, Howard: Fetal bradycardia after paracervical block, New Eng. J. Med. **279**:910, Oct. 24, 1968.

Kroger, Wm. S.: Childbirth with hypnosis, New York, 1961, Doubleday & Co., Inc.

Matthews, A. E. B.: Drugs in the first stage of labor, Nurs. Times **32**:20, May 19, 1967.

MacGregor, W. G.: Analgesia in childbirth, Nurs. Mirror **124**:1, June 23, 1967.

Obstetric anesthesia and perinatal morbidity, New Eng. J. Med. **279**:941, Oct. 24, 1968.

Perchard, Stanley: Hypnosis and the pregnant woman, Nurs. Mirror **124**:1, April, 1967.

Rosefsky, Jonathan, and Petersiel, Mel E.: Perinatal deaths and paracervical block anesthesia, New Eng. J. Med. **278**:530, March 7, 1968.

Smith, Bradley E.: Inhalation anesthesia ups risk of low Apgar score, Hosp. Top. **46**:88, March, 1968.

Walden, William D.: Anesthesia and analgesia. In Barber, Hugh R. K., and Graber, Edward A., editors: Quick reference to ob-gyn procedures, Philadelphia, 1969, J. B. Lippincott Co., chap. 10.

Yates, M. J.: Pudendal block in obstetrics, Nurs. Mirror **123**:556, March 17, 1967.

**For student's quick notes:**

# Chapter 15

# High-risk labor and delivery—I

A safe and happy childbirth is hoped for by all those involved. Unfortunately not all births terminate this way. You have learned that with good prenatal care more mothers can and do have a normal labor and delivery, but sometimes mishaps occur along the way. You are now ready to study about the risks associated with labor and delivery and the importance of observation for clinical signs and symptoms indicating deviation from normal progress.

## Premature rupture of the membranes

The membranes may rupture at any time during pregnancy. The woman may experience a gush of fluid from the vagina or she may be annoyed by a persistent trickle of fluid. If the perforation in the sac is small, it may seal over and the pregnancy will continue to term.

*Contributory factors.* Premature rupture of the membranes is substantially increased with (1) multiple pregnancies, (2) hydramnios, (3) fetopelvic disproportion, (4) breech presentation, and (5) occiput posterior. If the rupture occurs near term and the cervix is dilatable, the greater percentage of patients will deliver within 24 to 48 hours. If the rupture occurs when the cervix is closed, thick, and uneffaced, it may result in an inefficient type of labor (dysfunctional).

*Prognosis for the mother.* Prognosis for the mother is good unless she becomes infected. When the membranes are ruptured for more than 24 hours, the patient is considered potentially infected. Antibiotics given prophylactically to the mother will not protect the fetus and their value is still undetermined.

*Prognosis for the infant.* The prognosis for the infant depends on the period of maturity. Premature rupture of the membranes is a cause of intrapartal infection; when the presentation is footling, breech, or transverse, the cord may prolapse as the membranes rupture.

## Premature labor

A premature labor is one that occurs between the twenty-eighth and thirty-eighth week of gestation. A *spontaneous* premature labor (one where the presentation is normal) is generally of shorter duration than labor at term. However, complications do occur in more than 12% of premature deliveries and account for the high percentage of infant morbidity and mortality.

*Clinical pathological factors predisposing to onset of premature labor*

1. Acute urinary tract infections
2. Chronic hypertensive disease
3. Preeclampsia or eclampsia
4. Old cervical lacerations
5. Incompetent cervical os
6. Acute congenital infections
7. Blood dyscrasias

That nutrition plays a significant role is still only an hypothesis.

*Incidence of premature labors.* Premature labor occurs more often (1) in very young multigravidas, (2) in multiple pregnancies, (3) in first deliveries past the age of 40, (4) with a history of previous premature labors, and (5) in the Negro than in the Caucasian woman.

The doctor may order drugs in an effort to halt premature labor (Table 15-1); in other cases he may find it necessary to induce labor prematurely as treatment of certain complications, notably preeclampsia and diabetes.

During premature labor the fetal heart sounds should be taken every 15 minutes. When there are signs of fetal distress, 100% concentration of oxygen should be administered to the mother until the doctor arrives. The doctor tries to see the woman through labor with little or no sedation, taking into account that drugs decrease the infant's chance for survival. Phenergan and Sparine, 25 to 50 mg. intramuscularly, appear to have little effect on the fetal respirations. Doctors prefer regional anesthesia so that there will be no interference with fetal oxygenation.

*Effects on neonate.* Obstetrical trauma is a contributory factor in premature deaths.

The delicate tissue of the premature brain is not well protected and the doctor usually does a deep episiotomy to prevent resistance of a rigid perineum from traumatizing the infant's head.

If the infant is in good condition, the doctor may not clamp the cord until it stops pulsating, allowing placental blood to flow through the cord into infant's circulation. It has been stated by others that the cord should be clamped immediately after birth because the extra blood contributes to physiological jaundice. The liver of the premature infant cannot excrete the bilirubin formed from the excess blood received by the infant. The advantages or disadvantages of placental transfusion of blood have not been proved.

When resuscitation of the infant is necessary, the procedure must be gentle and minimal and should be administered by trained personnel.

A premature delivery holds physical hazards for the baby, but one must not forget the psychological hazards for the parents and family.

### Prolonged labor[2,4,6]

Formerly, a prolonged labor was defined as one extending beyond 24 hours, but with the progressive shortening in recent years

**Table 15-1.** Drugs used in an effort to halt premature labor[3,7]

| | |
|---|---|
| Lututrin (Lutrexin) | A nonsteroid uterine relaxing hormone isolated from ovary |
| | Unlike estrogen or progesterone |
| Progesterone U.S.P. (Lutocylin, progestin, Proluton) | Inhibits irritability of smooth muscles of uterus |
| Isoxsuprine hydrochloride (Vasodilan) | To be given before rupture of membranes; if given too late in labor, causes uterine inertia and postpartum bleeding |
| Relaxin (Releasin, Cervilaxin) | Synthetically prepared from ovarian extract of animals |
| Alcohol | 1.25 Gm. per kilogram of body weight |
| | May be given in 5% dextrose |
| | Alcohol locks release of oxytocin |

of the median in the duration of labor, 16 hours is now considered a prolongation of labor.

The time of onset of labor is often unknown or difficult to determine because of inaccurate information obtained from the patient. A prolonged labor is associated with the dystocias, but is not necessarily an abnormal labor.

*Contributory factors.* A prolonged labor is more likely to occur (1) in obese women, (2) when membranes rupture prematurely and the cervix is not dilatable, (3) when the cervix is displaced posteriorly, (4) after excessive doses of analgesics or sedatives, and (5) in malpositions (occiput posterior).

*Effects on the fetus and infant.* When the membranes rupture early and labor is prolonged, the fetus is likely to aspirate infected amniotic fluid; when there is interference with uteroplacental circulation, there is the possibility of intrauterine death; when the head has been compressed against the maternal pelvis, the infant is subjected to anoxia and cerebral damage.

## The dystocias

Dystocia may be defined as an abnormal labor, but not necessarily prolonged. The dystocias may be due to (1) anomalies in presentation, position, or development of the fetus, (2) some obstacle preventing normal progress of labor, or (3) deficiency in the power of uterine contractions.

### Anomalies in presentation, position, or development of the fetus

#### Contributory factors

1. Size and location of the placenta
2. Abnormal fetal attitude; extension instead of flexion of the head resulting in a brow or face presentation
3. A fetus with an anomaly such as hydrocephaly or anencephaly
4. Multiple pregnancy
5. Pendulous abdomen

*Occiput posterior.* When the occiput rotates to a posterior position instead of anterior, labor may be difficult and prolonged. When the head enters the pelvis with the occiput posterior, either R.O.P. or L.O.P., it is called *primary occiput posterior.* When the head engages as an occiput anterior and rotates to an occiput posterior, it is called a *secondary occiput posterior.* It is likely for the occiput to enter the inlet posteriorly or rotate posteriorly when there is some contraction of the pelvic inlet. In instances where the occiput fails to rotate spontaneously to anterior position, that is, it rotates to the direct occiput posterior position, it is termed *persistent occiput posterior* (P.O.P.). (See Fig. 15-1.) In cases where the head becomes arrested in a transverse position, it is called *deep trans-*

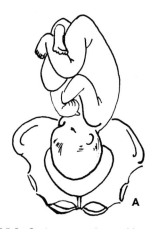 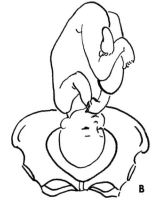

**Fig. 15-1.** Occiput posterior positions of fetus. **A,** Left occiput posterior. **B,** Right occiput posterior.

*verse arrest.* Occiput posterior positions may correct themselves with the occiput rotating to an anterior position. In such cases the second stage is usually prolonged. Since the presenting part remains high for a longer duration of time than when the occiput presents in an anterior position, the membranes tend to rupture early in labor. When the pelvic measurements are quite adequate and the fetus is not too large, it is possible for the fetus to be delivered in a posterior position. Otherwise, the doctor intervenes with operative procedures. He may apply forceps and rotate the occiput from posterior to transverse, then to anterior, remove the forceps, reapply them and deliver the infant in occiput anterior position (Scanzoni's maneuver). Kjelland's forceps are the choice of many obstetricians for this maneuver.

When the patient complains of constant, severe backache and contractions are irregular, the nurse may expect that the fetus is presenting with the occiput in a posterior position. When the position has been determined as a posterior, the nurse should encourage the patient to lie on the side opposite that toward which the fetus's back rests. Sacral pressure and massage affords some measure of relief. The fetal heart sounds are more likely to be heard loudest in the mother's right or left flank.

*Face presentation.* When the presentation is cephalic but the attitude is that of *complete* extension instead of flexion, the *face* will be the presenting part. The progress of the early part of labor may be somewhat delayed until the presenting part passes through the inlet, after which steady progress is made.

The majority deliver spontaneously, but where labor is prolonged, the diagnosis of face presentation is made by x-ray examination; the doctor may then decide to deliver the patient by cesarean section, or he may do a version and extraction.

Sometimes the presentation is not able to be determined by examination until the face has reached the perineum. The face is usually edematous and blue. This causes great concern to the parents, but they may be assured that in a few days the edema will disappear. This infant needs to be especially watched for the possibility of respiratory difficulties.

*Brow presentation.* Brow presentation differs from face in that the attitude is *partial* extension instead of complete extension. Spontaneous deliveries do not occur when the presentation is brow. The doctor may allow the patient a trial of labor to determine whether flexion can take place. If not, a cesarean section is performed.

*Transverse presentation.* A transverse lie occurs when the long axis of the fetus lies directly or obliquely across the mother's uterus. When labor starts, the shoulder frequently presents in the brim of the inlet. This presentation, therefore, is called *shoulder* and the denominator is the scapula (Sc.).

This abnormal presentation is more likely to occur in (1) multigravidas, (2) multiple pregnancies, (3) polyhydramnios, (4) fetal anomalies, and (5) low lying placenta. With this presentation the nurse will hear the fetal heart sounds more distinctly directly below the umbilicus. The membranes tend to rupture early with the possibility of a prolapsed cord, or descent of a fetal arm. Obviously it is not possible for the fetus to be delivered in this position, if its axis does not rotate. If determination of presentation is made before labor starts, the doctor may do an external version. If the patient is in labor, he may do an internal podalic version and extraction, or deliver the baby by cesarean section.

*Compound presentation.* When a fetal extremity such as a hand or foot enters the pelvis along with the head or breech, it is called a compound presentation. The etiological factor is usually something preventing the presenting part from fitting snugly in the pelvis, such as a low lying placenta. After examination the doctor may decide to deliver the patient vaginally or by cesarean section. (See Fig. 15-2.)

*Breech presentation.* Three percent of all full-term deliveries are breech presentations; they occur more frequently among the multigravidas and are likely to be repeated in the same women.

The prevalence of a breech presentation results from some interference with the mechanism of adaptation such as (1) high implantation of the placenta, (2) fetopelvic disproportion, (3) size of the fetus in relation to available intrauterine space, (4) hydrocephalus, and (5) multiple births.

*Varieties of breech* (Fig. 15-3)

COMPLETE. In the complete breech the legs are flexed on the thighs and thighs are flexed on the trunk with feet and buttocks presenting (5%) (A).

FOOTLING. This variety may present as single or double footling (25%) (B).

FRANK. The lower extremities are flexed on the trunk with the feet adjacent to the shoulders (70%) in a frank breech (C).

Prior to the onset of labor with membranes intact, the obstetrician may elect to do an external version, making the occiput the presenting part (cephalic version). This maneuver may be repeated several times, since the fetus may revert to the breech presentation after the version.

The first stage of labor progresses normally although the membranes are likely to rupture early and the presenting part may not descend until dilatation is complete. The second stage is generally longer, especially with the frank breech. Early rupture of the membranes is particularly dangerous for the fetus because of the possibility of intrapartal infection and of the cord prolapsing (p. 183).

The patient is usually moved to the delivery room when the cervix is fully dilated, and labor is allowed to continue as long as

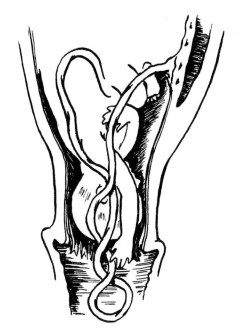

**Fig. 15-2.** Compound presentation with cord prolapse.

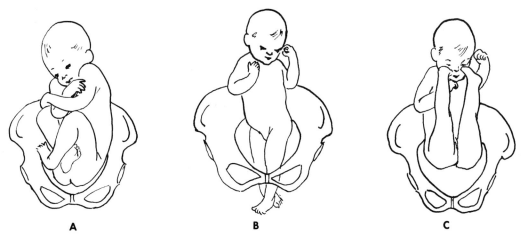

**Fig. 15-3. A,** Complete breech—fetus sitting in pelvis. **B,** Footling breech—may be single or double. **C,** Frank breech—buttocks presenting.

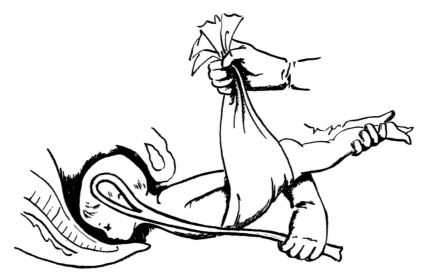

**Fig. 15-4.** Application of Piper forceps for delivery of after-coming head.

the heart sounds are within normal range. The nurse auscultates the fetal heart sounds in the area of maternal umbilicus. The breech is considered fully engaged when the buttocks are visible at the vulva, that is, indicates ample room for the head. As the umbilicus is born and the cord advances, the nurse monitors its pulsation. Application of the Piper forceps is indicated if pulsation of the cord becomes slow or irregular (Fig. 15-4). When force is required, it is applied from above as suprapubic pressure. This is known as Smellie-Veit, or Mauriceau maneuver.

*Prognosis for the mother.* The prognosis for the mother depends on the management of labor. She is subject to lacerations and postpartum hemorrhage from manipulations and exposure to deep anesthesia. The mortality rate, therefore, is slightly increased.

*Prognosis for the neonate.* The prognosis for the infant with breech presentation is not as good as if it were a vertex. Of the varieties, complete breech carries the best prognosis. As the result of pressure during frank breech extraction, it is more likely for fractures of the femur and skull, paralysis of the humerus, wryneck, or spinal cord injuries to occur than in the other varieties. Then, too, the after-coming head may compress the cord. If the infant is immature, it may not be able to withstand the trauma of delivery; subsequently anoxia and intracranial hemorrhage contribute to the mortality of a breech delivery. Epilepsy is more common among children delivered in breech birth than those born in spontaneous vertex.

The external genitalia will be quite edematous and the mother is certain to show concern when she examines her infant. The nurse can relieve the anxiety by explaining that the edema will disappear and the legs will assume their normal position in a short time.

*Anomalous development of the fetus.* The accumulation of cerebrospinal fluid in the ventricles of the brain results in a *hydrocephalic infant.* When there is gross disproportion between the head and pelvis, the breech accommodates better to the inlet and may present as such. Labor proceeds normally until the after-coming head cannot be delivered. In such cases the fluid is drained by perforating the skull. Hydrocephalus is sometimes suspected by palpation and the abnormality confirmed by x-ray examination. Hydrocephaly is hazardous to the mother. Since labor is obstructed, the lower uterine segment becomes distended and thin, and rupture may occur during labor or attempted delivery.

The *anencephalic* fetus may contribute toward dystocia, but it is not a common cause. The small head and soft mass is a poor dilator but may pass even through an incompletely dilated cervix.

An excessively large fetus may cause dystocia. Babies born of diabetic mothers are often in this category. Heredity also plays a part; large parents tend to have large babies. Here it is the size of the shoulders that often presents problems more than the weight. A short cord may also cause dystocia in that it may prevent the normal descent of the fetus.

## Obstacles preventing normal progress of labor

*Fetopelvic disproportion.* The dangers with fetopelvic disproportion are (1) delay in cervical dilatation, resulting in myometrial fatigue, (2) intrapartal infection from early rupture of the membranes and repeated vaginals, and (3) prolapsed cord.

Dangers for the fetus are (1) interference with uteroplacental circulation resulting in intrauterine asphyxia, (2) possible intracranial hemorrhage, and (3) cervical or brachial plexus damage.

Dystocia results if at any point during the mechanism of labor the pelvis is not adequate (even though the measurements may be normal). The size of the pelvis, then, is important only in relation to the size of the fetus.

When the head of the fetus cannot enter the true pelvis, the term *cephalopelvic* disproportion is used. Pelvic measurements may be normal, but the fetus may be excessive in size or have a congenital anomaly interfering with engagement.

When one or more of the pelvic measurements are abnormal, the patient is said to have a contracted pelvis. This may occur at any one of the important landmarks such as the inlet, midpelvis, or outlet. The contracture may be in the size or shape of the bones; it may be hereditary or a congenital anatomical defect. A "generally contracted

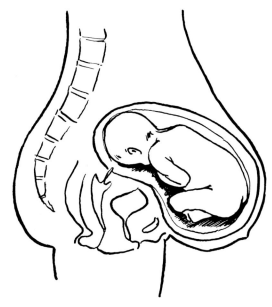

**Fig. 15-5.** Extremely pendulous abdomen in primigravida may signify fetopelvic disproportion and prevent engagement.

pelvis" is a small gynecoid pelvis. The head of the fetus as it passes through this type becomes greatly elongated along the occipitomental diameter. The fetus is more likely to present as breech or transverse in a woman with a contracted pelvis. A pendulous abdomen in the primigravida is usually evidence of disproportion (Fig. 15-5).

It is not for the nurse to know all of these abnormal types of pelves; her function is to understand the effect of pelvic disproportion on the progress of labor, the dangers to the mother and fetus, and how she can best administer to their welfare.

*Clinical progress.* The onset of labor is likely to be delayed because the presenting part cannot engage. In such cases the patient may develop dystocia. The membranes usually rupture early, with the possibility of the cord prolapsing.

In neglected cases where the mother is allowed to labor on with a contracted pelvis, she suffers maternal exhaustion and manifests this with clinical signs of temperature and pulse over 100, concentrated urine, dehydration, infection, and the possibility of rupturing her uterus.

The nurse may read on the patient's chart "borderline disproportion." This means that there is the possibility of a vaginal delivery. The obstetrician in such cases may give the patient a "test of labor," or a "trial of labor." He allows the patient to start labor spontaneously and once cervical dilatation is progressing, he may do an amniotomy to determine if progress can be improved. The length of a trial of labor is determined by maternal and fetal condition, not by a certain number of hours. A trial of labor continues to be successful just as long as the mechanism of labor continues to progress, that is, the cervix progressively thins, effaces, and dilates, and the presenting part progressively descends toward the perineum. A trial of labor fails when the mechanism of labor fails to progress beyond any given stage for a period of 1 hour. Then another solution must be found, usually cesarean section.

During this time, the doctor relies on the nurse's accuracy in observing strength, regularity, and frequency of contractions as well as how the patient and the fetus are withstanding the labor. Hydration needs to be maintained and the patient encouraged to void frequently.

**Cervical dystocia.** Even with regular strong contractions there are instances where normal effacement and dilatation of the cervix fail to take place. These cervical dystocias may be secondary to dysfunctional uterine action, malpresentations, fetopelvic disproportion, scar tissue formation, or growth. Women with severe cervical dystocia are usually delivered by cesarean section.

### Dysfunctional uterine powers

In Chapter 12 you studied about the normal physiological pattern of uterine activity—how the contractions were regular and increased progressively in frequency and intensity. When there is any interference with normal uterine activity, the patient is said to have dysfunctional labor.

**Classification.** Dysfunctional labor may be classified as *prolonged latent phase, protracted active phase,* or *abnormally rapid progress* (precipitate labor).

**Prolonged latent phase.** In the prolonged latent phase the tone of the uterus is hypertonic, spasms occur in some of the uterine muscles, and their activity is said to be uncoordinated.

*Etiology.* Etiology of the prolonged latent phase is attributed to excessive sedation or sedation given too early in labor (before the latent phase is terminated), or a thick, uneffaced, rigid cervix (usually in the elderly primigravida).

*Clinical progress.* Labor may be normal for a period of time, or it may be uncoordinated from the beginning. The first stage of labor is particularly long, and the condition is found almost entirely in primigravidas (90%). Cervical dilatation, if any, is slow and the advance of the presenting part is imperceptible. Fetal distress may occur early in labor. The patient complains bitterly of continuous pain, especially in the lumbar region, and the uterus is hypersensitive to palpation. The pain the patient experiences is out of proportion to the strength of the contractions.

*Treatment.* Treatment consists of rest and sedation. Ample rest is provided by use of a narcotic such as morphine to stop the abnormal contractions. Hydration is maintained by intravenous infusions. After this period of rest the contractions usually resume a normal pattern, the cervix dilates fully, and the fetus delivers spontaneously.

In cases where labor does not start spontaneously after the period of rest, the doctor may use oxytocin to stimulate labor, providing there are no contraindications. Amniotomy is not used as a means of stimulating contractions because of the danger of infection if labor is delayed.

**Protracted active phase.** In the protracted active phase the tone of the uterus is *hypotonic,* activity of the muscles is *coordinated,* but contractions are not strong enough to complete cervical dilatation. This type occurs mostly during the active phase but may continue on into the second stage.

*Etiology.* Etiology is often associated with malpositions, such as occiput posterior, cephalopelvic disproportion, overdistention of the uterus as in polyhydramnios, multiple pregnancy, congenital abnormalities of the uterus, or excessive sedation. Fetal distress does not usually occur with this type unless the patient becomes infected.

*Treatment.* The doctor orders x-ray pelvimetry, and if the cause is disproportion, the procedure is a cesarean operation. As long as there is no pelvic disproportion or fetal distress, the patient is allowed to continue labor and hydration is maintained. The doctor stimulates labor by amniotomy and oxytocin, 10 units in 1,000 ml. of 5% glucose in water (10 to 20 drops per minute).

*Nursing responsibilities.* The nurse's early recognition of a change in labor pattern will facilitate the doctor's intervention without delay, aid discovery of the cause, and institute treatment accordingly. When labor is prolonged, hydration must be maintained by intravenous infusions of glucose water, usually 2,500 ml. over a 24-hour period. This provides nourishment and prevents maternal distress and acidosis. Mental as well as physical exhaustion must be prevented. The patient realizes that she is not making progress and this adds to her mental anxiety. The nurse can contribute to the doctor's orders by providing comfort for the patient and by providing an environment conducive to rest and relaxation. She should encourage the patient to void at least every 3 hours to prevent distention of the bladder, since this only further impedes progress (Fig. 15-6). It is her duty to make every effort to protect the patient from intrapartal infection.

*Precipitate labor and delivery (abnormally rapid progress).* A precipitate labor and delivery occurs when myometrial contractions are too strong, and the woman delivers with only a few rapidly succeeding strong contractions and without sufficient time for preparation. She is usually unattended. It is defined as a labor completed in less than 3 hours. A precipitous labor and delivery may be as hazardous as a prolonged one.

Such a labor is more likely to occur when labor is induced by medical or mechanical means (oxytocin and amniotomy); multiparity may also influence the incidence. The mother is subject to the possibility of lacerations of the birth canal with subsequent postpartum hemorrhage. These forceful contractions may disrupt fetoplacental circulation and cause fetal anoxia. If the membranes rupture during one of these violent contractions, the rapid compression of the skull may cause subdural hemorrhage.

*Nursing responsibility.* Instructing the patient not to bear down is foolish because she cannot help but do so. The nurse's responsibility in such an emergency situation, that is, when there is no doctor in attendance, is to support the fetal head and perineum as the infant is delivered. A precipitate labor and delivery causes excite-

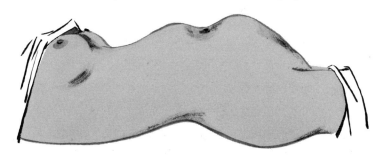

**Fig. 15-6.** Bladder distention, a cause of dystocia.

ment and mental anguish to the mother. It is important for the nurse to maintain her composure. The mother will recognize this and is more likely to cooperate when she feels the nurse knows what she is doing. The lives of the mother and baby are dependent on her actions until the doctors arrives.

### High-risk associated with multiple births[1,5]

In Chapter 8 you read about the high-risk associated with multiple pregnancies. Labor in multiple births, too, may be hazardous; it may be prolonged or terminate prematurely. The latter occurs in 80% of multiple pregnancies. When labor tends to be prolonged, various clinical factors contribtue to dysfunctional uterine action such as (1) overdistention of the uterus, (2) position or presentation (Fig. 15-7), and (3) size of the fetuses.

Complicating factors contributing to the high risk during the second stage are (1) after the birth of the first baby, with sudden reduction of intrauterine contents, placental separation is likely to occur before the second infant is born, (2) the second fetus may be in a transverse lie or some other malposition, increasing the possibility of a prolapsed cord, (3) the doctor may have to do a version and extraction to de-

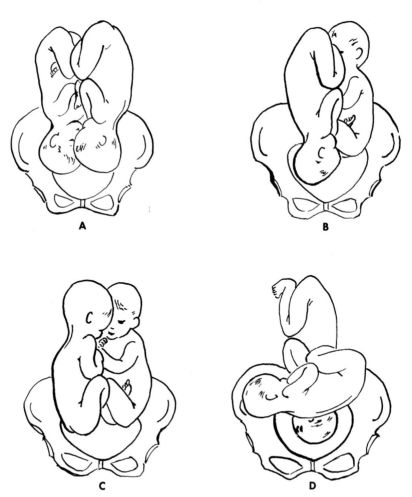

**Fig. 15-7.** Various positions that twins may assume. **A,** Both present as vertex. **B,** One presents as vertex, the other as breech. **C,** Both present as breech. **D,** One presents as vertex, the other as transverse.

liver the second infant, (4) the cervix may close and contractions stop before the second infant is delivered, and (5) postpartum hemorrhage is more likely, since the uterus is still distended or myometrial fibers are overstretched and cannot contract sufficiently. Loss of blood approximates twice the amount accompanying single births.

The doctor usually delays clamping of the cord to allow for transfer of as much blood as possible from the placenta to the baby. During this time oxygen is administered to the mother in case of intrauterine anoxia of the second baby.

The oxytocic is given after delivery of the second twin. If administered after the first twin is born, the second fetus may be trapped, or the placenta may separate before it is delivered. The outlook is more favorable when both present by the vertex.

*Prognosis.* Maternal morbidity is eight times greater than that of singleton vaginal delivery, and the mortality is slightly increased.

Perinatal mortality is higher after delivery of twins than for single births due to (1) prematurity, (2) anoxia of the second baby, and (3) prolapsed cord.

*Nursing responsibilities.* The nurse should monitor the fetal heart sounds of the second twin after delivery of the first baby and continue to do so every 3 to 4 minutes until it is delivered. She needs to give careful, constant watch over the patient during the fourth stage of labor by noting the tone of the uterus, pulse, blood pressure, and amount of bleeding. There is always a greater risk of postpartum hemorrhage after delivery of twins. The overdistended uterus contracts down with difficulty, and secondary inertia–type relaxation of the uterus occurs more readily because of the exhausting character of the second stage.

## Hemorrhage

Loss of over 500 ml. of blood during labor (including the fourth stage) is defined as hemorrhage. It is the leading cause of maternal mortality in the United States.

When hemorrhage occurs within the first 24 hours after delivery, it is called "early hemorrhage." When it occurs from 24 hours to 4 weeks postpartum, it is termed "late hemorrhage." The hemorrhage may be sudden and massive, or it may be slow and continuous.

### Etiology

The etiology of postpartum hemorrhage may be divided into five main groups: (1) uterine atony, (2) lacerations, (3) clotting defects (afibrinogenemia), (4) retained placenta, and (5) retained portions of cotyledons or secundines.

*Uterine atony.* Uterine atony is secondary to overdistention of the uterus when muscle fibers are stretched beyond their ability to contract and retract sufficiently to occlude the open blood vessels after delivery.

As stated on p. 154, control of hemorrhage after delivery is by contraction and retraction of fibers of the myometrium. When this myometrial function is disrupted, it is called *uterine atony*, meaning "lack of tone." Other causes are (1) deep and prolonged inhalation anesthesia that may reduce effectiveness of the contractions, (2) exhaustion from a prolonged labor, (3) operative deliveries such as versions and extractions, (4) mismanagement of the third stage of labor, and (5) precipitous labor and delivery, when the uterus empties so rapidly the muscle fibers cannot retract sufficiently.

The nurse should keep the following in mind: (1) Uterine atony is the most frequent cause of postpartum hemorrhage. Atony of the uterus causes steady bleeding with gushes of blood as muscles of the uterus make an effort to contract and retract. (2) In cases of uterine atony, the nurse's first duty is to grasp and massage the fundus *gently*. (3) Prevention is foremost in importance, since most maternal deaths from postpartum hemorrhage are preventable. (4) Prognosis depends on the extent of blood lost; therefore your early recognition of abnormal bleeding allows time for the doctor to determine the source of bleeding and institute treatment for control. (5) Anemia resulting from hemorrhage lowers the patient's resistance and predisposes to puerperal infection.

*Measures of treatment.* When the hemorrhage is due to hypofibrinogenemia, the blood loss is replaced and fibrinogen (Parenogen), 4 to 10 Gm., is given intravenously to bolster the clotting mechanism. The normal blood fibrinogen level during pregnancy is 250 to 500 mg. per 100 ml. of blood.

Ergotrate or Methergine, 1 ml. administered intravenously, or intravenous drip of 1 ml. oxytocin in 1,000 ml. of 5% dextrose, administered at the rate of 30 drops per minute, may be given.

When a blood transfusion is given, Pitocin may be added to this fluid instead of to a glucose solution. Dextran may be administered until blood is available. Dextran is a polysaccharide of high molecular weight that is used to maintain blood volume and blood pressure.

*Nursing responsibilities.* It is the nurse's responsibility to "be prepared"—to know what drugs are used in cases of postpartum hemorrhage and to have them at hand for immediate use. Fibrinogen should be on hand in *every* delivery room. The nurse monitors vital signs and keeps the doctor informed as to the pulse, blood pressure, and respirations of the patient. She guards the fundus, keeps her patient warm, and through her expert observation detects changes in clinical signs.

The nurse also needs to remember that the anemia resulting from hemorrhage lowers the patient's resistance and predisposes to puerperal infection.

*Lacerations.* After the third stage of labor is completed, the doctor inspects the vagina, perineum, and cervix for lacerations. The extent of vaginal and perineal lacerations is designated in degrees: (1) a *first degree* laceration involves mucosa and skin; (2) the *second degree* is deeper and involves disruption of muscular structures in the perineum; (3) the third degree involves the above plus the anal sphincter; and (4) the *fourth degree* involves the above plus the rectal lumen. Lacerations are caused (1) by precipitous deliveries, (2) at times by breech deliveries, (3) by large babies, and (4) when maternal tissues are friable (they are often unavoidable). The repair of such lacerations is called a perineorrhaphy.

Superficial lacerations of the cervix occur in almost every delivery. The "bloody show" is partly the result of such tears. These heal spontaneously. Deep cervical lacerations, on the other hand, are likely to bleed profusely, especially when the laceration extends into the uterine vessels in the lower uterine segment. The frequency of deep cervical lacerations are substantially increased in (1) precipitous labor and delivery, (2) scarred cervix, (3) breech extraction, and (4) forceful delivery of the infant through an incompletely dilated cervix. When the fundus is well contracted, but the patient has continuous bleeding, especially bright red, it is most likely due to an extensive cervical laceration.

***Retained or adherent placenta.*** As stated on p. 154 the placenta normally separates from the uterine wall and is expelled within a few minutes after the delivery of the infant. When the contractions that normally separate the placenta fail to occur, it is called an adherent, or retained placenta.

The placenta may separate but be retained within the uterus. This occurs when the cervix contracts and closes, or the muscle contractions fail to expel it spontaneously. Here the doctor may use the Brandt-Andrews maneuver for removal. (See p. 154.) If there is a partial separation, the attached part interfering with muscle retraction must be removed manually. This procedure may be traumatic to the uterus and result in uterine atony and consequent postpartum hemorrhage.

For such a procedure the nurse should have a sterile gown and gloves ready for the doctor. She should also anticipate his request for additional oxytocics and fluids for intravenous infusion.

*Placenta accreta.* Failure of placental separation may be pathological. The chorionic tissue grows directly into the myometrium. With this abnormal penetration, the placenta cannot separate and is called a placenta accreta. With manual removal of a placenta accreta, there is further danger of postpartum hemorrhage. And if the placenta cannot be finger dissected away from the myometrial wall, an emergency hysterectomy must be resorted to as a lifesaving measure.

### Rupture of the uterus

Rupture of the uterus is a serious complication. The incidence is about one per 2,000. The rupture may be *complete* or *incomplete*. It may occur spontaneously, traumatically, or as a rupture of a previous caesarean section scar.

*Etiology*
*Spontaneous rupture*
1. Injudicious use of oxytocics
2. Cephalopelvic disproportion
3. Abnormal presentations
*Traumatic rupture*
1. Delivery through an undilated cervix
2. Forceful breech extraction
3. Difficult forceps delivery
4. Internal podalic version, with extraction
*Postcesarean rupture.* This is more likely to occur during subsequent pregnancy, and the tear is usually at the site of the previous incision.

*Clinical picture.* When rupture occurs during labor, it is most often in the lower segment. Any obstacle interfering with progress of normal mechanism of labor may cause powerful traction to be exerted on the lower uterine segment, drawing the contraction ring of Bandl to a higher level than usual (may reach level of the umbilicus). This gives the impression that the bladder is full, but after catheterization, the contraction ring becomes thicker and more pronounced. As the contractions increase in

frequency and intensity, the lower segment becomes extremely sensitive; this causes excruciating pain. These signs and symptoms should alert the nurse to notify the doctor, since they indicate that rupture is imminent. Her ability to function adequately in such an emergency may save the life of the mother and fetus. (See Fig. 15-8.)

When the uterus ruptures, the patient screams from the pain, and uterine contractions cease, as does fetal activity and heart action. The patient may say the pain is less, but she shows anxiety. Directly then, the symptoms of shock will appear—hypotension, rapid, weak pulse, and pallor. Vaginal bleeding may be noted.

When the rupture occurs during hard labor (tetanic contractions), the fetus may be forced through the vaginal canal or extruded into the abdominal cavity.

In cases when the rupture is incomplete, the fetus is not extruded into the peritoneal cavity. When rupture occurs in lower segment, blood accumulates in the broad ligaments and forms a subperitoneal hematoma. Diagnosis may not be made until signs of shock appear.

Treatment is an emergency laparotomy.

*Prognosis.* When the rupture occurs through a scar from previous section, it is usually less extensive and, if treated immediately, the mortality for the mother and fetus is much lower than with a complete rupture. When the rupture is complete,

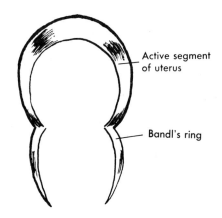

**Fig. 15-8.** Bandl's or pathological retraction ring.

Active segment of uterus

Bandl's ring

the fetal mortality is practically 100%. Maternal mortality depends on prompt therapy. The obstetrician determines whether the uterus should be sutured or removed.

## The cardiac patient in labor[8]

For the cardiac patient, labor is an added burden on the heart. Labor normally imposes acceleration of the pulse (especially during a uterine contraction) and increases the oxygen consumption and the cardiac work. If the pulse goes over 110 and the respirations above 24 during the first stage of labor, the nurse should notify the doctor. A persistent pulse increase above 110 to 120 per minute, dyspnea, and pulmonary congestion may be the earliest signs of heart failure. Demerol is the drug of choice during labor; in addition to relieving pain, it relieves pulmonary edema and helps the patient to rest. Scopolamine is not given because it increases the heart rate.

A quiet environment and a cheerful nurse in constant attendance, with genuine concern for her patient's welfare, are conducive to rest and can certainly alleviate anxiety.

A vaginal delivery is preferable to the cesarean section, since the cardiac patient does not tolerate major surgery very well. The fetus is usually delivered by forceps to avoid bearing down efforts and to shorten the second stage of labor. Pudendal, caudal, or epidural block is the regional anesthetic method of choice. Oxytocics are avoided unless absolutely necessary. They constrict all the blood vessels in the intraabdominal organs and force too much blood back to the heart at one time. As the infant is being delivered, the nurse applies pressure to the abdomen to avoid vascular collapse from rapid abdominal decompression. Sandbags are sometimes used for this purpose.

**STUDY QUESTIONS**
*Matching*

Match the terms in the first column with their appropriate definitions in the second column:

(a) Posterior occiput — Retraction ring of muscle fibers; warning sign of impending rupture of the uterus

(b) Breech — Version whereby the doctor makes the feet the presenting part

(c) Dystocia — Head of fetus cannot enter the pelvis

(d) Primary occiput posterior — Head enters pelvis with occiput posterior

(e) Secondary occiput posterior — Evidence of disproportion

(f) Cephalic — Laceration involving rectal lumen

(g) Podalic — Fetal heart sounds are more likely to be heard loudest in area of mother's umbilicus when fetus is in this position

(h) Pendulous abdomen in primigravida — Version whereby doctor makes occiput the presenting part

(i) Small gynecoid pelvis — Abnormal labor, not necessarily prolonged

(j) Dysfunctional labor — Extreme molding of the head

(k) Precipitous labor — Head engages anteriorly and rotates to posterior position

(l) Fourth degree laceration — Discomfort experienced by patient is out of proportion to strength of contractions

(m) Third degree laceration — Labor completed in less than 3 hours

(n) Bandl's ring — Lacerations involving muscular structure of perineum and anal sphincter

(o) Cephalopelvic disproportion — Fetal heart sounds are more likely to be heard loudest in mother's right or left flank when fetus is in this position

*Multiple choice*

1. When the doctor determines the fetal position to be posterior, the nurse will encourage the patient to:
   (a) lie on side opposite that toward which the fetus's back rests.
   (b) lie flat on her back.
   (c) lie on side toward which the fetus's back rests.
2. The doctor notates on the patient's chart "borderline disproportion." The nurse should interpret this as meaning:
   (a) the patient will have to be delivered by cesarean section.

(b) there is the possibility of a vaginal delivery.

(c) the patient has a platypeloid pelvis.

3. In multiple births the outlook for the infants is more favorable when:
   (a) both present as vertex.
   (b) both present as breech.
   (c) one presents as vertex, the other breech.

4. The most frequent cause of postpartum hemorrhage is:
   (a) internal versions.
   (b) prolonged inhalation anesthesia.
   (c) uterine atony.

5. Within the first hour of birth it is normal for the newborn's respirations and heart rate to average:
   (a) respirations 40 to 80, heart rate 130 to 140.
   (b) respirations 30 to 40, heart rate 100 to 120.
   (c) respirations 40 to 60, heart rate 130 to 140.

6. The first sign of intrauterine anoxia is:
   (a) a temporary increase of fetal heart rate between contractions, then a slowing.
   (b) slowing of fetal heart rate between contractions.
   (c) slowing of fetal heart rate during contractions.

7. The nurse knows prolonged labor is more likely to occur in:
   (a) obese women.
   (b) instances where the mother was given excess analgesics.
   (c) in the very young primigravida.
   (d) the multigravida more than in the primigravida.
   1. a and b    2. b and c    3. c and d

8. The nurse will suspect that the patient has a posterior presentation when:
   (a) she complains of severe, constant backache.
   (b) contractions are irregular.
   (c) fetal heart sounds are heard loudest in mother's right or left flank.
   (d) all of these.

9. When certain complications exist it may be necessary to induce labor prematurely. Among these would be:
   (a) lack of engagement of presenting part.
   (b) diabetes.
   (c) severe preeclampsia.
   (d) polyhydramnios.
   1. a and c    2. b, c, and d    3. a and d

10. Fetal mortality rate for twins is especially high among those born to:
    (a) the primigravida.
    (b) mothers at age 45 and over.
    (c) the very young mother.
    (d) mothers between age 25 and 30.
    1. a, b, and c    2. b only    3. c and d

11. When the parturient patient has a temperature and pulse over 100, concentrated urine, and dehydration, the nurse knows the patient is:
    (a) going into shock.
    (b) suffering from maternal exhaustion.
    (c) suffering from a renal shutdown.

*True or false*

(T) (F) 1. Premature rupture of the membranes predisposes to intrapartal infection.

(T) (F) 2. Acute urinary tract infection is a factor predisposing to premature labor.

(T) (F) 3. Prolonged labor is defined as lasting more than 48 hours.

(T) (F) 4. A cervix displaced posteriorly may contribute to prolonged labor.

(T) (F) 5. A prolonged labor is always an abnormal labor.

(T) (F) 6. A pendulous abdomen may be a factor contributing to a posterior position.

(T) (F) 7. A low lying placenta may be a factor in the fetus presenting transversely.

(T) (F) 8. Breech presentations occur more frequently among primigravidas.

(T) (F) 9. The second stage of labor is more likely to be longer with a frank breech than with a footling.

(T) (F) 10. Of breech varieties the complete carries best prognosis.

(T) (F) 11. Excessive sedation may be a factor in dysfunctional labor.

(T) (F) 12. Loss of blood with multiple birth approximates twice the amount accompanying a single birth.

(T) (F) 13. Maternal morbidity is eight times greater with multiple birth than with single vaginal delivery.

(T) (F) 14. Postpartum hemorrhage predisposes to puerperal infection.

(T) (F) 15. An abruptio placentae might result from an internal version.

**REFERENCES**

1. Beck, A. C., and Taylor, E. Stewart, editors: Obstetrical practice, ed. 8, Baltimore, 1966, The Williams & Wilkins Co., pp. 282-287.
2. Fell, M. R.: Prolonged labor, Nurs. Mirror **126:**29, March 22, 1968.
3. Fuchs, Fritz: Stopping premature labor with alcohol, Briefs **30:**59, April, 1966.
4. Grimm, Elaine: Uterine dysfunction or pro-

longed labor. In Richardson, Stephen, and Guttmacher, Alan, editors: Childbearing: its social and psychological aspects, Baltimore, 1967, The Williams & Wilkins Co., p. 14.

5. Montagu, M. F. Ashley: Prenatal influences, Springfield, Ill., 1962, Charles C Thomas, Publisher, p. 417.

6. Oxorn, Harry, and Foote, Wm. R.: Human labor and birth, New York, 1964, Appleton-Century-Crofts, chap. 32.

7. Rodman, Morton J., and Smith, Dorothy W.: Pharmacology and drug therapy in nursing, Philadelphia, J. B. Lippincott Co., p. 551.

8. Rovinsky, Joseph, editor: Medical, surgical, and gynecologic complications of pregnancy, Baltimore, 1965, The Williams & Wilkins Co., p. 29.

**SELECTED READINGS**

Beck, A. C., and Taylor, E. Stewart, editors: Obstetrical practice, ed. 8, Baltimore, 1966, The Williams & Wilkins Co., chaps. 17 and 19.

Brown, David: The history of blood transfusion, Nurs. Mirror **126**:19, June 14, 1968.

Diddle, A. W.: Postpartum hemorrhage, Hosp. Med. **4**:91, June, 1968.

Humphrey, Arthure: Avoidable factors in maternal deaths, Nurs. Mirror **126**:22, March 29, 1968.

Oxorn, Harry, and Foote, Wm. R.: Human labor and birth, New York, 1964, Appleton-Century-Crofts, chap. 29.

Russell, Keith: Bony pelvic dystocia, Hosp. Med. **5**:37, July, 1969.

**For student's quick notes:**

# Chapter 16

# High-risk labor and delivery—
# II. Operative obstetrics

In this chapter you will learn about the procedures classified as operative obstetrics and about your responsibilities in preparing patients for and in assisting the doctor with operative procedures.

## The episiotomy
### Indications

The term episiotomy is used synonymously with perineotomy. An episiotomy is used widely today because (1) lacerations are thereby prevented, (2) such an incision heals better and is easier to repair than a ragged tear, (3) it allows for easier, safer egression of the head, thereby preventing possible brain damage, (4) if performed before tissues are overstretched, it may reduce incidence of prolapse in subsequent deliveries, (5) it shortens the second stage of labor, and (6) it may prevent painful hemorrhoids. It is performed for a majority of forceps deliveries.

It has been stated that the injection of hyaluronidase, a tissue-softening enzyme, into the perineum may ease childbirth or avert the need for a perineotomy.

### Types

*Median incision.* The median incision is made directly downward in the midline almost to the anal sphincter. With this type, there is less bleeding, and discomfort during the healing process is minimal. It is not used where episiotomy must be extensive. (See Fig. 16-1, *B.*)

*Mediolateral incision.* The mediolateral incision is made downward and outward in direction of lateral margin of the anal sphincter. This type is preferred where the baby is large and where the perineum is short. The doctors choice of right or left incision depends on position of the presenting part. (See Fig. 16-1, *A.*)

## Induction of labor

Commencing labor by artificial methods if referred to as induction of labor.

### Maternal indications

1. Preeclampsia not controlled by medical therapy
2. Chronic hypertension
3. Prolonged labor due to hypotonic uterine inertia
4. Delayed onset of labor after 24 hours of rupture of the membranes
5. Rh sensitization
6. Polyhydramnios

### Fetal indications

1. Postmaturity
2. Excessive size of the infant
3. Fetal death
4. Maternal diabetes after thirty-sixth week of gestation

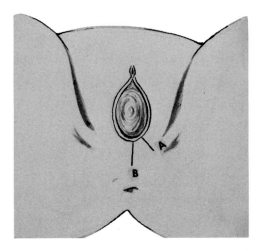

**Fig. 16-1.** Episiotomy. **A,** Area of incision for mediolateral episiotomy. **B,** Area of incision for median episiotomy.

## Elective induction of labor

The term elective induction of labor is used when the doctor of his own accord decides to induce labor. He may do this when the patient has a history of precipitate labors and lives a distance from the hospital or for convenience of the mother or himself. He examines the patient to be certain that there is no fetopelvic disproportion, that the presentation and position are normal, and that the cervix is dilatable.

## Methods of induction

Methods of induction may be surgical, medical, or hormonal. A forthcoming method is by electrical stimulation. See reference 1.

*Surgical induction.* Artificial rupture of the membranes is said to be a relatively safe method of induction for women *at or near term.* It may be combined with medical induction. Rupture of the membranes allows descent of the fetal head; this pressure shortens muscle bundles of the myometrium and brings about good reflex stimulation, but it does carry the risk of danger to the mother and the fetus. The presenting part may be displaced to an abnormal position or the cord may prolapse.

When the doctor wishes to do an am-niotomy, the nurse prepares the patient for a sterile vaginal examination. If the bed is kept in Fowler's position after the amniotomy, it facilitates drainage of the fluid. Contractions normally start within 48 hours.

*Medical induction.* One means of medical induction is the administration of castor oil and quinine sulfate. The patient is given 1 ounce of castor oil (causes irritability of smooth muscles of the intestines and uterus), followed by quinine sulfate, 60 mg., every 30 minutes for three doses (stimulates smooth muscles of the uterus). A soap and water enema is given after the first dose of quinine sulfate.

*Hormonal induction.* Induction of labor was performed as early as the 1600s, by surgical method (amniotomy). This same method is in use today, in many instances, along with use of oxytocin. See "Induction of labor by use of hormones," p. 202.

## Risks associated with induction of labor

### Maternal risks

1. Rupture of the uterus from tumultuous labor
2. Lacerations
3. Hemorrhage (separation of the placenta) as a result of uterine spasm

### Fetal risks

1. Prematurity
2. Fetal hypoxia
3. Central nervous system injury

### Nursing responsibilities

The nurse should be in constant attendance. It is her responsibility to record frequency, strength, duration of the contractions, and their effect on fetal heart sounds. She should check the blood pressure every 30 minutes and note tone of uterus during and between contractions. If at any time the contractions occur at less than 2-minute intervals, and the duration is long sustained, there will be interference with the transfer of adequate oxygen to the fetus, with subsequent fetal anoxia. The nurse should stop the infusion and notify the

## INDUCTION OF LABOR BY USE OF HORMONES

**Generic name:** Oxytocin injection, U.S.P.
**Trade names:** Pitocin,* Syntocinon, Uteracon, Pitocin citrate

| Route | Action | Dosage |
|---|---|---|
| Intravenously | The drug is used to initiate uterine contractions and overcome uterine inertia and produces clonic, rhythmic contractions. It acts quickly but contractions are not sustained.<br><br>Too rapid administration can cause a continuously contracted uterus and risk fetal anoxia. | Ten units are placed in 1,000 of glucose solution. Initial flow is usually 10 to 15 drops per minute with increase every half hour until patient is in labor.<br><br>Dosage must be individualized since oxytocin acts differently in different women. |
| Intramuscularly | It has been stated that this method should be abandoned since there is no way of terminating action if the contractions become tetanic.<br><br>Magnesium sulfate solution, 10 ml. of 20%, should be at hand for relaxant action on the myometrium. | At 30- to 45-minute intervals 0.03 ml. (½ minim) is given. |
| Intranasally | Cotton pledgets moistened with Pitocin solution are inserted into nasal cavity. | |
| Buccally | Pitocin citrate tablet is placed under tongue. This is repeated every 30 minutes until labor is established. | |

*"The plasma of pregnant women near term contains an enzyme, pitocinase, in such high concentration that half of an intravenously given dosage of Pitocin is destroyed in about 90 seconds. Thus, within 2 or 3 minutes of shutting off an intravenous infusion, the oxytocic activity has ceased." (From Oxorn, Harry, and Foote, Wm. R.: Human labor and birth, New York, 1964, Appleton-Century-Crofts, p. 382.)

**Generic name:** Diethylstilbestrol
**Trade name:** Stilbestrol in oil (a synthetic estrogen)

| Action | Dosage |
|---|---|
| Sensitizes uterine musculature to become more reactive to natural posterior pituitary oxytocins. | 5 mg. intramuscularly, q. 4 hr. for 6 doses. |

**Generic name:** Sparteine sulfate
**Trade name:** Tocosamine, Spartocin (a plant derivative)

| Action | Dosage |
|---|---|
| Induces labor and overcomes uterine inertia. | 1 ml. (150 mg.) intramuscularly, repeated hourly, if necessary, up to 4 doses. |

doctor. He should be available for immediate call.

## Obstetrical forceps

Forceps are instruments designed to (1) *rotate* the head from an abnormal position to one that will facilitate delivery and (2) *extract* the fetus from the birth canal. Forceps are classified according to the level of the presenting part in the pelvis (station).

*Low forceps.* Low forceps are used when the skull has reached the perineum and is visible during a contraction (station +3), when progress is slow, and when the mother is becoming exhausted.

*Mid forceps.* When the biparietal diameter of the fetal head has passed through the inlet and the skull has reached the ischial spines (station +1 to +2), midforceps are used.

*High forceps.* The head has entered the pelvis but is unengaged. Application of high forceps at this station is traumatic to both mother and fetus. They are seldom used in obstetrics today.

*Prophylactic (outlet) forceps.* When presenting part is on the perineum and the caput is visible, prophylactic (outlet) forceps are applied. Here the doctor elects to shorten labor to avoid pounding of the head on the perineum and to save the mother from exhaustion.

*Piper (after-coming head) forceps.* In a breech presentation, after the body is born, the head may be delivered with Piper forceps. They are designed to fit the after-coming head. (See Fig. 15-4.)

### Clinical factors indicating application of forceps

#### Maternal factors
1. When the patient has a rigid perineum (The forceps shorten the bearing-down phase, thereby eliminating pressure of the fetus's head on the perineum. This is combined with an adequate episiotomy.)
2. Rotation when there is an arrest of the head—Scanzoni's maneuver (p. 186)
3. Prevention of lacerations
4. When contractions of the second stage are ineffectual
5. Complications such as bleeding or oncoming maternal exhaustion

#### Fetal factors
1. Irregular heart rate
2. Passage of meconium in cephalic presentation

### Risks involved with application of forceps

#### Maternal risks
1. Injury to the bladder or rectum
2. Lacerations of the vagina and cervix
3. Hemorrhage
4. Infection

#### Fetal risks
1. Facial or branchial palsy
2. Cord compression
3. Intracranial hemorrhage

Before the obstetrician applies the forceps, the nurse will observe that he (1) catheterizes the patient, (2) ruptures the membranes, (3) determines that the cervix is fully dilated, and (4) makes accurate examination for position of presenting part (head).

## Versions

A version is an operative procedure in which the presenting part is maneuvered to substitute another presentation. The obstetrician may perform this operation externally by manipulating the fetus through the abdominal wall. This is usually done during the last month of pregnancy. He may do an internal version by introducing his hand into the uterus. This procedure is not performed while the patient is in early labor. It is usually done for the delivery of a second twin.

### External cephalic version

External manipulation brings the *head* down and into the pelvic brim as from a transverse lie or turns a breech presentation into a cephalic presentation. The dangers of external version are (1) interference with uteroplacental circulation and (2) induction of premature labor.

## Internal podalic version

The obstetrician inserts his hand inside the uterus, grasps the feet, and turns the fetus to a footling breech. Internal versions are always podalic.

### Indications for internal version
1. When the umbilical cord is prolapsed
2. A transverse lie
3. Delivery of second twin
4. Compound presentation

### Dangers of internal version
1. Uterine atony as a result of deep anesthesia required for the version
2. Lacerations of the cervix
3. Abruptio placentae
4. Infection
5. Fetal anoxia from deep anesthesia or compression of the cord

*Nursing responsibilities.* The nurse's responsibility is to have the patient empty her bladder previous to the operation and to check fetal heart sounds before, during, and after the procedure. The nurse also needs to guard the uterus with special vigilance during the fourth stage of labor.

## Cesarean section

The cesarean section is an operative procedure by which the fetus is delivered through an incision in the abdominal wall and the uterus.

Hendrick van Roonhuyze was credited with having performed several cesarean sections with success as early as 1663. The modern era for performing a cesarean section is said to have started about 1882, when Max Sänger refined the method of suturing the uterine wall. In America John Lambert Richmond performed the first cesarean section at Newton, Ohio, on April 22, 1827. The low (cervical) cesarean section, originated by H. Sellheim in 1908, was perfected and popularized by Joseph De Lee in 1916.

Today the cesarean section is a safe surgical procedure for the mother, but the fetal mortality doubles that of a normal vaginal delivery. The perinatal survival has improved in that the procedure avoids difficult forceps procedures, prolonged labors, and internal versions. However, the perinatal mortality and morbidity after a cesarean section is still higher than with a normal vaginal delivery. Predisposing factors in the mother, such as diabetes and antepartal bleeding, lead to anoxic conditions in the fetus and to prematurity. Prematurity of the infant in the elective cesarean is a definite factor in perinatal morbidity and mortality. Therefore the high mortality associated with cesarean sections is attributed to these complications rather than to this method of delivery. The most serious complications after the section are hemorrhage and infection.

### Maternal indications
1. Fetopelvic disproportion
2. Chronic nephritis
3. Uterine dystocia
4. Placenta previa or abruptio placentae when vaginal delivery is not feasible
5. Previous uterine surgery
6. Severe preeclampsia
7. The elderly primigravida
8. Essential hypertension

### Fetal indications
1. Rhesus incompatibility
2. Diabetes where labor cannot be induced successfully
3. Fetal distress

### Types

*Classical section.* The uterus is incised in the midline (corpus of the uterus). The advantage is that it can be done more quickly than the other types. This is an important factor when the mother or the fetus is in danger. It is also more applicable when the fetus is in a transverse lie. The disadvantage is that there is more danger of rupture of a uterine scar in subsequent pregnancies; the risk of hemorrhage is also greater.

*Low segment type (laparotrachelotomy).* In low segment type of cesarean section the incision is made in the low cervical segment of the uterus. The advantages are (1) less danger of infection or hemorrhage,

(2) less likelihood of rupture of the uterus in subsequent pregnancies, and (3) better healing of the wound.

*Elective section.* The term elective is used when the cesarean section is performed at a scheduled time prior to the onset of labor, such as with a known fetopelvic disproportion. The patient is usually admitted to the hospital the day prior to the surgery. This allows time for laboratory studies and provides an opportunity to rule out presence of infection.

*Extraperitoneal section.* In the extraperitoneal section the lower segment is approached by separating the bladder from the uterus, not entering the peritoneal cavity. The danger of infection is reduced, but it is a technically difficult procedure.

*Cesarean hysterectomy.* This is also known as the Porro operation and involves removal of the uterus after the classical cesarean section is done.

• • •

There can be no set rule as to who is delivered by cesarean section. Each patient is an individual and should be managed as such. If the patient is delivered by cesarean section because of inadequate pelvic measurements, there is no alternative but cesarean section with subsequent pregnancies. It has been stated that in cases where the initial cesarean section was done because of complications that need not recur in subsequent pregnancies, such as hemorrhage, such patients may be delivered vaginally. They are observed carefully as they progress and may be delivered vaginally despite uterine scars. The nurse's responsibility in caring for these patients is to be extra diligent in her observation as the labor progresses.

When the patient is informed that she is to be delivered by cesarean section, it certainly has its psychological impact on her. This may be the first experience with surgery; in addition there is always great concern as to the outcome for the infant. The nurse can help by assuring the patient that surgical procedures are safe and that it is being performed in her best interest. When the nursing staff is informed that there is to be an emergency cesarean section, there seems to be an aura of hurry and excitement; this can permeate to the patient and should be avoided.

### Neonatal response

Maternal complications such as antenatal bleeding and diabetes contribute to a higher incidence of respiratory difficulties. Because of the pressure on the fetal thoracic cavity during the normal birth process, secretions from the upper respiratory tract are more likely to be expelled than when delivery is by cesarean section. It has been cited that cesarean babies make better adjustments to their postnatal environment than instrument-delivered babies, except when they have suffered anoxia.[2]

### STUDY QUESTIONS
*Multiple choice*

1. If the uterus becomes tetanic as the result of oxytocin administration, the nurse would have the following drug at hand because of its relaxant action on the myometrium.
   (a) 20% magnesium sulfate.
   (b) 1 ml. relaxin hormone.
   (c) 1 ml. Cervilaxin.
2. If a patient has an occiput posterior presentation, and the doctor states his intention of doing a rotation, the nurse would expect him to ask for the:
   (a) Kjelland forceps.
   (b) Piper forceps.
   (c) outlet forceps.
3. An elective cesarean section means that it will be performed:
   (a) at a scheduled time prior to the onset of labor.
   (b) before 38 weeks' gestation.
   (c) as soon as labor starts.
4. It is not unlikely for the placenta to separate prematurely after delivery of the first of twins due to:
   (a) sudden reduction in intrauterine contents.
   (b) profound drop in blood pressure.
   (c) presentation of the second fetus.
5. The most serious complication after cesarean section is:
   (a) hemorrhage and infection.
   (b) paralytic ileus.
   (c) adhesions.

6. Another term for the after-coming head forceps is:
   (a) Kjelland.
   (b) Piper.
   (c) Elliot.
7. A cesarean section would most likely be performed on a patient with the history of:
   (a) fetopelvic disproportion.
   (b) two previous sections.
   (c) hypertension.
8. Rotating the head from a posterior to anterior position is termed:
   (a) Scanzoni's maneuver.
   (b) Ritgen's maneuver.
   (c) Brandt-Andrews maneuver.
9. The following complications are indications for cesarean section:
   (a) essential hypertension.
   (b) chronic nephritis.
   (c) infection of the birth canal.
   1. a and b    2. a and c    3. all of these

*True or false*

(T) (F) 1. One of the dangers of an external version is induction of premature labor.
(T) (F) 2. Fetal and infant mortality is greater following a cesarean section than a normal vaginal delivery.
(T) (F) 3. All lacerations need to be repaired.
(T) (F) 4. Malpositions are frequently associated with small pelves.
(T) (F) 5. The pain caused by stretching of the cervix is felt mainly in the back.
(T) (F) 6. Versions and extractions are the main causes of traumatic rupture of the uterus.

*Matching*

Match the terms in the first column with their appropriate definitions in the second column:

(a) Pitocin — Repair of lacerated cervix
(b) Mediolateral episiotomy — Danger of infection is reduced with this type cesarean section
(c) Ergotrate — Valuable in cases of prolonged labor due to hypotonic uterine inertia
(d) Stilbestrol in oil — Cesarean hysterectomy
(e) Compound presentation — Type episiotomy done where the perineum is short; leaves only a slight scar
(f) Extraperitoneal section — Produces sustained tetanic contractions of uterine muscles
(g) Low-segment section — Synthetic estrogenic preparation used to stimulate uterine contractions
(h) Median episiotomy — Acts quickly to produce contractions of the uterine musculature but is rapidly inactivated
(i) Porro operation — Indication for an internal version
(j) Perineotomy — Less blood loss with this type episiotomy, and less danger of its extending through sphincter ani
(k) Perineorrhaphy — Danger of hemorrhage is reduced with this type section
(l) Induction of labor — Surgical incision of the perineum

**REFERENCES**

1. Fields, Harry: Induction of labor: methods, hazards, complications and contraindications, Hosp. Top. 46:63, Dec., 1968.
2. Hurlock, Elizabeth: Child development, New York, 1964, McGraw-Hill Book Co., p. 86.

**SELECTED READINGS**
*Induction of labor*

Beckman, Harry: Pharmacology—the nature, action and use of drugs, ed. 2, Philadelphia, 1961, W. B. Saunders Co., p. 81.
Fell, M. R.: Inductions of labor, Nurs. Mirror 122:35, April 8, 1966.
Friedman, Emanuel: Inductions. In Greenhill, J. P., editor: Obstetrics, ed. 13, Philadelphia, 1965, W. B. Saunders Co., chap. 24.
Rodman, Morton J., and Smith, Dorothy W.: Pharmacology and drug therapy in nursing, Philadelphia, 1968, J. B. Lippincott Co., chap. 39.

*Cesarean section*

Gunn, Alexander: Caesarean section, Nurs. Times 63:425, March 31, 1967.
Montagu, M. F. Ashley: Life before birth, New York, 1964, New American Library, Inc., chap. 12.
Montagu, M. F. Ashley: Prenatal influences, Springfield, Ill., 1962, Charles C Thomas, Publisher, p. 412.
Oxorn, Harry and Foote, Wm. R.: Human labor and birth, New York, 1964, Appleton-Century-Crofts, chap. 37.
Reis, Ralph A.: Hazards of cesarean section reduced after 34 weeks' gestation, Hosp. Top. 46:88, March, 1968.
Russell, J. K.: Caesarean section, Nurs. Times 64:1158, Aug. 30, 1968.

**For student's quick notes:**

**UNIT III**

# The postpartum period

With the familiar phrase "mother and baby doing well," the new mother approaches the last phase of the maternity cycle—the time between arrival of the baby and return of the generative structures to the prepregnant state. This phase of the maternity cycle is called the *puerperium.* The word is from the Latin, "having brought forth a child." These changes are involuntary, orderly, and involve about 6 weeks, with one exception, lactation. Preparation for this task which started during pregnancy, now begins to function fully and may continue beyond the 6-week period.

Chapter 17

# The normal puerperium

The woman you instructed during pregnancy and supported during labor and delivery continues to be a challenge to your nursing skills, for all is not over after the birth of the infant.

The maternity nurse of today is aware of the *continued* needs of the new mother, who must be instructed concerning physical changes in her body, for they often cause concern, especially to the primipara.

It takes time for some mothers to cope with the additional demands of being a new mother. The psychological components of the puerperium are intricate and involve numerous emotional responses. The maternity nurse is aware of this and of problems that may be encountered as the mother adapts to parental responsibilities.

The adaptive changes from apprehension and anticipation to realization of parenthood were discussed in the first part of Chapter 2. The changes in body systems as each in its own intricate mechanism contributes to full restoration of the mother's normal physiology are now discussed under physiological and clinical aspects.

It is true that nature directs the mother's recuperation, but the nurse, through teaching and guidance, can contribute to the physical and mental health of the mother.

## Psychological aspects

After completion of the fourth stage of labor, the mother is transferred to the postpartum unit. After a refreshing bath she is usually ready to settle down to a much needed rest. Some mothers are ravenously hungry and cannot rest until after light nourishment.

It is common knowledge that the newborn needs love, but so does the new mother, especially the expression of her husband's love and his display of interest in the baby. The nurse will provide an appropriate environment whereby they may be alone together. The new mother has strong feelings of dependency, and the new father's protection will sustain her above all else.

Some new mothers are willing and eager to take over their new responsibilities; others cling to their own mothers and shift their new responsibilities to them. The woman you instructed during her labor and delivery is suddenly aware that her anticipation is now a reality. As the hours pass there is a rising curve of emotional strain and tension for most new mothers. During the period of waiting, the mother-to-be was the center of attention, but now she must share this with her new-born. She recalls birth as wonderful, yet distressing. She experiences a deep, abiding pleasure in the thought of being needed, but this is disturbed by the feeling of manifold responsibilities. Family patterns need to be rearranged; problems may seem overwhelming as little doubts creep in. Conflicts between new responsibilities and personal interests, for example, having her freedom restricted, may cause her to wonder about her capacity to be a good mother. Conflicting opinions of well-wishers who press their advice on her add to the dilemma. All of these factors, in addition to glandular changes, give rise to anxiety and contribute to the phenomenon of "postpartum blues."

The student may find it difficult to understand the new mother's periods of weeping after observing her enthusiasm and joy, but as a nurse she needs to be aware of the emotional instability associated with puerperal physiology: that depression does occur and can be transient or become critical. She learns to recognize signs and symptoms and be prepared to provide the emotional support the mother needs. She can help by being a good listener when the mother wants to talk because some women require verbal expression. Other mothers find strength by retreating within themselves. Here the nurse can help by quiet understanding.

This disillusionment and depression must be differentiated from developing puerperal psychosis. Doctors tell us that a familial predisposition to mental illness *may* be involved; the stress accompanying labor and delivery or the realities to be faced after the infant is born can trigger a recurrence if there has been a history of mental depression. Other doctors disagree, believing that postpartum depression is not necessarily a product of previous emotional instability but a combination of many factors. Patients with puerperal psychosis manifest insomnia, dejection, loss of interest, wide mood swings, and undue concern. The symptoms seldom appear before the first week. Many patients recover within 3 to 6 months with therapy, but those with schizophrenic tendencies do not have a good prognosis.

## Physiological, clinical, and nursing aspects
### The uterus

At the time of transfer from recovery room, the uterus should be palpable as a firm, rounded mass, with the fundus in the midline and in the area of the umbilicus. Its outline may be seen through the abdominal wall.

On p. 156 you learned that at the site

**Vital signs**

| | |
|---|---|
| **Temperature** | The temperature generally remains normal during the puerperium. A slight rise may point to dehydration or excitement. |
| **Pulse** | The pulse rate is more labile than the temperature. The nurse may expect the pulse to be somewhat slower, averaging between 60 to 70. It may fall to as low as 40, which is considered a transient phenomenon. |
| **Blood pressure** | The temporary rise in blood pressure after delivery slowly dissipates, and by the time the patient is admitted to the postpartum unit it is again stabilized. |

where the placenta was attached, the blood vessels are torn and bleeding, protected by superficial thrombi at the narrowed openings of the placental vessels, and that the intricate arrangement of muscle fibers is so designed as to close off these bleeding vessels and prevent hemorrhage. As the muscle fibers contract and retract to check the bleeding, another mechanism is taking place—*involution* of the uterus. This bulky organ is getting smaller and back into normal contour. This is brought about slowly by catabolism of tissue, atrophy of muscle fibers, and reduction of edema. Glandular epithelium proliferates readily and reestablishes the endometrial surface. This is analogous to the regenerative phase of the menstrual cycle. The use of oxytocics stimulates the muscle contraction, but has little effect on normal course of involution. (See Fig. 17-1.)

Along with this is a third change; as muscle fibers contract, the decidua separates and is expelled. This disintegrating layer is cast off in the vaginal discharge called *lochia* and is usually shed by the third day.

Measurement of the height of the fundus through the abdominal wall and observation of the vaginal discharge (lochia) give the nurse an index to normal progressing involution and healing of the endometrium. The rate of involution is determined by daily palpation of the fundus of the uterus, using the umbilicus as a guideline. The first day the fundus can be palpated in the area of the umbilicus. By daily palpation the nurse will note that it involutes quite rapidly, and at about the tenth day, the uterus has descended into the pelvis and can be no longer palpated. This tends to occur more rapidly in the primipara and in women who nurse their babies. Within 1 or 2 weeks the entire endometrium is restored, except that area where the placenta was attached. This area resumes normal physiology after another 3 weeks.

After delivery the empty, bulky uterus weighs approximately 2 pounds, but in the

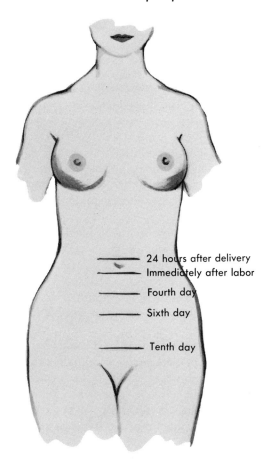

24 hours after delivery
Immediately after labor
Fourth day
Sixth day
Tenth day

**Fig. 17-1.** Involution of uterus.

6-week period through the process of involution the uterus will have attained its prepregnant position and its weight will be between 1 and 2 ounces. Delay in involution may be caused by retention of clots, tissue, distended bladder, or full rectum.

After delivery the cervix is edematous, relaxed, and congested, but as minute tears heal, new muscle fibers form and within a few weeks the internal os closes, but the external os appears as a mere transverse slit, never closing completely.

### The vagina

The vagina also undergoes a process of involution and regains its tonicity fairly rapidly. The labia lose their cushion of fat and may become quite flabby. Rectocele, urethrocele, and cystocele are not infrequent. The vagina even undergoes some relaxation after delivery by cesarean section.

### Lochia

As the result of sloughing of decidua from the uterus the woman has a vaginal discharge for approximately 2 to 3 weeks after delivery. This discharge is a blood stained fluid consisting of red and white blood cells, microbes, mucus from the cervical glands, and epithelial cells from the vaginal canal, in addition to the decidual tissue.

The initial flow is chiefly blood from the vessels at the site of the placenta mixed with shreds of decidua. Clots are abnormal and should be reported. Lochia is bright red in color and called *rubra*. This initial flow is usually shed by the third day. As the vessels thrombose the amount becomes less and appears as a sanguine-serous discharge called lochia serosa, which changes to pink or brown because of an increase in white blood cells and bacteria. By the tenth day the color is yellow to white, now called lochia alba, due to further increase in white blood cells. Normally it decreases in amount to a gradual spotting by 3 to 4 weeks.

Lochia varies in amount, type, odor, and length of time before discharge ceases. It is said to be less profuse in mothers who nurse their infants, although there may be a temporary increase in the amount of blood in the lochia while the infant nurses. Length of time of discharge is also said to be shorter in women who ambulate freely and are active, in those delivered by cesarean section, and in women who had an elevated temperature. Women who have prolonged labors tend to have increased lochia discharge. The odor varies with the type of bacteria present.

When lochia rubra persists or reoccurs after the lochia alba stage, involution may not be progressing normally. Bits of cotyledons may be retained along with tissue and, if not expressed, can develop into placental polyps. On discharge the mother should be instructed to contact her doctor should this occur, since it may be due merely to fatigue.

### The perineum

A period of 6 to 8 weeks elapse before the tone of these pelvic muscles is restored. This can be understood when we consider the immense stretching these structures were subjected to during parturition. While ambulation is important, the nurse needs to interpret this intelligently for the mother and instruct her to avoid standing for any length of time because of the weight of pelvic structures on these muscles.

*Perineal care.* The nurse gives perineal care to the mother at the time of the admission bath. Methods are variable, but all involve an aseptic technique and keeping the area clean and dry. In addition she teaches the mother according to the method she was taught by her instructor, stressing the principles of perineal hygiene. Thereafter the mother cares for herself. However, the perineum should be inspected daily by the nurse. With adequate perineal care, an incision usually heals in about 1 week.

*Perineal discomfort.* Perineal discomfort is the most common complaint of mothers. This is understandable when one considers the immense stretching of the birth canal and of the perineal structures and the swelling of tissues involved in the episiotomy.

The discomfort caused when sitting down can be relieved if the mother is instructed to squeeze her gluteal muscles, since this will prevent stretching and pulling on the sutures. Perineal sutures are absorbed in about a week or 10 days. Ointments and analgesic preparations in the form of sprays, moist pads such as Tucks, sitz baths, and infrared light are all measures used to relieve this discomfort.

### Afterpains

On p. 156 you learned about the physiological phenomenon whereby the uterine muscles contracted and retracted to prevent hemorrhage. In the primiparous woman this mechanism takes place without causing too much discomfort, but the uterus of the multiparous woman lacks muscle tone and during this process of involution it does not remain contracted but relaxes at short intervals and gives the mother the sensation of cramplike pains called afterpains. There are other reasons why mothers experience afterpains, such as (1) oxytocic drugs were given to increase the contracted state of the muscle fibers, (2) the infant's sucking stimulates the sympathetic nervous system to release oxytocin, which in turn stimulates uterine contractions, (3) muscles were subjected to much distention such as multiparity or polyhydramnios, and (4) particles of cotyledons and blood clots remain in the uterus. The discomfort is experienced for 2 to 4 days and may be relieved by analgesic medications.

### The abdominal wall

The abdominal wall is distended and relaxed after delivery. In some mothers the muscle tonicity is regained quickly, in others this is not so. The degree of restoration of tone depends a great deal on the muscle tone and body posture from early childhood. If as a child, during youth, and prenatally the mother had ample protein in her diet and practiced good posture and proper exercise, it is likely that she will regain strong, sturdy abdominal and breast muscles.

In some mothers the abdominal wall is so lax, especially in the midline, that the recti muscles separate. This is known as

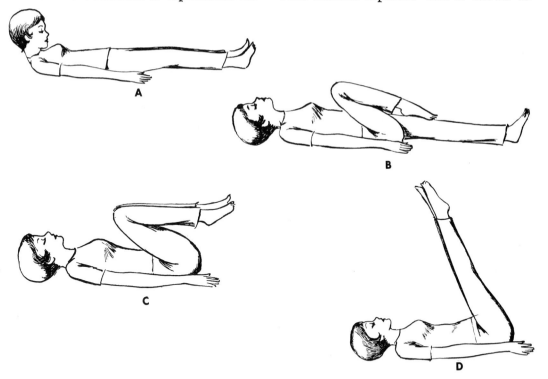

**Fig. 17-2.** Various exercises to be practiced during puerperium. **A,** The woman raises her head from the supine position and tries to touch her chin to her chest without moving any other part of the body; this aids in strengthening abdominal muscles. **B,** Lying in supine position, woman bends one knee at a time on the abdomen and tries to touch buttocks with her heel; this strengthens gluteal muscles. **C,** Making the effort to keep her back flat and arms at side of her body, while trying to touch chest with knees, will strengthen both abdominal and gluteal muscles. **D,** The woman raises both legs at one time, raising them up as far as possible without lifting the head or bending the knees; this strengthens abdominal and leg muscles.

"diastasis of the recti muscles." Predisposing causes may be (1) polyhydramnios, (2) multiple gestation, (3) a very large baby, and (4) grand multiparas. The doctor prescribes good body mechanics, ample rest, and exercises to restore muscle tone.

The use of abdominal binders has been almost completely abandoned, since it is no longer believed that binding the abdomen helps restore muscle tone. This is better accomplished by postpartum exercises. However, women who are accustomed to wearing a girdle may continue to do so after delivery.

The striae of pregnancy along the abdomen and thighs lose their purplish red color and become silvery irregular lines.

### Exercises

Not all women need to exercise to restore tone to their muscles, but some women do. The aim of exercises is (1) to tone skeletal muscles, especially those stretched during labor and delivery such as the abdominal and perineal, (2) to improve physique, (3) to reduce excessive fat, (4) to improve tone of breast muscles, and (5) to correct posture that was altered during pregnancy.

The new mother should discuss exercising with her obstetrician and abide by his decision regarding when to start exercises and the type he wishes her to practice. While in the hospital she is usually advised or permitted to do simple exercises such as those shown in Fig. 17-2.

### Tub baths[4]

What type of bathing facilities are recommended for the new mother? There are pros and cons among the doctors regarding the value or advisability of tub bathing. Few maternity units are equipped with adequate facilities for tub baths and thus the shower is recommended. Those doctors in favor of tub bathing during the early puerperium stress the following advantages: (1) lochia and dried blood are better cleansed from the perineum, (2) discomfort of hemorrhoids is relieved, (3)

bladder function improves, (4) a nervous, tense mother becomes relaxed, and (5) the woman feels more refreshed after a soak in warm water.

The belief that tub baths predispose to infection are unfounded, since simple tests with starch and iodine proved that bath water does not enter the vagina.

### Early ambulation

While the mother is confined to bed (immediate hours postpartum), she should assume the position most comfortable to her. Changing position does facilitate drainage of the lochia. Slight elevation of the head and knees will contribute to free circulation of blood to the lower extremities.

The mother should have assistance on the first trip to the bathroom. Having her dangle for a few minutes with feet placed on a chair before stepping out of bed may prevent a light feeling in the head. The mother should be told that there will likely be a free flow of blood at this time because the blood does not drain as readily through the vagina when the mother is in the recumbent position. Otherwise this can be a frightening experience for her as she feels the sudden gush of blood.

The modern approach to early ambulation for the maternity patient is given full recognition and its value not disputed, but a *gradual* approach to full activity should be explained to the mother. Early ambulation does improve bladder and bowel function, improves circulation, especially in the lower extremities and reduces the tendency toward blood clot formation and thrombophlebitis.

Although many mothers are ready to care for their own needs within hours of delivery, they should be advised not to overload their temporarily reduced physical resources. The mother who requires more nursing care should not be forced too rapidly in adapting to hospital routines. The nurse should provide an environment of flexibility for her so that she can adapt to her new role in her own way. By observing her and talking with her, the nurse quickly learns how much help she needs and plans accordingly.

## Weight loss

When the mother is ambulatory, one of her first visits is to the scales. Even prior to ambulation she may inquire of the nurse how much weight the mother ordinarily loses. The nurse may inform the mother that the weight loss generally equals that of the products of conception, including blood volume and amniotic fluid (18 to 20 pounds). Eight to 9 pounds of this is the immediate weight loss, and as tissue fluid is eliminated and involution proceeds, further decrease may be noted. Weight gained in excess of this will be deposited as fat.

## Diaphoresis

Diaphoresis is normal during the puerperium. Some mothers experience "night sweats" for weeks after delivery. Glands of the skin respond to changes in metabolism and help the body rid itself of excess tissue fluid. The nurse should encourage daily bathing because it enhances activity of the skin and helps the mother relax.

## Bladder function

It is important that the patient empty her bladder within 8 to 10 hours after delivery. The majority of mothers can do so with a positive approach and encouragement from the nurse. Every effort should be exerted to avoid catheterization, since there is evidence this procedure contributes to postpartum bacteriuria. It is possible for the bladder to be distended without the mother being aware of it. When the bladder becomes overdistended, it causes temporary displacement of the uterus, pushing it to either side and causing it to relax, with subsequent hemorrhage.

There are reasons why spontaneous voiding may be impossible after delivery. These include (1) anesthesia may affect the nerve supply to the bladder, (2) perineal injuries may delay her ability to relax the urethral sphincter, and (3) the urethra or bladder wall may have been so traumatized during labor and delivery that she does not have the sensation of a full bladder and experiences no discomfort.

It is also important that the nurse note whether the mother is voiding sufficient amounts. Voiding in small quantities (less than 100 ml.) indicates that she is not emptying her bladder. This residual urine predisposes to infection (cystitis). Acute pyelonephritis is not uncommon after prolonged labors with deep anesthesia.

Normally the mother has marked diuresis between the second and fifth day. This is nature's way of restoring normal water balance. It is not unusual for lactose to be present in the urine due, of course, to establishment of lactation. Proteinuria may also be present but should disappear by the third day.

## Bowel function

Delay in bowel function for a few days after delivery is to be expected. There are a number of reasons for this: (1) the mother is usually given an enema or suppository at the beginning of labor, (2) she may not have eaten for a number of hours, (3) less fluid is in the intestinal tract due to puerperal diuresis, (4) abdominal muscles are flaccid, (5) pressure exerted by the gravid uterus is withdrawn, (6) she may be apprehensive about tearing sutures, and (7) if she has hemorrhoids, defecation may be delayed because of discomfort involved.

The physician may order a laxative or rectal suppository to be given the second evening. Some mothers tend to restrict fluid intake, believing it will decrease breast engorgement, but this is not so. The nurse should encourage the mother to drink fluids freely and again establish a regular time for defecation.

Tympanites is also normal during this time and may produce some discomfort.

## Hemorrhoids

Painful hemorrhoids are a common complaint during pregnancy and the puerperium. Blood becomes trapped in the rectal veins due to pressure of the presenting part of the fetus during the last weeks of pregnancy and commonly follows pressure and straining efforts during labor and delivery. If the mother had hemorrhoids before pregnancy, they are certainly aggravated during the birth process.

The discomfort is relieved by the sitz bath, anesthetic sprays, and witch-hazel compresses. The nurse may suggest that the mother assume the Sims' position while in bed, since this relieves some of the pressure from the congestion in the veins.

### Physiology of lactation[1] (Fig. 17-3)

*Engorgement.* As the lactogenic hormone prolactin (luteotropic, LTH) contributes to lacteal secretions, there will be a stasis of veins and lymph ducts in the breasts, resulting in engorgement of these structures.

Regardless of whether the woman breast feeds or not, her breasts will go through this physiological change. It usually occurs about the second day in the primipara and about the third day in the multipara. The breasts become tense and painful. The engorgement may even extend to lymph nodes in the axilla. This congestion usually subsides within 24 hours if the mother is breast feeding. The mother may ask you to pump her breasts, thinking the discomfort is due to overdistention with milk. She needs to be told that this is not so, but that pumping the breasts would only aggravate the condition.

If the mother is not to nurse her infant, the process of engorgement can be inhibited to some extent with the use of parenteral steroids (estrogen-androgen preparations). Among these drugs are diethylstilbestrol (stilbestrol, Stilbetin), chlorotrianisene (Tace), or methallenestril (Vallestril). Deladumone OB may be ordered as a single intramuscular injection (2 ml.) to be given while the mother is in labor or immediately after delivery. This prevents engorgement and eliminates taking medica-

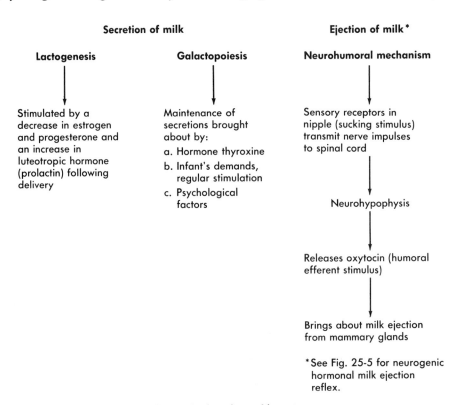

Fig. 17-3. Physiology of lactation.

tions during the puerperium. The nurse may inform the mother that these drugs may increase the flow of lochia and cause irregular periods of bleeding after cessation of the therapy. Not all doctors order hormone preparations; they are of the opinion that proper breast support and cold compresses, along with analgesic medications, are all that is required.

*Care of the breasts.*[3] During the period of engorgement the infant may have difficulty grasping the nipple. Instructing the mother how to use the electric breast pump for 1 or 2 minutes before placing the infant to the breast usually puts enough traction on the nipple so that the infant can grasp it without difficulty. When the electric pump is not available the hand pump may be used, but it is not as satisfactory. A nipple shield may also be used. The nurse shows the mother how to express colostrum from the breasts into the shield and then place it tightly over the nipple. This prevents the infant from sucking in air as he draws the mother's nipple into the shield. In most instances 1 or 2 minutes on the shield are sufficient to pull the nipple out, at which time the infant may be placed directly to the breast nipple.

If the nipples do become tender, the nurse should not ignore the complaint. There are usually standard p.r.n. orders for preparations such as tincture of benzoin, balsam of Peru, or lanolin to be applied as preventive measures in avoiding fissures or bleeding. The doctor may recommend that the mother use the shield for a few feedings until the tenderness in the nipple subsides.

The mother should be instructed (1) to wash her hands before handling her breasts and (2) to keep her breasts clean by daily use of soap and water and by drying thoroughly after this care.

Whether the mother breast feeds her infant or chooses the artificial method, she needs to be advised concerning proper support for her breasts. The mother may be more comfortable in a brassiere a size larger than she usually wears. This is ad-

vised when the mother is breast feeding. A constricting brassiere interferes with free circulation of fluid to and from the breasts. The breasts should be supported in the cups in the direction of body midline and not compressed against the chest. The nurse might remind the mother that proper support will relieve some of the discomfort of engorgement and prevent undue sagging of the breasts.

In general, if the mother is given adequate instructions by the nurse in preparation for nursing and care of her breasts and if the mother abides by these instructions, there should be little or no discomfort experienced by the nursing mother. Indeed, it should be the time she enjoys most with her infant.

The nurse should instruct the mother to wash the inner removable pads of her nursing brassiere with soap and water and rinse well. A brassiere soiled with colostrum or milk makes a good medium for the growth of bacteria.

*Relation of lactation to ovulation.* That lactation is associated with delay in ovulation (attributed to lack of FSH and LH hormone) is a well known fact, but this is not a safe contraceptive method, since mothers often do become pregnant while nursing (p. 235).

*Diet during lactation.*[2] The energy requirement of the mother is variable, but the recommended caloric intake is between 2,800 and 3,000 calories. Intake of one and one-half quarts of milk daily is recommended because it furnishes a good percentage of essential nutrients. The amount of milk secreted depends on glandular activity and regular stimulation of the breasts, not on increasing fluid intake as the layman erroneously believes. However, the mother should have ample fluids (2,500 ml.) per day to aid the kidneys in ridding the body of metabolic wastes. Her own demands of thirst are her guide. See Fig. 17-4 and review Fig. 6-3 for the recommended increase of nutrients.

*Instructions to the mother.* Instructing the mother concerning her diet during lac-

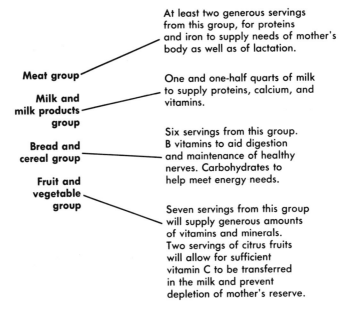

Meat group — At least two generous servings from this group, for proteins and iron to supply needs of mother's body as well as of lactation.

Milk and milk products group — One and one-half quarts of milk to supply proteins, calcium, and vitamins.

Bread and cereal group — Six servings from this group. B vitamins to aid digestion and maintenance of healthy nerves. Carbohydrates to help meet energy needs.

Fruit and vegetable group — Seven servings from this group will supply generous amounts of vitamins and minerals. Two servings of citrus fruits will allow for sufficient vitamin C to be transferred in the milk and prevent depletion of mother's reserve.

**Fig. 17-4.** Diet during lactation

tation is simply this: she may eat any food that agrees with her, but we want her to maintain a good, balanced diet.

## REFERENCES

1. Huffman, John W.: Breast changes during and after pregnancy, Redbook 127:28, Aug., 1966.
2. Meyer, Herman: Infant foods and feeding, Springfield, Ill., 1960, Charles C Thomas, Publisher, p. 52.
3. Porter, Dorothy: Care of the puerperal breast, Hosp. Top. 45:103, March, 1967.
4. Smith, Reginald Armitage, and Hodgson, Jane E.: Study affirms benefits of postpartum tub baths, Hosp. Top. 44:101, Oct., 1966.

## SELECTED READINGS

*Postpartum exercises*

Findlay, Eleanor: Figure control for your postpartum patient, RN 32:38, Jan., 1969.
Liley, H. M. I.: Modern motherhood, New York, 1966, Random House, Inc., pp. 221-225.
Smith, Christine Spahn: Maternal-child nursing, Philadelphia, 1963, W. B. Saunders Co., pp. 191-195.
Wiedenbach, Ernestine: Family-centered maternity nursing, New York, 1968, G. P. Putnam's Sons, p. 305.

*Physiological aspects*

Bergstrom, N. I.: Ice application to induce voiding, Amer. J. Nurs. 69:283, Feb., 1969.
Brown, Louise S.: Effectiveness of nursing visits, Canad. Nurse 63:45, Jan., 1967.
Christine, Sister Marie: Postpartum nursing care, Canad. Nurse 61:29, Jan., 1965.
Eastman, Nicholson J., and Hellman, Louis M., editors: Williams' obstetrics, ed. 13, New York, 1966, Appleton-Century-Crofts, chap. 19.
Greenhill, J. P., editor: Obstetrics, ed. 13, Philadelphia, 1965, W. B. Saunders Co., chap. 26.
Hogan, Aileen: The role of the nurse in meeting the needs of the new mother, Nurs. Clin. N. Amer. 3:337, June, 1968.
Menning, Emilie, Henning, Emilie, Martoglio, Gilda, Quita, Maria, Reinbrecht, Janet, and Strickland, Marie: A dynamic nursing appraisal of the puerperium. In Lytle, Nancy, editor: Maternal health nursing, Dubuque, Iowa, 1967, William C. Brown Co., pp. 153-163.
Nedbor, Pearl, and Averette, Henry: Hospital institutes program for self-perineal care, Hosp. Top. 46:81, May, 1968.
Redman, T. F.: After the birth is over, Nurs. Mirror 125:267, Dec. 15, 1967.
Sine, Idamae Kelii, and Cameron, Joyce: Relief of afterpains, Nurs. Clin. N. Amer. 3:327, June, 1968.
Streshinsky, Shirley: The truth about those new mother blues, Parents' Magazine 64:56, April, 1969.
Williams, Bryan: Forty-eight hour maternity discharge-good or bad? Nurs. Mirror 127:33, Oct. 11, 1968.
The womanly art of breast feeding, Franklin Park, Ill., 1958, LaLeche League of Franklin Park, Inc., chap. 3.

*Psychological aspects*

Astrachan, John: Puerperal emotional disturbance, Hosp. Top. **45**:73, Dec., 1967.

Auerbach, Aline: Meeting needs of new mothers, Child Family **6**:9, Winter, 1967.

Baker, A. A.: Psychiatric illness in parents, Nurs. Mirror **128**:37, April, 1969.

Bakwin, Harry, and Bakwin, Ruth: Clinical management of behavior disorders in children, ed. 3, Philadelphia, 1966, W. B. Saunders Co., pp. 53-55.

Brandt, Yanna: What doctors now know about depressed young mothers, Redbook **130**:69, March, 1968.

Brecher, Edward, and Brecher, Ruth: Why some mothers reject their babies, Redbook **127**:49, May, 1966.

Chappel, John N., and Daniels, Robert S.: Puerperal psychosis, Hosp. Med. **5**:11, June, 1969.

Dunbar, Flanders: Psychology of the puerperium. In Greenhill, J. P., editor: Obstetrics, ed. 13, Philadelphia, 1965, W. B. Saunders Co., pp. 480-487.

Gordon, Richard, and Gordon, Katherine: Factors in postpartum emotional adjustment, Amer. J. Orthopsychiat. **37**:359, March, 1967.

Green, Sidney, and Nathan, Paul: New mother's blues, Parents' Magazine **40**:40, May, 1965.

Grimm, Elaine: Relationship of personality variables to postpartum adjustment and attitudes toward the child. In Richardson, Stephen A., and Guttmacher, Alan F., editors: Childbirth: its social and psychological aspects, Baltimore, 1967, The Williams & Wilkins Co., pp. 29-31.

Hartman, Carol: Psychotic mothers and their babies, Nurs. Outlook **16**:32, Dec., 1968.

Hemphill, R. E.: Infanticide and puerperal mental illness, Nurs. Times **63**:1473, Nov. 3, 1967.

Liley, H. M. I.: Modern motherhood, New York, 1966, Random House, Inc., pp. 83-87.

Lock, Frank R.: How husbands can help with pregnancy blues, Redbook **125**:48, Oct., 1965.

Meek, Lucille: Maternal emotions and their implications in nursing, RN **32**:38, April, 1969.

Meeroll, Joost A.: Mental first aid in pregnancy and childbirth, Child Family **5**:11, Fall, 1966.

Riker, Audrey: New parent blues, Child Family **6**:10, Spring, 1967.

Williams, Barbara: Sleep needs during the maternity cycle, Nurs. Outlook **15**:54, Feb., 1967.

The womanly art of breastfeeding, Franklin Park, Ill., 1958, LaLeche League of Franklin Park, Inc., chap. 3.

**For student's quick notes:**

# Chapter 18

# Conditions contributing to a high-risk puerperium

Nursing measures are aimed at protection against the development of complications. Despite this, there are predisposing factors that serve as avenues for invasion of disease-producing bacteria during the puerperium. The most common ones are discussed in this chapter.

## Puerperal infections

When reading about the history of obstetrics you were introduced to the works of Ignaz P. Semmelweis, Oliver Wendell Holmes, and Louis Pasteur, whose untiring efforts eventually unfolded the etiology and sources of puerperal infection. The name of Charles White from Manchester, England, should also be added as a contributor, for he is given credit for presenting methods of preventing puerperal infection as early as 1773.

In past decades epidemic forms of puerperal infection were caused by beta-hemolytic streptococci, but with progress in obstetrics and maternity nursing, prenatal care, better management of patients during parturition and puerperium, and with the advent of antibiotics, serious infections are seldom encountered today. This does not mean that we can neglect our vigilance and rely on antibiotics because indiscriminate use of these agents may stimulate growth of resistant strains of bacteria. Puerperal infection is still an important cause of maternal morbidity and mortality in the United States.

Puerperal infections are wound infections of the birth canal. They may be local

or transmitted by blood and the lymphatic system and involve the uterus and adjacent structures. If the mother has a temperature elevation to 100.4° F. (oral) on any 2 of the first 10 days after delivery, exclusive of the first 24 hours, she is classified as being morbid. Fever, then, is the first cardinal symptom, which is sometimes preceded by a chill. Along with this is the elevated pulse rate. However, fever is not essential for the diagnosis of puerperal infection. Fever in the parturient woman may be caused by kidney, bladder, or upper respiratory infection.

If you will think of the empty uterus as a large, open wound with an edematous, bruised area where the placenta was attached and, in addition to this, of an edematous cervix with possible minute tears, then you can readily understand just why such areas provide an ideal environment for growth of pathogenic bacteria.

### Modes or sources of infection

Nearly all bacteria that cause puerperal fever are exogenous; such sources include droplet infections of attendants, bacteria from other puerperal women, contaminated linens or equipment, and innumerable other sources so prevalent in a hospital. The predominating organism is the anaerobic streptococci, although the staphylococci are the most common cause of vaginal and perineal infections, such as abscesses in the area of the episiotomy and in tears of the vaginal mucosa.

The anaerobic streptococci as well as many other microorganisms are normal inhabitants in the vagina of most women, but their pathogenicity may be influenced by numerous factors favorable to their growth or by conditions unfavorable to the mother's natural defensive mechanism. She ordinarily has a white cell count of 20,000 to 30,000 per cubic millimeter for 1 or 2 days after delivery, especially after a prolonged labor, so that this is not necessarily a sign of infection. Predisposing causes of puerperal infection are (1) postpartum hemorrhage (adequate replacement of blood loss as indicated is an important factor in prevention of puerperal infection, (2) trauma such as prolonged labor with intrauterine operative manipulations, (3) preexisting anemia lowers resistance, (4) prolonged rupture of the membranes, and (5) placental fragments retained within the uterus.

### Endometritis

The offending organism may lodge in the endometrium (endometritis), usually at the placental site, or extend to the inner muscle layer (endomyometritis).

The severity depends on (1) mother's resistance, (2) virulence of the organism, and (3) extent of trauma during parturition. In mild cases there will be slight elevation of temperature (under 101° F.), the pulse is under 100, and the mother will complain of headache and general malaise. *Adequate drainage* for escape of placental fragments or bits of tissue may be the only treatment required. The doctor usually orders the patient kept in Fowler's position to establish such drainage. Oxytocic drugs may be ordered to stimulate uterine contractions and promote drainage. The nurse should provide a quiet environment and

encourage free intake of fluids. Breast feeding need not be discontinued.

In more serious cases the temperature may rise to 103° to 104° F., ushered in by chills, and the pulse will be 120 or over. The patient will complain of severe "afterpains." On palpation the uterus is tender and boggy, and involution is retarded. The lochia may be copious, with foul odor (putrefactive bacteria), or it may be scant and odorless; the latter occurs where there is some obstruction to drainage (lochiometra) and in some severe streptococcal infections. This is considered more dangerous than the odorous type discharge.

*Treatment.* A penicillin and streptomycin combination or the tetracyclines are effective treatment against most of the pathogenic organisms. The mother should be isolated. This not only protects other mothers but also provides a restful environment for the mother. If the process does not extend further than the endometrium, the temperature falls and by 10 days the infection subsides.

### Pelvic cellulitis (parametritis)

If the organism extends along the blood vessels and lymphatics, cellulitis (parametritis) involving the peritoneum and broad ligament results. Generally it follows infected cervical lacerations or is a continuation of the original endometrial infection.

*Clinical course.* Patient has a sustained, persistent high temperature (104° F.), and the uterus is extremely tender. This confines her to bed for a considerable time.

*Treatment.* Antibiotics are ordered according to results of culture and sensitivity tests.

### Cervicitis

The cervix is easily subjected to trauma —minute tears to deep lacerations. The serosanguineous drainage from the uterus forms a pool of media in which pathogenic microorganisms increase. This is especially so when the mother's resistance to infection is low and she has deep cervical lacerations. This can be detected on the 6-week postpartum examination and treated by conization.

### Thrombophlebitis

After delivery of the placenta, bleeding from open sinuses is controlled by contraction and retractions of muscles as well as by increased fibrinogen with formation of thrombi within the sinuses. These thrombi act as barriers against invading organisms. However, if predisposing factors are present, such as preexisting varicosities where blood flow is sluggish, infections such as endometritis, and trauma inflicted during labor and delivery, pyogenic organisms may invade the uterus, and the inflammatory process may continue along the walls of the blood vessels and attack the pelvic veins (thrombophlebitis). This is the most common mode of extension of puerperal infection and the most likely offender is the anaerobic streptococci.

Two groups of veins involved are (1) uterine, ovarian, and hypogastric, which lead to pelvic thrombophlebitis and (2) femoral, saphenous, and popliteal, which lead to femoral thrombophlebitis. An older term for this type is "phlegmasia alba dolens" or "milk leg."

*Symptoms.* Symptoms of thrombophlebitis do not usually appear while the mother is in the hospital, that is, before 7 to 10 days after delivery. The condition is preceded by a low grade infection of the birth canal. When the organism attacks the femoral vein, the mother complains of pain in the groin or calf of the leg, and along the course of the vein. The onset is abrupt with chills and high fever (103° to 104° F.), rapid pulse, severe pain, and swelling of the extremity. The edema starts in the foot and then gradually involves the leg and thigh. Thrombi formation in the pelvic veins leads to spasms of femoral artery and causes the edema and severe pain of the extremity involved.

The arterial spasms also produce a bluish white pallor of the skin over the tensely swollen area. The course of the disease is prolonged 2 to 3 weeks. When the mother is permitted to ambulate, a recurrence is likely in the other leg.

*Treatment and nursing care.* The affected leg is elevated on a pillow and pressure of bed clothing is relieved by a cradle over the leg. An ice bag along the affected vein helps control the swelling. While giving nursing care, protect the involved leg and handle it with extreme gentleness. The patient is on complete bed rest while febrile. If the mother is on anticoagulant therapy to prevent extension of the clot, the nurse notes character and amount of lochia. The dosage of heparin or Dicumarol is determined by daily prothrombin levels. Since the convalescent period is prolonged (2 to 3 weeks), the nurse encourages the mother to eat nourishing food and does all she can to bolster the morale of the patient. She prevents spread of infection by proper disposal of drainage and through washing of her hands. When the patient is permitted to ambulate, an elastic stocking may be ordered to help control the swelling.

Phlebothrombosis differs in that there is little pain or inflammatory reaction. The mother may have a slight elevation of temperature and little pain, but dorsiflexion of the foot and pressure over the deep veins will cause pain in the calf of the leg (Homan's sign). The danger involved is that the thrombi may break loose and result in pulmonary embolism.

## Other complications
### Delayed postpartum hemorrhage

Delayed or late postpartum hemorrhage was defined on p. 193 as the loss of over 500 ml. of blood after the first 24 hours after delivery. Retained particles of cotyledons and pieces of fetal membrane are the most likely cause. Early recognition and prompt referral to the physician may prevent serious delayed hemorrhage.

Placenta polyps occasionally develop from such retained fragments. In this case the patient must be readmitted to the hospital, since the hemorrhage may be profuse and prolonged. Treatment consists of uterine curettage.

### Puerperal hematomas

Hematomas are the result of injury to blood vessels and are more likely to occur after rapid spontaneous delivery or after prolonged pressure during labor and delivery. A predisposing factor may be large varicosities in the pelvic area. They may also occur within the episiotomy if a vein is pricked during repair. (See Fig. 18-1.)

When the mother complains of *severe* pain in the perineal area and the feeling of pressure on the rectum and bladder, the nurse should inspect the area. The skin will likely show discoloration and swelling.

The doctor usually orders cold compresses and analgesics to relieve the pain. Small hematomas are absorbed. The larger ones must be incised and vessels ligated.

### Subinvolution

When the normal process of involution is retarded, it is called *subinvolution*. Normal involution may be interfered with when the following are present: (1) inadequate drainage, (2) retained pieces of cotyledons or tissue, (3) uterine fibroids, and (4) infections such as endometritis. The mother has a prolonged period of lochial discharge and may complain of a dragging sensation in the pelvic area and of irregular bleeding.

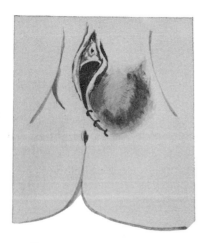

Fig. 18-1. Perineal hematoma.

On examination the doctor will determine the cause and treat accordingly. Subinvolution may be a cause of late postpartum hemorrhage.

### Mastitis

Mastitis is an infection in the breasts. *Staphylococcus aureus* is the common offender, gaining access through fissured nipples. It does not, as a rule, occur before the third or fourth week after delivery. The first sign is chills, then follow elevation of temperature and an increase in pulse rate along with extremely swollen, tender breasts.

Prophylaxis involves measures such as (1) reminding the mother not to permit the infant to nurse too long at any one feeding, (2) instructing the mother of the importance of washing her hands before handling her breasts (the nurse, too, must certainly remember this when assisting the mother and infant in nursing), (3) inserting a portion of areola into infant's mouth so that his jaws compress the milk pockets instead of the tip of the nipple, and (4) teaching the proper method for releasing nipple from the infant's mouth.

*Treatment.* Proper support for the breasts, antibiotics such as novobiocin, and hot or cold packs are the usual orders. Some doctors permit the mother to continue nursing the infant, believing it is advisable to remove excess milk and reduce stasis. Other doctors discontinue feeding on the affected breast until the infection subsides. If treatment with antimicrobial drugs is instituted before abscess formation, the infection can be controlled within 48 hours.

### Puerperal cardiac patient

On p. 108 you read about the importance of adequate medical supervision for the cardiac patient during pregnancy. What about the puerperal phase of her maternity cycle? The first 12 hours after delivery are the most critical due to physiological changes, such as the sudden rise in cardiac output because blood that would have gone to the placenta and uterus now goes into general circulation and the right side of the heart carries an overload. Delay of diuresis also plays a part.

The doctor usually keeps the patient on bed rest for a week or more. It is the nurse's responsibility to observe the patient for signs of pulmonary congestion and for edema and to use every precaution to avoid infection. Even visitors should be restricted, for they are often carriers of respiratory tract infections. Before the patient is discharged, explicit instructions should be given to the family that the patient must be relieved of all domestic functions until doctor permits the patient to resume her responsibilities.

## SELECTED READINGS

Beck, A. C., and Taylor, E. Stewart, editors: Obstetrical practice, ed. 8, Baltimore, 1966, The Williams & Wilkins Co., chap. 38.

Diddle, A. W.: Postpartum hemorrhage, Hosp. Med. 4:91, June, 1968.

Eastman, Nicholson, J., and Hellman, Louis M., editors: Williams' obstetrics, ed. 13, New York, 1966, Appleton-Century-Crofts, chap. 36.

Graber, Edward A., and Loizeaux, Leon S.: Postpartum pelvic hematomas. In Barber, Hugh R. K., and Graber, Edward A., editors: Quick reference to ob-gyn procedures, Philadelphia, 1969, J. B. Lippincott Co., p. 105.

Greenhill, J. P., editor: Obstetrics, ed. 13, Philadelphia, 1965, W. B. Saunders Co., chap. 75.

Rodman, Morton J.: Drugs that affect blood coagulation, RN 32:59, June, 1969.

Stevens, Bette A.: Postpartum eclampsia, Nurs. Mirror 123:331, Jan., 1967.

**For student's quick notes:**

# Chapter 19

# Integrated mother-baby care

The mother's active participation in the care of her infant provides an opportunity for her to recognize his needs and administer to them as they occur. This not only brings pleasurable satisfaction to the infant, but it contributes to development of her motherliness. This early integrated care is the birth of security and trust in the infant's world.

It is the opinion of many doctors and nurses that it is unnatural to separate an infant from its mother at birth. In fact it is only in the American culture that this is done. We need to establish more programs of integrated care for the mother and her newborn. This simply means that the mother may have her baby with her when she desires and with an opportunity for more frequent periods of actual contact. It is a natural response of a mother to want to respond to her infant's cry, rather than to observe the baby "crying it out" in a central nursery.

With such a feasible plan the new mother discovers her infant's needs and recognizes the care "her" baby requires. She can bathe her baby when he is awake and feed him when he is hungry. As the mother handles the infant she feels a sense of achievement, not defeat, anxiety, and resentment that many experience while they observe nurses "taking over" the care they would like to administer. (See Fig. 19-1.)

As she cares for her infant and administers to his needs, she recognizes his helplessness and dependence on her; this in itself may develop her self-confidence, evoke mother love and help her respond

in a meaningful way. The gentleness with which she holds and soothes him, the rocking chair, the warmth of her body, and the tone of her voice all transmit security to the infant. This not only elicits tender feelings within the mother but are necessary for healthy emotional development of her infant. She learns his pattern of behavior and by the day of discharge she feels quite capable of handling her infant. This integrated care provides an environment conducive to the father visiting with his wife and the new member of the family. This provides an early intimacy between the three.

The traditional rigid scheduled nursery procedures are not usually the nurse's choice. Infants must be awakened for morning care and taken to their mothers for feeding to comply with standard feeding schedules, ignoring a plan that would be most beneficial to the mother and infant. If the infant is asleep when taken to the mother, he will not feed well. This is as frustrating to the mother as it probably was to the infant when his earlier need to be fed was ignored. The mother feels deprived of her right when a little later she stands at the observation window and sees the nurse feeding her baby. The

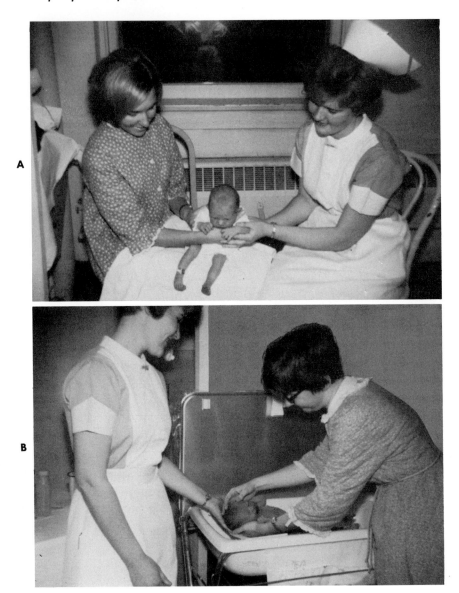

Fig. 19-1. A, Student nurse assists new mother in learning art of burping infant. B, On day of discharge from hospital, student instructs the new mother in bathing infant. C, Father shares the joy of becoming acquainted with his infant as mother looks on. D, One objective of the maternity nurse is to send home a healthy, contented mother and baby.

mother returns to her room feeling defeat because she could not give gratification to her infant. We observe this stress in the infant by scratched faces, excoriated knees, and finally exhaustion.

In situations when such an integrated plan of care is optional and the mother hesitates, it is usually due to the fact that she does not understand the plan. She may believe she "must" take complete care of the infant. She needs to be informed that the services of a professional nurse are always available to her and that she may care for the baby as she likes. Integrated care must not be forced on her. Some mothers are overanxious and tense.

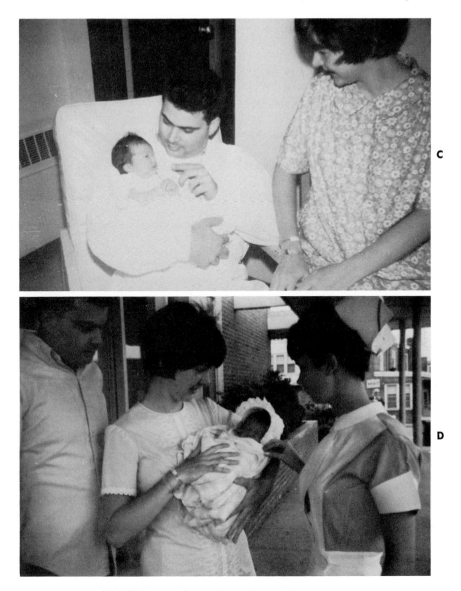

**Fig. 19-1, cont'd.** For legend see opposite page.

There are those mothers who shift their responsibilities on others to care for the infant and display no interest in mothering their infants. Others need to be stimulated and encouraged in wanting to care for the infant. They accept this helpless creature with open arms, but then what! When doctors and nurses fail to see the psychological benefits derived from the plan, they do not encourage the participation, and the mothers are more likely to have negative attitudes also. Success of an integrated plan of care is dependent on interest of nursing personnel and adequate orientation of all involved. Maternity nurses need to be trained in the task of guiding mothers to develop positive rather than negative attitudes toward enjoying motherhood. The nurse needs to give recognition for her efforts as well as encouragement and praise. It is difficult to provide supportive nursing care unless we provide an environment with sufficient opportunity for personal contract between mother and infant.

When the day of discharge arrives, she will not leave with a "strange bundle" but with feelings of confidence because she has proved her capabilities of caring for the infant and derived great satisfaction in observing her infant's reactions to her love. Assisting the mother in meeting this real situation is indeed a nursing skill. The maternity nurse experiences a feeling of true reward and satisfaction as she observes the mother's pleasure in caring for her newborn. All new mothers should therefore be encouraged to participate in such care of their infants.

**SELECTED READINGS**
*Integrated mother-baby care*

Blake, Florence G., and Wright, F. Howell: Essentials of pediatric nursing, ed. 7, Philadelphia, 1963, J. B. Lippincott Co., p. 157.

Coome, Barbara: Rooming-in brings family together, Canad. Nurse **65**:46, June, 1969.

Finbarr, Sister Mary: Family-centered maternity program in a general hospital, Child Family **6**:3, Summer, 1967.

Gettys, Elaine, and Stephan, Frances: We've found a compromise rooming-in plan, RN **28**:81, April, 1965.

Newton, Niles: Maternal emotions, New York, 1955, Paul E. Hoeber, Inc., chap. 7.

Pederson, Frank A., and Robson, Kenneth S.: Father participation in infancy, Amer. J. Orthopsychiat. **39**:466, April, 1969.

Waltner, Elma: Intensive care for newborns enhanced by "mothering-in," Hosp. Top. **44**:104, Sept., 1966.

**For student's quick notes:**

# Chapter 20

# Preparation for discharge

In this part you have learned about the demands made on the new mother, both physiological and psychological. Each day of the early puerperium, you gave her support and encouragement as she developed confidence while adapting to her new role. Now that she is ready for discharge she needs instructions concerning continued care of herself. This chapter outlines such a regimen.

## Postpartum examination

Some doctors do a pelvic examination on the patient before discharge; others wait until the 6-week examination in their office. The purpose of the examination is to (1) inspect the perineum, (2) note the condition of vaginal canal and cervix, (3) note the degree of involution, and (4) note the condition of the breasts and nipples.

Before the mother is discharged, the nurse should impress on her the importance of the 6-week examination, and if she is a clinic patient, see that she receives her appointment card before she leaves the hospital for home.

## Regimen for self-care at home

Mimeographed forms handed to the patient for self-care at home are of little, if any, value unless the nurse explains the purpose and importance of adhering to the instructions.

### First week

1. Care for her baby and herself only
2. Rest greater part of the day and avoid fatigue
3. Stair climbing restricted—remain on one floor for the first week

4. May continue with exercises practiced in the hospital
5. Tub bathe in warm water at least once a day and shampoo hair at any time.
6. May walk out of doors provided she does not have to climb stairs
7. Encourage mother to eat high protein foods, fruits, vegetables, and milk products; vitamin and mineral supplement should be the same as during pregnancy
8. Encourage mother to drink fluids freely
9. Should wear brassiere constantly
10. Vaginal discharge should decrease in amount and be yellowish white

### Second week

1. May go up and down stairs
2. Abstain from coitus for at least 1 month, allowing time for episiotomy to heal
3. Gradually assume light household tasks, such as preparing simple meals
4. At least 8 to 10 hours of sleep with rest periods of 1 hour twice daily is recommended
5. May drive a car if she so desires

6. Continue exercises, adding a few new ones if desired
7. Continue wearing brassiere constantly
8. Check breasts for presence of tenderness; lactation should gradually subside if infant is on artificial type of feeding
9. Lochia should be quite scant

*Third week*

1. Assume normal activities, but avoid lifting and undue fatigue
2. Continue rest periods during the day
3. Lochia will likely subside this week
4. Assume normal household duties, again avoiding fatigue

During this time the mother should have returned to her approximate prepregnant weight. If she has acquired excess fat, she can discuss this with the doctor when she returns for her examination. The breasts should have stopped lactating by this time. If she notices reestablishment of lactation, she might bind her breasts with a simple towel, bringing the breasts to the midline. Such a binder might furnish more firm support than the brassiere cup.

## Return of the menses

Her first period will be heavier and more prolonged than her usual menses. First ovulation usually occurs within 6 weeks if she is not lactating; if lactating she may not ovulate or menstruate until she weans the infant. A small percentage of mothers ovulate, but they do not menstruate or ovulate and menstruate while lactating. In some mothers the first menses are irregular and even simulate beginning of the menarche.

**STUDY QUESTIONS**
*Multiple choice*

1. In checking Mrs. D, who is 6 hours postdelivery, you find her blood pressure to be 126/96, and her uterus is somewhat boggy and located to the left of the midline. Her bleeding is moderate in amount. The first thing you will do is:
   (a) gently massage the fundus until it becomes firm.
   (b) call the doctor for an order to give Mrs. D an oxytocic.
   (c) notify your supervisor.
2. Your next measure will be to:
   (a) give Mrs. D perineal care and make her comfortable.
   (b) take her temperature.
   (c) encourage Mrs. D to empty her bladder.
3. Credit for having discovered the organism causing puerperal infection was earned by:
   (a) Ignaz Semmelweis.
   (b) Louis Pasteur.
   (c) Oliver Wendell Holmes.
   (d) Charles White.
4. You would advise a new mother not to drive her car until:
   (a) the completion of the puerperium.
   (b) at least the second week of the puerperium.
   (c) lochia discharge has ceased.
5. Which one of the following patients would most likely be predisposed to thrombophlebitis?
   (a) one with preexisting varicosities.
   (b) one delivered by cesarean section.
   (c) one having a prolonged labor.
6. Afterpains are more likely to be experienced when:
   (a) the labor and delivery was precipitous.
   (b) the mother is breast feeding.
   (c) the mother is taking oxytocics.
   (d) the mother was delivered by cesarean section.
   1. b only   2. a, b, and c   3. all of these
7. Mrs. T had a history of severe preeclampsia. She was delivered of twins, one weighing 6 pounds 3 ounces, and the other 5 pounds. The second twin was delivered by Scanzoni's maneuver. Mrs. T was transferred to postpartum unit 3 hours after delivery. Due to prenatal complications and trauma during parturition, this mother should be observed carefully for the following:
   (a) signs of infection.
   (b) hemorrhage.
   (c) convulsions.
   (d) subinvolution.
   1. b only  2. a, b, and c  3. all of these
8. A late postpartum hemorrhage is one that occurs:
   (a) within 12 hours after delivery.
   (b) after the first 24 hours.
   (c) at the end of the puerperium.
9. Mrs. F has the diagnosis of endometritis and is on complete bed rest. She asks you if she should assume any particular position in bed. You will:
   (a) tell her to assume the position most comfortable.

(b) make her comfortable in the Fowler's position.

(c) have her lie flat in bed.

10. Mrs. E delivered a 6-pound baby girl spontaneously. She had a right mediolateral episiotomy. Six hours after delivery she complains of pain in the perineal area with pressure on the rectum and bladder. This is most likely due to:

(a) edema from the episiotomy.

(b) trauma from the delivery.

(c) a developing hematoma.

11. While you are assisting in the clinic with the 6-week postnatal examinations, a patient questions you as to the stretch marks on her abdomen and thighs, inquiring when they will disappear. Your answer should be:

(a) they lose their purplish red color but remain as silvery irregular lines.

(b) they will disappear as time goes by.

(c) they will remain as they are at this time.

12. After 5 hours of labor, Mrs. T delivered spontaneously. When you admit her to the postpartum unit, her vital signs are temperature 99.4° F., pulse 46, respirations 20, blood pressure 116/70. This slight elevation of temperature is most likely due to:

(a) dehydration.

(b) developing infection.

(c) excitement following delivery.

13. Mrs. B and Mrs. C are rooming together. Mrs. B is bottle feeding her baby and Mrs. C is breast feeding. After Mrs. B hears your discussion with Mrs. C concerning breast feeding, she states; "I suppose it is too late for me to breast feed after having the baby on the bottle for 2 days." The most appropriate answer for you to give Mrs. B would be:

(a) Yes, it is too late. You are receiving medication to suppress lactation. Perhaps the next time you have a baby you would like to try breast feeding.

(b) If you truly wish to breast feed, the medication can be discontinued and with regular nursing, the flow of milk will be reestablished.

(c) Because Mrs. C is successful does not mean you will be. Your baby is doing well on the formula.

14. Mrs. D had a prolonged labor due to uterine dysfunction. She was delivered under deep anesthesia with forceps. Although Mrs. D was observed carefully in the recovery room, it is your nursing responsibility to continue close observation of Mrs. D because with prolonged labor and operative intervention, you know she is more likely to:

(a) develop uterine atony.

(b) develop a vulvar hematoma.

(c) have difficulty voiding.

(d) all of these.

15. You may also expect Mrs. D to:

(a) develop postpartum blues.

(b) have difficulty initiating *early* breast feeding.

(c) be ordered on complete bed rest for several days.

*True or false*

(T)  (F)  1. Striae gravidarum fades but never disappears.

(T)  (F)  2. Afterpains rarely last longer than 4 days.

(T)  (F)  3. Oxytocins are important in aiding involution.

(T)  (F)  4. During the first day after delivery the nurse will expect the lochia to be mixed with large blood clots.

(T)  (F)  5. A low pulse rate (40) during the early puerperium needs to be reported to the doctor immediately.

(T)  (F)  6. Lochia is increased in women delivered by cesarean section.

(T)  (F)  7. Lactose is normally present in urine of puerperal women.

(T)  (F)  8. Leukocytosis is normal during the early puerperium.

(T)  (F)  9. Subinvolution frequently accompanies endometritis.

(T)  (F) 10. Subinvolution may be a cause of late postpartum hemorrhage.

(T)  (F) 11. Proteinuria occurs in a percentage of women after parturition but disappears by the third day.

(T)  (F) 12. Involution of the uterus is more rapid in the primipara and in mothers who nurse their babies.

(T)  (F) 13. A full bladder predisposes to postpartum hemorrhage.

(T)  (F) 14. A sudden rise in temperature on the third day after delivery would likely be due to mastitis.

(T)  (F) 15. Secretion of milk is inhibited in the febrile mother.

**For student's quick notes:**

UNIT IV

# The neonate

When the student begins her clinical experience in the nursery, she is likely to view the newborn as an uncoordinated, helpless creature, but she soon learns that this is not so; within each neonate are the potentialities for physical, mental, and psychological growth and development, which will be influenced by heredity and environment.

This unit will acquaint you with the physiological and psychological changes in the newborn as he adapts to extrauterine environment. The time that it takes the newborn to make this stable adjustment to his environment is called the *neonatal period* and usually involves 4 weeks.

In addition to administering to his transitional needs, you will learn how to care for and protect this creature of God. First you will study about his normal behavior and his characteristic variants, and then you will learn to recognize deviations from the normal.

Opportunities for teaching are manifold. This is not only a period of adjustment for the newborn, but the new mother also needs time to become acquainted with her baby. The nurse guides her as she learns about his behavior patterns and instructs her in his development and neonatal care prior to discharge.

Chapter 21

# The recovery nursery

The ideal nursery arrangement provides a unit where the *immediate* newborn can be observed and given constant attention. Chapter 21 of this unit deals with just such a plan. Here you will learn of the hazards involved during the transitional period after birth and how stabilization of respirations and temperature helps the newborn make a more satisfactory adjustment to his extrauterine environment.

## Importance of careful, constant observation

The transition from intrauterine to extrauterine environment—the infant's first attempt at independent existence is the time of highest neonatal morbidity and mortality. Birth is traumatic and there is no doubt that the infant needs help and time as well to recover from the experience. Therefore immediate, careful, and constant observation is a necessity until the transition has been satisfactorily made. The nurse must be thoroughly familiar with oxygen therapy, infant resuscitation, and stabilization of respirations and temperature to meet his immediate needs. She must also be aware of other possible problems he may present as he makes these early adjustments.

When he is transferred from the delivery room, the nurse should determine if he needs to be placed in the Isolette with oxygen or into an incubator for additional warmth. If the infant is placed in an Isolette, no clothing should be applied so that vital signs can be more accurately observed. When a diaper is applied, care should be used to see that it is pinned lightly to avoid pressure on the diaphragm.

The infant's color may indicate respiratory problems, bleeding, or other symptoms from which a nursing diagnosis of possible problems could be made. There is an interval of time between the birth of the infant and the first examination by the pediatrician and it is during this interval that the nurse has the important function of observing closely to diagnose tentatively.

## Problems during transitional period
### Stabilization of temperature

For the newborn, external warmth is basic to survival. Since the infant comes from a liquid environment, his wet body is subject to drastic decrease in thermal temperature. His meager subcutaneous fat provides little, if any, insulation. Full-term infants, but not the premature, increase their rate of metabolism on exposure to cold, but the rate of heat loss is nevertheless greater than its production.

At birth the temperature of the newborn is approximately 0.5° C. above that of the mother's and drops on an average of 3° C. within the first hour. As heat production increases during the first 2 to 3 days, the respiratory rate decreases, but it is about a week before the infant regulates his own body temperature.

Our aim is to produce an environmental temperature in which the infant will be able to minimize the energy he exerts in his effort to maintain heat regulation. Regulating the abdominal skin temperature between 96.8° and 98.6° F. is most likely to meet this need. Increase and decrease in environmental temperature must be adjusted according to each infant's metabolic needs. Skin temperature may be measured frequently and changes in control adjusted accordingly. The Servocontrol to monitor abdominal skin temperature is ideal for it measures the energy exchange between infant and his environment. Since infants have an inadequate sweating mechanism, temperature must be monitored carefully to avoid hyperthermia. It should not exceed 99° F.

The neutral thermal environment for term infants is 32° to 34° C. (89.6° to 93.2° F.), with 40% to 60% humidity. Such an environment not only keeps him comfortable but also aids body metabolism. Since it would not be practical to work in such a temperature and most nurseries are air conditioned, the infant needs to be protected by warm blankets. When the environmental temperature drops below body temperature, metabolism increases and, therefore, the need for oxygen is increased. The newborn will, therefore, show restlessness when the environmental temperature is too low for his comfort.

### Stabilization of respirations

The nurse monitors respirations every 15 minutes for the first hour after birth, and then every 30 minutes for the next 2 hours. Many times he has difficulty ridding his air passages of oral mucus. An aspirating bulb should be a part of the equipment of every unit. Analgesia and anesthesia administered to the mother will certainly show their depressing effect on the infant's respirations.

Normally the newborn's breathing is largely diaphragmatic and irregular in depth and rhythm. The infant in distress shows an entirely different pattern, such as described on p. 168. Infants whose respirations are normal in the first hour and then show progressive increase to 60 or more per minute within 36 hours have a high mortality rate. If the infant is kept on his side (preferably the right side), ordinary mucus will drain from the respiratory passages and favor lung expansion. Large amounts of mucus interfere with respirations and produce a feeling of suffocation. In such cases the infant is unable to signal his distress. Suction should be gentle, but adequate. A plug of mucus may cause respiratory distress or even sudden death. Early observation to detect onset of symptoms and prompt action on the part of the nurse mean early and appropriate therapy by the doctor.

The nurse observes any cyanosis, constant or intermittent. Intermittent attacks are seen in intracranial hemorrhage. Persistant cyanosis is seen in cardiac anomalies.

The nurse must also be alert to other signs and symptoms of respiratory distress such as (1) sternal retraction with expiratory grunts, (2) overinflated chest, (3) flaring of the nostrils, (4) chin lag, (5) cyanosis, (6) a heart beat over 160 per minute for over a 1-minute duration, (7) respirations over 60 per minute, and (8) weak, limp, and exhausted infant.

The nurse observes the infant for abdominal distention. Any gastric distention interferes with respirations and expansion of the lungs. Abdominal distention suggests meconium ileus; a scaphoid abdomen may indicate a diaphragmatic hernia. She is first to recognize the high-pitched cry so characteristic of the infant suffering intracranial hemorrhage. She knows that pallor is not normal and may represent anoxia, anemia, or shock.

### Hemorrhage[1,2]

The possibility of a tendency to hemorrhage should be kept in mind, for although the infant's prothrombin level is elevated at birth (from the mother), it declines until about the sixth day when the liver is able to function in the formation of prothrombin.

Vitamin K is an essential precursor of prothrombin and much of it is supplied to the baby from the lumen of the intestine where it is made by bacteria, especially *Escherichia coli.* Since bacterial flora are

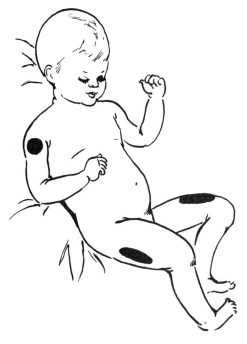

**Fig. 21-1.** Sites for intramuscular injection.

necessary for its synthesis and the infant's intestines are sterile at birth, this may be the reason for the decline of the prothrombin level (physiological hypoprothrombinemia).

For this reason the administration of synthetic vitamin K to prevent hemorrhage is the routine order in many newborn nurseries. The doctor may even order it given to the mother prior to delivery. Vitamin K, of course, can only be useful in preventing bleeding caused by a lowered prothrombin. There are several other factors involved in coagulation that may be responsible for bleeding if they are deficient.

The analogues that are water soluble are the usual preparations used (dose of 0.5 to 1 mg. of phytenadione [$K_1$]) and are adequate as a prophylactic. Jaundice in the newborn has been reported after parenteral administration of large doses of these water-soluble vitamin K analogues. The natural fat-soluble form of this vitamin (phytenadione [$K_1$]) apparently does not cause this condition. (See Fig. 21-1.)

### Other problems

During the infant's stay in the recovery nursery the nurse may observe the following signs and symptoms; the possible causes are also given.

| **Observation** | **Possible causes** |
|---|---|
| 1. Stained vernix | 1. Fetal distress |
| 2. High-pitched cry | 2. Central nervous system damage |
| 3. Expiratory grunting | 3. Respiratory distress syndrome |
| 4. Mouth breathing | 4. Choanal atresia; also present in mongoloids |
| 5. Lips and torso cyanotic | 5. Cardiac, neurological, or respiratory anomaly |
| 6. Constant drooling | 6. Tracheoesophageal atresia |
| 7. Scaphoid-shaped abdomen | 7. Diaphragmatic hernia |
| 8. Abdominal distention | 8. Meconium ileus |
| 9. Aggravated cyanosis with crying | 9. Cardiac anomaly |
| 10. Slow, shallow, and irregular respirations | 10. Central nervous system damage |
| 11. Lethargy | 11. Excess analgesia or anesthesia given to the mother, cerebral damage, or infection |
| 12. Hyperactivity | 12. Cerebral damage, hypoglycemia, or hypocalcemia |

| **Maternal complication** | **Observe infant for** |
|---|---|
| 1. Premature rupture of the membranes<br>2. Rapid labor and delivery<br><br>3. Prolonged labor with heavy sedation and anesthesia<br><br>4. Polyhydramnios<br>5. Oligohydramnios<br>6. Blood discrepancy | 1. Infection<br>2. Respiratory distress and signs of intracranial hemorrhage<br>3. Signs of central nervous system damage; expect infant to be weak, limp, exhausted, and disinterested in feeding<br>4. Signs of intestinal obstruction<br>5. Abnormalities of the kidneys<br>6. Early appearance of jaundice |

Further scrutiny of the infant is necessary when the mother had a history of the above.

## Transfer of neonate to regular nursery

When it is determined that the infant has made satisfactory adjustment to the environment, such as stabilization of temperature and respirations, it may be transferred to the regular nursery.

### REFERENCES
1. Smith, Carl: Blood diseases of infancy and childhood, ed. 2, St. Louis, 1966, The C. V. Mosby Co., p. 103.
2. Wefring, K. W.: Hemorrhage in the newborn and vitamin K prophylaxis, J. Pediat. 63:663, 1963.

### SELECTED READINGS
*Recovery nursery*
Arnold, Helen, Putnam, Nancy, Barnard, Betty Lou, Desmond, Murdina, and Rudolph, Arnold: The newborn. Transition to extra-uterine life, Amer. J. Nurs. 65:77, Oct. 1965.
Avery, Mary Ellen: The lung and its disorders in the newborn infant, Philadelphia, 1964, W. B. Saunders Co., p. 31.
Babson, Gorham S., and Benson, Ralph C.: Primer on prematurity and high-risk pregnancy, St. Louis, 1966, The C. V. Mosby Co., pp. 81-87.
Desmond, Murdina, Rudolph, Arnold, and Phitaksphraiwan, P.: The transitional care nursery, Pediat. Clin. N. Amer. 13:651, Aug., 1966
Editorial: News about the newborn and unborn, J.A.M.A. 208:686, April 28, 1969.
Guyton, Arthur C.: Textbook of medical physiology, ed. 3, Philadelphia, 1966, W. B. Saunders Co., p. 1172.
James, L. S.: The importance of observations of the newborn infant at birth. In Lytle, Nancy A., editor: Maternal health nursing, Dubuque, Iowa, 1967, William C. Brown Co., pp. 97-106.
Latham, Helen, and Heckel, R. V.: Pediatric nursing, St. Louis, 1967, The C. V. Mosby Co., p. 14.
Montagu, M. F. Ashley: Prenatal influences, Springfield, Ill., 1962, Charles C Thomas, Publisher, pp. 481-492.
Parsons, Coleen J.: The intensive care obstetrical nursery, Canad. Nurse 61:35, Jan., 1965.
Siegel, Dorothy: A better start for all babies, Parents' Magazine 63:53, Nov., 1968.
Smith, Robert M.: Temperature monitoring and regulation, Pediat. Clin. N. Amer. 16:643, Aug., 1969.

**For student's quick notes:**

Chapter 22

# Admission of the neonate to the nursery

Just what does the nurse do for the newborn on admission to the nursery?
This chapter discusses your responsibilities and the variants so
characteristic of the newborn.

## Physical findings and
## nursing responsibilities
### The admission bath

When the newborn is admitted to the
regular nursery, the nurse in charge receives a report on his progress while in
the recovery nursery—if his respiratory and
circulatory mechanisms are functioning
adequately and whether he has voided
and passed meconium. She now takes over
the responsibility for his continued care.
She continues to observe his respirations
at intervals and is alert for oral mucus.
Observation to prevent obstruction of the
respiratory tract is still important because
respiratory distress is not always present
at birth; it may develop gradually and
manifest itself hours or even days later.

The nurse bathes the infant (according
to the routine she was taught). Preferences
vary as to whether the infant is to be
bathed with soap and water, pHisoHex,
or other antibacterial preparations. Whatever the method, she remembers to keep
the infant warm to avoid thermal shock.
As she bathes him she will notice that the
superficial vessels are prominent. This plus
a high hemoglobin and, in some instances,
pressure during the birth process give a
ruddy appearance to the entire body.

### The skin

The skin texture of the neonate varies,
but it tends to be dry and lacking in natural oils. Some newborns show cracks,
fissures, and peeling. For these infants,
water baths act as an irritant. The pediatrician may approve or disapprove the use
of oils and baby ointments. Some doctors
believe that such preparations are a good
media for growth of bacteria, especially if
not applied properly.

### Erythema toxicum neonatorum

Erythema toxicum neonatorum or urti-
carial skin lesions are believed by some
doctors to be the result of hypersensitive
skin. In some infants these lesions may
be seen immediately after delivery; in others they appear during the first few days
of life and disappear within 1 week. The
lesions are especially prominent on the infant's back and chest.

### Capillary hemangioma

*Stork's beak marks.* Stork's beak marks
produce small, reddened areas in the skin,
particularly on the eyelids, nave, and upper
lip. They blanch on pressure and are more
common among light-complected neonates.
They become more noticeable during periods of crying and tend to disappear by
the end of the first year.

*Nevi vasculosus (strawberry mark).* Nevi
vasculosus are of a bright or dark red
color, with raised, rough surfaces. They
are not usually present at birth but appear
during the first or second month. This

type of birthmark is seen more in the premature infant. The majority disappear between the ages of 7 and 8 years.

*Nevi flammeus (port-wine stain).* Nevi flammeus are red to purple in color. They do not blanch on pressure and do not disappear spontaneously.

### Mongolian spots

Mongolian spots are macular areas of dark blue- to purple-colored pigmentations that are distributed over the lumbar, sacral, and gluteal regions. They are more pronounced in the Negro infant; they have no anthropological significance and tend to disappear during the first or second year of life.

Birthmarks should be identified for the mother, since she is certain to be concerned about them after she brings the infant home. It is difficult to allay her anxiety because of the deeply imbedded superstitious convictions she may have; many a mother feels that she has "marked" her infant and may experience a sense of guilt because of her infant's blemish.

Rarely the nurse may observe harlequin color change. A line of demarcation appears down the midline of the body. The skin involving the entire right or left side is quite red, whereas the other half side is normally pink. This is due to a temporary vasomotor disturbance and disappears after a few hours or days.[1]

She may also notice a white, caseous, cheesy substance adherent to the skin. This is called vernix caseosa and is most prominent in the creases and folds of the skin. These areas need gentle, meticulous care because they are excellent sources of entry for infectious agents. The infant may have much, little, or no vernix. Opinions vary as to whether the vernix should be removed or allowed to remain on the skin. It is believed by some doctors to have beneficial properties in protecting the infant from superficial infection. It will be shed spontaneously in about 2 days.

Lanugo is a fine downy hair appearing over the body, which is more evident on the back and shoulders. It is more abundant in the premature infant and is lost during the first few weeks of life.

Whether or not a dressing should be placed around the umbilical cord is optional.

Until the newborn's nervous system has matured enough to control his body temperature, each infant should be clothed according to his specific requirements. A diaper, shirt, and soft receiving blanket prove sufficient in an environmental temperature of 80° F. Temperature returns to normal in 6 to 7 hours after birth.

On p. 167 you read that after the initial response to birth, the infant relaxed and fell asleep. After this period of rest he manifests a period of reactivity—kicking, stretching, and making random movements of his extremities. His cry is lusty and he usually shows signs of hunger, such as sucking on his fingers or little fist. In cases where the mother was heavily sedated during labor and under deep anesthesia for delivery, the nurse cannot expect this pattern of response.

### Acrocyanosis

Peripheral circulation is somewhat sluggish; for this reason the nurse will observe acrocyanosis, or cyanosis of the extremities, for several hours after birth. The sweat and sebaceous glands have little function during the neonatal period, which is an important factor in regulation of body temperature.

### The head

The nurse will note that the head is the largest part of the body, which comprises about one fourth of his size. The circumference averages 13 to 14 inches. The crown-rump measurement (sitting height) equals the head circumference.

The bones of the skull are held together by membranes called sutures. Openings at the junction of the skull bones are called fontanels. There are six fontanels at birth —anterior, posterior, two sphenoid, and two mastoid. The nurse should be able to palpate both the anterior and posterior fontanels. The anterior fontanel normally closes between the ninth and sixteenth month and the posterior between 8 to 10 weeks (Fig. 11-6). When the nurse assists the doctor with the physical examination on a newborn, she will note that he palpates the anterior fontanel. A depressed fontanel may indicate dehydration; a bulging fontanel may indicate intracranial hemorrhage, hydrocephalus, or congestive heart failure. The level of the fontanel is an indication of pressure within the central nervous system.

The skull bones are relatively soft and the head may appear elongated. This is termed *molding*. It may be caused by the intrauterine position or during passage through the birth canal. It is particularly noticeable in firstborns and when labor was prolonged. At birth the infant's bones are relatively soft and the joints quite elastic. This to some extent eases passage through the birth canal. (See Fig. 22-1.)

The mother is often concerned about the shape of her infant's head and should be told that the head will be symmetrical within the first year (p. 286). She is also likely to be concerned if her infant has a facial asymmetry. This occurs when the infant's head remains in a lateroflexed position in utero because the shoulder is pressed into the neck against the mandible.

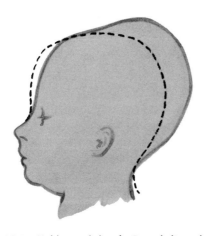

**Fig. 22-1.** Molding of head. Dotted line shows normal shape.

She may be told that this distorted appearance will gradually disappear.

### The chest

The chest is rounded; measurement is slightly smaller than that of the head and averages 12 to 13 inches. The contour of the trunk is normally cylindrical. By 6 months the circumference of the head and chest are approximately equal.

### The abdomen

The contour of the abdomen is cylindrical and relatively prominent. There are various factors that influence the general appearance of the newborn, such as race, size of the parents, and health of the mother.

### Weight

The range of birth weight and height is quite variable but on the average, full-term male infants are slightly larger (overall) than females. Their average birth weight is 7½ pounds, and the average length is 20 inches. "Total body water [is] 70-75% of body weight."[*]

A number of factors play a part in the size of the offspring: (1) the first born tends to weigh less at birth than later siblings, (2) mothers who smoke excessively tend to have smaller babies than mothers who do not smoke, (3) age and size of parents, and (4) interval between pregnancies.

The infant loses approximately 10% of his birth weight during the first few days of life. The greater loss is fluid rather than tissue, and the larger infant loses a greater proportion of his birth weight.

When the weight loss is more marked, symptoms of inanition fever are likely to appear. Temperature may elevate between 103° and 104° F. This may be avoided if the nurse will offer the infant sufficient fluids.

By the fifth day his weight becomes

---

[*]From Hughes, James G.: Synopsis of pediatrics, ed. 2, St. Louis, 1967, The C. V. Mosby Co., p. 171.

stable and by the tenth day, he regains his birth weight. The infant doubles his birth weight in five months and triples it in 12 months, all other factors being normal. New mothers tend to be overly concerned about their infant's weight. This need not be so if the nurse explains about their early adjustments and the reasons why they lose weight such as (1) small intake of fluids, (2) adjustment to formula, and (3) loss of meconium from the bowels and urine from the bladder.

### The mouth

The mouth is normally pink. Along the lower gums one may note gray-white lesions (inclusion cysts) that are frequently thought to be teeth. Extending beneath the tongue is a fold of tissue (frenulum linguae) that connects the tongue to the floor of the mouth. In some infants it extends to the tip of the tongue. Such infants have difficulty in nursing at the breast, especially when the mother's nipples are short or flat. When an infant has difficulty sucking, the nurse might examine the tongue, and if the frenulum is the cause, she should report this to the doctor. He may decide to clip the tip of the frenulum.

In examining the mouth the nurse may note the accumulation of epithelial cells (Epstein's pearls) over the posterior portion of the hard palate. They disappear in about 2 weeks.

### The eyes

At birth the eyes are a slate gray color. They assume their permanent color by 6 to 12 months.

*Subconjunctival hemorrhage.* When the infant opens his eyes, one may observe subconjunctival hemorrhages that are caused by congestion and rupture of capillaries during the birth process. These hemorrhages disappear in about 2 weeks.

*Incoordinate eye movements.* Poor neuromuscular control of orbital muscles results in random movements of the eyes (transient strabismus). Orbital muscular

control is gained gradually during the first 3 to 4 months of life.

*Setting-sun sign.* Poor neuromuscular control may also produce a downward displacement of the eyes that is called the *setting-sun sign.* This sign is also noted with hydrocephalus and kernicterus.

*Chemical conjunctivitis.* Chemical conjunctivitis occurs as the result of irritation induced by silver nitrate solution instilled into the eyes in the prophylaxis of gonorrheal ophthalmia. In addition to edema of the eyelids, the nurse will note a purulent discharge. The reaction is noticed within an hour or so after birth. See p. 287 for a discussion on bacterial conjunctivitis.

*Tearing.* The lacrimal glands do not function at birth, and tearing is not usually seen before 8 weeks. If the nurse does observe tearing, it may be due to blockage of the lacrimal ducts by exudate resulting from the irritation of silver nitrate.

### The genitals

In the female infant the labia minora are quite prominent and protrude over the labia majora. Within folds of the labia is a white substance called *smegma,* and a mucoid vaginal discharge may also be noted. This may be blood tinged—a physiological manifestation of maternal hormone transfer.

In the male infant the prepuce is usually adherent to the glans. Removal of this foreskin (circumcision) is recommended by most doctors. The testicles are usually in the scrotum. In some infants they remain in the inguinal canal. This is known as cryptorchidism. The nurse explains to the mother that in some infants the descent is delayed, especially in the premature.

### Posture

Variations in posture of the newborn are associated with uterine presentations. In a cephalic presentation the posture of the newborn is one of partial flexion with the chin resting on upper part of the sternum. As the days go by, this posture relaxes more and by the end of the neonatal period the infant tends to assume the tonic neck attitude when lying supine. He may keep the legs fully extended or they may remain elevated toward the chest. When the infant presents as a frank or complete breech, the mother should be informed that it may take several weeks before the legs will assume the usual posture. The feet are characteristically dorsiflexed.

### Neonatal bilirubinemia (physiological jaundice)[2]

At birth there is a gradual drop in the red blood cell count to an average of 5 million per cubic millimeter by the end of the second week. It is the function of the spleen to break up the hemoglobin from the worn out red cells. This pigment (end product) is released into circulation as indirect bilirubin (unconjugated or insoluble). It circulates to the liver and there an enzyme, glucuronyl transferase, catalyzes and transforms it to a soluble or direct bilirubin. Only after it is acted on

by this enzyme can it be excreted by the liver into the intestines and by the kidneys into the urine.

Physiological jaundice is due to hepatic immaturity because the liver may not be able to secrete sufficient glucuronyl to change the insoluble bilirubin to soluble form. This indirect bilirubin then accumulates in the tissues and results in symptoms of jaundice (bilirubinemia).

Physiological jaundice does not ordinarily appear before 36 hours after birth because it takes this amount of time for enough bilirubin to accumulate to stain the tissues.[*] By the third day the bilirubin level reaches 5 to 7 mg. per 100 ml., but it is considered normal if it is not in excess of 12 mg. per 100 ml. in the absence of hemolytic disease.

The deficiency of this enzyme is greater in the low birth weight infant, that is, they have more difficulty conjugating bilirubin. This is the reason why the jaundice

---

[*]Normal levels are 0.25 to 0.75 mg. per 100 ml.

| Mother's concern | Nurse's response |
|---|---|
| 1. Pink, papular rash on the body | 1. Erythema toxicum—etiology unknown; may be due to a response to the milk proteins |
| 2. Pinpoint papules over bridge of the nose and chin | 2. Milia—caused by overdistended sebaceous glands; tends to disappear spontaneously |
| 3. Swelling of the scalp | 3. Molding—skull bones overlap as head passes through birth canal; shape of the head will be normal within a few days |
| 4. Brick-red color to urine | 4. Limitation of kidney function; substance (uric acid crystals) excreted in the urine |
| 5. Red marks on infant's face | 5. Traumatized area from the birth process; usually forceps marks |
| 6. Soft spot on infant's head | 6. Area allowing for brain growth |
| 7. Hiccups | 7. Nerve stimuli—full stomach pushes against liver and diaphragm causing irritation |
| 8. Strabismus | 8. Immaturity of eye muscles |
| 9. Tremors or quivering of the lower jaw | 9. Uncontrolled response to stimuli |
| 10. Tremors of extremities | 10. Insufficiency of sufficient parathyroid hormone secretions to regulate calcium-phosphorus balance |

is evident *earlier* and *persists* longer in these infants.

When the nurse observes clinical jaundice in the newborn she may check the laboratory report and find that the plasma bilirubin level has reached 4 to 5 mg. per 100 ml. She may observe this icterus in the sclerae and in the posterior gum margins along with the skin, especially of the face and chest.

The infant so affected will show lack of interest in feeding and appear somewhat listless, but this jaundice requires no treatment. Clinically, it can no longer be detected by the seventh day.

Jaundice appearing within the first 24 hours of birth almost always indicates a blood incompatibility. See discussion on hyperbilirubinemia, p. 288.

There are a number of variants in the newborn that cause unnecessary apprehension in the mother. With simple explanation, the nurse can allay her anxieties.

## STUDY QUESTIONS
### Matching
Match the terms in the first column with their appropriate definition in the second column:

(a) Rapid respirations     __Gray-white lesions along lower gum margin

(b) Suture lines     __Scaphoid-shaped abdomen

(c) Lacrimal     __Caused by enzyme deficiency in the liver of the newborn infant

(d) Inclusion cysts     __Type respirations accompanying dyspnea

(e) Retinal hemorrhages     __Name of opening at junction of skull bones

(f) Physiological jaundice     __These glands do not function before eighth week after birth

(g) Milia     __Caused by over distention of sebaceous glands

(h) Fontanel     __Caused by rupture of capillaries during birth process

(i) Diaphragmatic hernia     __Name of membrane separating bones of the skull

### True or false
(T) (F) 1. Physiological jaundice in the newborn does not ordinarily appear before 72 hours after birth.

(T) (F) 2. First born infants are somewhat heavier on the average than later siblings.

(T) (F) 3. Smaller babies lose a proportionately greater amount of their birth weight than do the larger ones.

(T) (F) 4. An infant with erythema toxicum should be isolated.

(T) (F) 5. Jaundice appearing within the first 24 hours after birth almost always indicates a blood incompatibility.

### Multiple choice
1. One of the specific nursing measures of the recovery room nurse is that she maintain infant's temperature between:
   (a) 96.8° and 98.6° F.
   (b) 96° and 98° F.
   (c) 99° and 99.4° F.

2. The metabolism of the newborn infant, full-term and premature, is least at an environmental temperature of:
   (a) 89.6° to 93.2° F.
   (b) 93.5° to 94.2° F.
   (c) 95.6° to 89.6° F.

3. A mother questions you about the mongolian spots on her baby. Your response will be:
   (a) they are skin pigmentations with no anthropological significance.
   (b) they tend to disappear by the end of the second year.
   (c) they are permanent skin pigmentations.

4. When the environmental temperature is too low the infant will:
   (a) become listless.
   (b) become restless.
   (c) not respond to stimuli.

5. On exposure to cold:
   (a) the full-term infant can increase his rate of metabolism.
   (b) the full-term and premature infant can increase their rate of metabolism.
   (c) the sweat glands are active and help increase rate of metabolism.

6. Normally the full-term infant's respirations are:
   (a) largely diaphragmatic, irregular in depth and rhythm.
   (b) largely abdominal, irregular in depth and rhythm.
   (c) largely diaphragmatic, irregular in depth but regular in rhythm.

7. Full-term, healthy newborn infants normally:
   (a) regain birth weight by the tenth day.
   (b) regain birth weight by end of the second week.
   (c) double their birth weight by end of the neonatal period.

8. Physiological jaundice appears:
   (a) earlier and persists longer in the low birth weight infant.

(b) later but persists longer in low birth weight infants.

(c) earlier but persists longer in the full-term infant.

9. While caring for the infant with physiological jaundice, the nurse will expect him to:
   (a) be listless.
   (b) show little interest in feeding.
   (c) have a subnormal temperature.
   1. a only    2. a and b    3. all of these

10. The infant in respiratory distress will:
    (a) be limp and weak.
    (b) be hyperactive.
    (c) always have a high-pitched cry.

## REFERENCES

1. Schaffer, Alexander: Diseases of the newborn, Philadelphia, 1965, W. B. Saunders Co., p. 860.
2. Smith, Carl: Blood diseases of infancy and childhood, ed. 2, St. Louis, 1966, The C. V. Mosby Co., chap. 8.

## SELECTED READINGS

Blake, Florence, and Wright, F. Howell: Essentials of pediatric nursing, ed. 7, Philadelphia, 1963, J. B. Lippincott Co., chap. 7.

Eastman, Nicholson J., and Hellman, Louis M., editors: Williams' obstetrics, ed. 13, New York, 1966, Appleton-Century-Crofts, chap. 20.

Holt, L. Emmett, McIntosh, Rustin, and Barnett, Henry: Pediatrics, ed. 13, New York, 1962, Appleton-Century-Crofts, pp. 95-100.

Hughes, James G.: Synopsis of pediatrics, ed. 2, St. Louis, 1967, The C. V. Mosby Co., chap. 10.

McKay, R. J., Jr., and Smith, Clement A.: The physical examination. In Nelson, Waldo E., editor: Textbook of pediatrics, ed. 8, Philadelphia, 1964, W. B. Saunders Co., pp. 339-344.

Schaffer, Alexander: Diseases of the newborn, Philadelphia, 1965, W. B. Saunders Co., chaps. 96, 108, and 109.

**For student's quick notes:**

# Chapter 23

# The mother, the neonate, and the nurse

The mother and her infant need to become acquainted with each other because they both have adjustments to make. Chapter 23 gives you insight into normal and abnormal responses and will help you understand the mother's various reactions.

## Infant's initial visit with the mother

It is not "natural" to separate a mother from her baby. In doing so we add to the emotional tension and anxiety experienced during parturition. After admission procedures are completed, the infant should be taken to the mother. It may be that she saw the infant in the delivery room, but if she was delivered under anesthesia, it is likely that her first view of the baby was rather vague. It relieves anxiety and tension if the mother is permitted to examine her baby, while the nurse stays by the bedside and answers any immediate questions she might have concerning him. Such thoughtful simple gestures mean a great deal to the new mother and no nurse can be too busy to extend this courtesy.

All mothers-to-be dream about what their infant will be like. Reality may be quite different from a 9-month fantasy and when she first looks on her infant she begins to realize that the baby is far from what she expected. With time on her hands, she wonders about her motherliness and her feelings toward the infant. These thoughts contribute to the emotional lag discussed on p. 211. She needs someone to talk with, and who but the nursery nurse should recognize this and take time to discuss these responses with the mother.

## Factors influencing various early responses to neonate

The normal attitude of parents toward the offspring is acceptance manifested in love and affection. Variables in response to the newborn are manifold and are attributed to a host of influences. The new parents must be given time to become reconciled to their status of parenthood; for some persons this may be a tremendous responsibility. One or both may be struggling to adjust to parenthood according to their cultural background.

Parturition has its psychological affects on the mother as well as physiological. Giving birth is an abrupt interruption of unity between the mother and her fetus, and in some women it takes time for "maternal feelings" to develop. Actually, the new mother has a strong need to be mothered herself. When her husband and close family members provide emotional support, she can better adjust to the new role.

### Effects of labor

Women who have difficult labors and require deep anesthesia for delivery are more likely to experience an emotional lag in responding to their newborn. They are not ready to "mother" the infant as early in the postpartum period as is the mother who required little sedation or who participated in the birth. These mothers respond with open arms whereas those who were deeply anesthetized experience little gratification or fulfillment and describe their feelings as "empty" or "inadequate."

*Overanxiety*

The nurse should recognize overanxiety. This is more likely to occur when the woman has had a previous stillbirth, or there has been a death among siblings. Overanxiety may even occur when the infant is rejected.

A mother cannot enjoy her infant if she is filled with fear. She needs a supportive nurse to help her become familiar with the patterns of her infant's behavior and to explain the characteristic variants. She is likely to be concerned about his irregular breathing, his reflexes, especially the startle reflex, rashes, mucus, and crying. The nurse, while explaining these normal reactions, should put stress on the infant's positive characteristics such as good muscle tone and good sucking reflex.

*Rejections*

One new mother may complain because the infant is brought to her so soon after birth, while another repeatedly asks to see her newborn. Not all mothers "yearn" to care for their babies. Attitudes of rejection are more likely to be observed in the following situations: (1) there is marital discord; (2) the infant has a defect; (3) the pregnancy is premarital; (4) the parents were raised in a home where children were a burden; (5) either one or both parents are disappointed in the sex of the infant; (6) the new mother experienced emotional deprivation during her childhood, and (7) the woman is deeply involved in a profession.

## The neonate's emotional response[1,2]

It is the general agreement that meeting the physical needs of infants is not sufficient.

Neonates differ in response to emotional stimulation. Some infants need to be picked up and mothered frequently. Their distress is relieved only when soothed and held close. Other neonates display stress reactions when handled frequently. The newborn may lack sensitivity to the world about him, but he certainly responds to the warmth and security of mothering. His response to this manifestation of love is the foundation of all behavior patterns. Meeting the neonate's early emotional needs is step "one" in the formation of his personality. Some authorities question whether this security is important to him during the first few days of life, but there is little doubt that the tactile sensations which the newborn experiences as you hold him, comfort him, and feed him convey this feeling of security.

*Crying*

Very early the infant learns that comfort and security can be restored on demand. During the neonatal period, the mother learns to interpret whether the cry is an emotional response to hunger, discomfort, or pain. The mother also learns that her baby's cry is different from cries of others and that the cry varies in intensity with his need, whether it is hunger, pain, or the need to be cuddled.

*Sleep and activity*

Each infant has his own adaptive, self-regulatory pattern for sleep and activity. By observation the nurse soon learns that each infant is a unique individual. He behaves according to his needs and responds as they are satisfied. Some infants do not require as much sleep as others; they are awake for longer periods of time and are more active. Others sleep from one feeding to another and when awake appear quite content, showing little sensitivity to stimuli.

The nurse may expect the infant to be quite sleepy or inactive for 1 or 2 days after birth, especially if the mother was heavily sedated during labor and under deep anesthesia for the delivery. Some of these infants are problems and develop inanition fever. In contrast there are those who seldom seem to relax; they are irritable and hyperactive. The thought has been expressed that this may be due to hyperactivity of the mother during pregnancy. These infants startle easily and tend to rub off the superficial layers of the skin of their heels, knees, and toes, and they have disturbed sleep patterns. They do, indeed, need the security of mothering. They should never be left to "cry it out." When the infant signals distress, he deserves attention. The busy nurse will find that if she wraps the infant securely in a soft, warm blanket and places him gently in the corner of his bed, he will relax and fall asleep. The feeling of the blanket certainly does not replace the security of the mother's or nurse's arms, but it does quiet and help the infant rest when the nurse has many others to care for.

## REFERENCES

1. Bakwin, Harry, and Bakwin, Ruth: Clinical management of behavior disorders in children, ed. 3, Philadelphia, 1966, W. B. Saunders Co., pp. 10-11.
2. Blake, Florence, and Wright, F. Howell: Essentials of pediatric nursing, ed. 7, Philadelphia, 1963, J. B. Lippincott Co., p. 140.

## SELECTED READINGS
*Factors influencing responses of the neonate*

Bakwin, Harry, and Bakwin, Ruth: Clinical management of behavior disorders in children, ed. 3, Philadelphia, 1966, W. B. Saunders Co., pp. 53-54.

Carey, Wm.: Maternal anxiety and infantile colic. Is there a relationship? Clin. Pediat. 7:590, Oct., 1968.

Chess, Stella: Individuality in children, its importance to the pediatrician, J. Pediat. 70:676, Oct., 1966.

Deutsch, Helen: The psychology of women, New York, 1945, Grune & Stratton, Inc., chaps. 7 and 8.

Hurlock, Elizabeth B.: Child development, ed. 4, New York, 1964, McGraw-Hill Book Co., pp. 98-99.

Newton, Niles: Maternal emotions, New York, 1955, Paul E. Hoeber, Inc., chap. 5.

Paradise, Jack L.: Do tense mothers tend to have colicky babies, RN 30:107, Jan., 1967.

Robson, Kenneth: The role of eye-to-eye contact in maternal-infant attachment, Mental Health Digest, p. 12, Jan., 1968.

Rosenblum, Leonard A., and Kaufman, J. Charles: Variations in infant development and response to maternal loss in monkeys, Amer. J. Orthopsychiat. 38:418, April, 1968.

Scheinfeld, Amram: Your heredity and environment, ed. 4, Philadelphia, 1965, J. B. Lippincott Co., p. 34.

Smitherman, Colleen: The vocal behavior of infants as related to the nursing procedure of rocking, Nurs. Res. 18:256, May-June, 1969.

Taylor, Ann: Deprived infants: potential for affective adjustment, Amer. J. Orthopsychiat. 38:835, Oct., 1968.

Watson, E. H., and Lowrey, G. H.: Growth and development of children, ed. 5, Chicago, 1967, Year Book Medical Publishers, Inc., p. 170.

**For student's quick notes:**

Chapter 24

# Growth and development
# of the neonate

Growth and development of the neonate occur at a rapid pace. You may be astonished at both the physiological and psychological changes that occur during this period, and at how variable their needs are, even during the few days the infant is in your care. Chapter 24 deals with this growth and development.

### Sensory status

The structure of the sense organs is well developed at birth, but response is not very acute. Even as early as the first day, infants will respond differently to external stimuli. These differences are probably transient and have little or no bearing on future behavior. (See Fig. 24-1.)

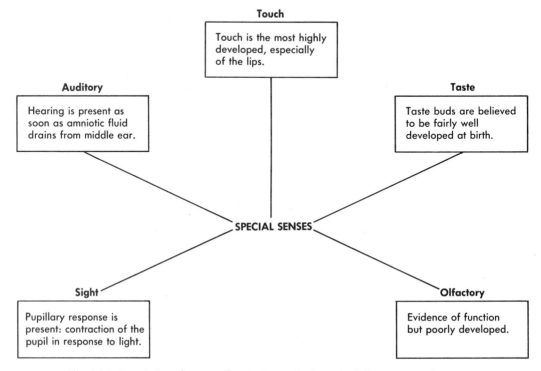

Fig. 24-1. Description of sensory functioning at birth in the full-term, normal neonate.

# Development of reflex behavior

Eye blinking  ——————→
> Blink response is positive. It may be induced by stimulating the sucking reflex.

Sucking  ——————→
> The healthy, normal newborn will suck on response to oral stimuli. This reflex can be observed as the infant sleeps.

Rooting or mouthing  ——————→
> The infant will turn his head in the direction of the stimuli when the cheek is lightly touched. If the infant's cheek is placed against the mother's breast he will "root" for the nipple and move his lips in preparation for sucking. By the second day the sucking and rooting for the nipple should be quite acute. This is a good sign of alertness of the infant. It disappears between the sixth and twelfth month.

Moro  ——————→
> This reflex may be elicited by a sharp bang on the table. One will note an abduction and extension of the arms, hands open with "C" position of the fingers, and movement of the legs. This reflex disappears within 6 to 8 weeks. Persistence beyond 4 months may indicate neurological damage.

Startle  ——————→
> This reflex may be elicited by sudden tapping of the sternum or by a loud noise; the elbow will flex and the hand remain closed. Should not be confused with Moro reflex.

Extrusion reflex  ——————→
> This reflex causes infant to extrude any substance placed on anterior portion of the tongue. Reflex diminishes about the fourth month and facilitates ingestion of semisolid foods.

Deglutition reflex  ——————→
> The deglutition reflex permits swallowing of fluids. Immaturity of this reflex is one of the reasons some infants regurgitate so frequently.

Walking reflex  ——————→
> Flexion and extension of the legs, simulating walking, can be elicited by supporting infant in an upright position with soles of feet against flat surface. This reflex disappears after 4 to 6 weeks. (See Fig. 24-2.)

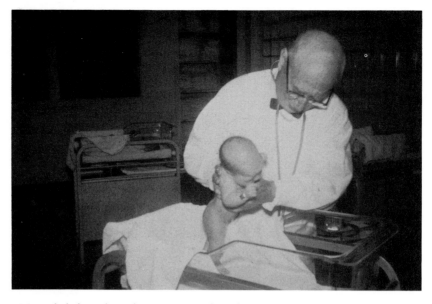

**Fig. 24-2.** Included in physical examination of newborn infant is testing of reflexes. This illustrates the "walking reflex."

Crying reflex      ⟶

> It has been hypothesized that crying is a reflex in response to physical or psychological stimulation that signals the need for attention. Hunger and discomfort will elicit this reflex.

Babinski reflex      ⟶

> The infant will extend big toe and flex other toes when the sole of the foot is stroked.

Grasp suspension or palmar reflex      ⟶

> This reflex may be elicited by placing a thin object in palm of infant's hand. The fingers will flex and grasp the object. As traction is applied, the arm can be drawn upward until the infant hangs from the fingers momentarily. Reflex is strongest at 40 weeks' gestation and disappears in most infants by 3 months.

Tonic neck reflex or fencing position      ⟶

> When the infant is in supine position and quiet, he lies with his head turned to one side, with the arm extended on the same side, and with the other arm bent. This reflex appears late in the neonatal period. It disappears in the normal infant between second and third month. In cerebral palsy the reflex tends to persist.

## Body systems
### Circulatory system

Within a few minutes after birth the structures functioning in fetal circulation are occluded, and circulation of the pulmonary system is established, with oxygenated blood circulating throughout the infant's body. The nurse may observe a bluish tinge to pink color of some newborns during the first day of life. This is due to intermingling of arterial and venous blood.

The red blood cell count and hemoglobin level are high at birth, averaging 6 million per cubic millimeter and 12 to 22 grams per 100 ml., respectively. The hematocrit averages 52%. Even though the mother may be anemic, the infant usually has a normal hemoglobin concentration at birth, but he may quickly develop anemia.

The red blood cell count decreases to between 3 and 4 million by 6 weeks, a temporary anemia that disappears by the sixth month as bone marrow activity becomes established. The hemoglobin declines gradually and by 2 weeks of age the infant starts to use reserve iron stored in his liver. Blood volume approximates 10% of the infant's weight, but the volume averages more if blood is allowed to flow from the placenta into the infant (equivalent to 25%).

The white blood cell count is variable but averages 15,000 to 20,000 per cubic millimeter at birth, and then declines to approximately 12,000 per cubic millimeter by the end of the first week.

### Digestive system

Although the digestive system is immature at birth, absorption and utilization of nutrients are satisfactory, except for fats. The neonate requires more nourishment in proportion to his weight than does the

### NORMAL INFANT STOOLS

| Stools of breast fed infant[2] | Stools of artificially fed infant |
|---|---|
| 1. Feces soft<br>2. Fermentive flora high in *L. bifidus* (no pathogens); produces acid media and inhibits growth of putrefactive organisms; low pH 4 to 6<br>3. Inoffensive odor result of fermentation instead of putrefaction<br>4. Greenish yellow color<br>5. More frequent due to ease with which feces pass through colon | 1. Feces more firm<br>2. Mixed flora (coliform, putrefactive); some putrefactive organisms are pathogens; high pH, 6 to 8<br>3. Putrefactive bacteria cause strong odor to feces<br>4. Brownish yellow color<br>5. Less frequent |

### ABNORMAL INFANT STOOLS

| Signs and symptoms | Probable cause |
|---|---|
| 1. Clay-colored stool<br>2. Large amount of mucus<br>3. Tarry stools | 1. Indicates abnormality of the bile duct<br>2. Irritation of the intestines<br>3. May be the result of blood swallowed during passage through the birth canal, or bleeding into the intestinal tract; Downey-Apt test will differentiate maternal from fetal hemoglobin |

adult, but the quantity and quality must coincide with his ability to assimilate the nutrients. The infant who is artificially fed does not always tolerate the formula prepared for him, and consequently digestive disturbances occur that result in refusal to feed, vomiting, and diarrhea.

The gastric glands are functioning at birth. Hydrochloric acid and the two enzymes pepsin and rennin are important in contributing to digestion in the stomach. Casein is acted on by rennin and precipitates as a large curd in artificial preparations, whereas the protein in human milk (lactalbumin) precipitates as a fine, soft curd contributing to ease of digestion.

The stomach of the infant receiving breast milk empties in 2 to 3 hours; when artificially fed, emptying time is longer.

As in the adult, the greater part of digestion takes place in the duodenum and small intestines. Protein not acted on by gastric chemistry is subjected to pancreatic and intestinal secretions; the resultant amino acids are converted into body proteins or burned. What part do the large intestines contribute? Primarily, they absorb water, although sugars reaching the intestines are fermented by the bacteria that multiply rapidly as food is given. The high lactose content in breast milk is acted on by the *Lactobacillus bifidus* and converted into lactic acid, a medium that hinders the growth of pathogens.

The liver is relatively large in the newborn. This is understood when we recall that it served as an important organ in blood formation during fetal existence. If the mother's diet was adequate in iron, the infant will have a sufficient amount stored in his liver to aid in hemoglobin formation for the first 5 months of his life.

The first functioning of the digestive system is evidenced by passage of the meconium plug and then meconium stools. The meconium plug is a mass of meconium formed in the terminal part of the rectum during fetal existence. It differs from meconium in that it is lighter in color, thicker in consistency, and covered by a pseudo-membranous sac. On rare occasions this plug may interfere with the first defecation and the anal ring may have to be dilated by digital examination (meconium plug syndrome).[1,3] This stimulates peristalsis and contributes to the mass being passed spontaneously.

Meconium is a sticky, greenish black, odorless material secreted during intrauterine life and consists of bile pigments, mucus, vernix, lanugo, hormones, enzymes, and carbohydrates. The first stool is normally passed within 24 hours of birth. An infant who does not pass a stool by this time should be seen by the doctor. It may be due to lower bowel obstruction, meconium ileus, or imperforate anus.

After the infant starts digesting formula or breast milk, the meconium is replaced by the typical transitional stool that is greenish brown and soft in texture. It may contain remnants of meconium. About the fourth day the stools become yellow in color. The number of stools per day is variable and is affected by amount and type of formula and by the muscle tone of the gastrointestinal tract. As food enters the stomach, it stimulates peristalsis in the lower intestinal tract. The nurse may notice that the infant usually has a bowel movement after each feeding. This is called *physiological diarrhea.*

The pediatrician is interested in the character of the feces; it gives evidence of the physiology of the infant's digestion.

### Endocrine system

Endocrine disturbances in the mother may be reflected in the neonate. Hypertrophy of the islands of Langerhans (seen in infants born of diabetic mothers) and congenital exophthalmic goiter in neonates whose mothers have history of hyperthyroidism may appear.

***Hypocalcemic tetany.*** Hypocalcemic tetany is an increased neuromuscular irritability that results from lack of calcium. The normal blood calcium level is 9 to 11 mg. per 100 ml. If it is below 8.0 mg. per 100 ml. and the phosphorus blood level is above 7.0 mg. per 100 ml., the nurse may expect symptoms of hypocalcemia and observes the infant for jerky movements of the extremities and, in some cases, periods of cyanosis.

Postnatal hypocalcemia is likely to be seen the first day of life when the mother had a difficult labor and delivery, in infants born of diabetic mothers, and in premature infants. Tetany of the newborn is usually not observed clinically until days after birth or even 1 or 2 weeks postnatally. It is manifested more in the artificially fed infant due to difference in the calcium: phosphorus ratio of cow's milk (increased phosphorus, decreased calcium concentration). The recommended calcium:phosphorus ratio for the neonate's diet is 1.5:1. Calcium chloride, 1 to 2 grams, or calcium lactate, 3 to 4 grams, may be added to the formula each day in divided doses to prevent or to treat hypocalcemic tetany.

Hypocalcemic tetany is also attributed to poor clearance of phosphorus by the immature kidneys, physiological hypofunction of the parathyroid glands, and alkalosis resulting from hyperventilation.

Maternal endocrine physiology may be manifested in the neonate. Two examples of this are (1) pseudomenstration and (2) breast hypertrophy.

*Pseudomenstruation.* Because of the sudden withdrawal of estrogen in the uterine endometrium, the female infant may exhibit slight vaginal spotting called *pseudomenstruation*. The mother certainly needs to know that it regresses rapidly and that it is no cause for concern.

*Breast hypertrophy.* The nurse may note breast hypertrophy in both sexes, with minute secretions resembling colostrum called *witch's milk*. This is due to the presence of maternal hormones in the infant. The mother should be instructed not to manipulate the breasts, since this may predispose to mastitis. Hypertrophy recedes spontaneously with a few days.

Endocrine disturbances in the mother may also be reflected in the neonate. Ex-

amples of this are hypertrophy of the islands of Langerhans in infants born of diabetic mothers and congenital exophthalmic goiter in nonates whose mothers have a history of hyperthyroidism.

### Hemopoietic system

The liver and spleen are important organs of blood formation during fetal life, and they retain the ability to make blood cells for sometime after birth (p. 262). The life-span of the infant's red blood cells is between 60 and 100 days.

### Nervous system

The newborn has the ability to signal his needs and the capacity to respond to those who mother him. At birth the brain is well advanced structurally but not functionally. The cerebral areas are slower in developing; hence, they are not ready to function to any great extent at this early period of adaptation. The newborn's early response depends on neuromuscular development. He functions, therefore, on a reflex level, and minutes after birth one may observe movements such as sucking and blinking that will later be followed by sneezing, stretching, and hiccuping. His perception of the world is a slow, gradual process. By the end of the neonatal period one may observe the first sign of cerebration—he begins to watch his mother when she speaks to him.

### Urinary system

The infant does well without fluids for the first few hours after birth, since he has ample water in his tissues (35% of body weight). The nurse will note a negative physiological response for approximately the first 24 hours; that is, he may not void for that period of time even though urine is usually in the bladder at birth. To handle excretion of the metabolic wastes, ample water is needed. This is met during the neonatal period if he nurses regularly or receives an adequate amount of formula. Some pediatricians recommend glucose water between feedings to aid tubule resorption and to prevent dehydration and the development of jaundice. This is especially so during the summer months or if the infant is febrile.

The glomeruli of his kidneys are mature, but the tubules are limited in their ability to function adequately. They are unable to maintain water and electrolyte balance (resorb water and selected solutes) until about 6 weeks after birth. Urine is hypotonic with low clearance of sodium, chloride, and urea. The kidneys are also limited in their ability to respond to an abnormal fluid balance such as in diarrhea or with improper feedings. He may go from one extreme to the other—from dehydration to edema.

## STUDY QUESTIONS
### Matching
Match the terms in the first column with their appropriate definitions in the second column:

(a) Meconium ileus    ___This reflex disappears in most full-term infants by 3 months of age

(d) Tetany    ___Most highly developed of the five special senses

(c) Grasp reflex    ___Permits swallowing of fluids

(d) Irritation of intestines    ___Abdominal distention is a prominent sign of this abnormality

(e) Abnormality of bile duct    ___Increased neuromuscular irritability

(f) Touch    ___This reflex normally disappears by the twelfth month

(g) Deglutition reflex    ___Large amount of mucus in the stools

(h) Rooting reflex    ___Clay-colored stool

### True or false
(T) (F) 1. Persistance of the Moro reflex beyond 3 months may indicate neurological damage.

(T) (F) 2. Hemoglobin and hematocrit are higher in the newborn than in the adult.

(T) (F) 3. The first sign of cerebration occurs between fifth and eighth week of life.

(T) (F) 4. Bile in the newborn infant's stool is not normal.

(T) (F) 5. Kidney tubules are limited in their ability to function adequately at birth.

(T) (F) 6. Tremors of the extremities may be due to insufficient parathyroid hormone.

(T) (F) 7. The immediate newborn is not capable of responding emotionally.

(T) (F) 8. Emotional deprivation during a woman's childhood may be a reason for maternal rejection.

(T) (F) 9. Women who are not ready to "mother" their infants at birth lack maternal instinct.

(T) (F) 10. All healthy mothers yearn to care for their babies.

(T) (F) 11. Attitudes of mothers toward their newborn tend to be unstable the first few days of life.

(T) (F) 12. The tonic neck reflex tends to persist in an infant with cerebral palsy.

## REFERENCES
1. McKay, R. J., Jr., and Smith, Clement A.: Meconium plug. In Nelson, Waldo E., editor: Textbook of pediatrics, ed. 8, Philadelphia, 1964, W. B. Saunders Co., p. 378.
2. Meyer, Herman: Infant foods and feeding, Springfield, Ill., 1960, Charles C Thomas, Publisher, p. 66.
3. Schaffer, Alexander: Diseases of the newborn, Philadelphia, 1965, W. B. Saunders Co., p. 390.

## SELECTED READINGS
Bakwin, Harry, and Bakwin, Ruth: Clinical management of behavior disorders in children, ed. 3, Philadelphia, 1966, W. B. Saunders Co., pp. 7-9.
Broadribb, Violet: Foundations of pediatric nursing, Philadelphia, 1967, J. B. Lippincott Co., chap. 7.
Illingworth, R. S.: The development of the infant and young child, ed. 3, Baltimore, 1966, The Williams & Wilkins Co., p. 117.
McKay, R. J., Jr., and Smith, Clement A.: Physiology of the newborn infant. In Nelson, Waldo E., editor: Textbook of pediatrics, ed. 8, Philadelphia, 1964, W. B. Saunders Co., p. 330.
Schaffer, Alexander: Diseases of the newborn, Philadelphia, 1965, W. B. Saunders Co., p. 497.
Silberstein, Richard, and Dolgin, Joseph: The cephalic reflex: an aspect of the rooting reflex, Clin. Pediat. 6:305, May, 1967.
Watson, E. H., and Lowrey, G. H.: Growth and development of children, ed. 5, Chicago, 1967, Year Book Medical Publishers, Inc., p. 297.

**For student's quick notes:**

# Chapter 25

# Feeding the neonate

Whether the mother chooses the feed her baby the "natural" way or the "artificial" way is her decision to make. You will learn about the various factors contributing to her choice, and how you can be a source of help to her. You will learn about the neonate's nutritional requirements, and how you can assist the mother in learning about the feeding habits of her infant.

## Meditation

As you set your lips to the source of
   your strength and growth
Even so I, my son, turn my heart to
   the source of mine.
Your nourishment is more than a chemical
   accomplishment,
And my provision for you is more than
   milk.
Drink deeply, my son, for we are
   building a man—
You and I and God, in this mystical,
   maternal moment.
"As a child quieted on its mother's breast
   As a child that is quieted is my soul."

*Mary Fritz*
SAN JOSE, CALIFORNIA

## Nutritional requirements
### Caloric needs

Utilization of food is another transition the newborn must make. The newborn grows rapidly during infancy; his metabolic rate is greater (twice that of the adult), and therefore his caloric requirement per unit of weight is higher during this time. At 10 days he requires 50 to 55 calories per pound of body weight.

The average requirement of the healthy newborn (at about 10 days) is 2½ ounces of "mature" breast milk, equivalent to 50 calories per pound of body weight per day,

supplemented with vitamin D and, in some instances, vitamin C. This is a guide, but it must be kept in mind that nutrient needs may vary markedly for infants of the same age and weight. Weight gain averages 5 to 8 ounces per week. As the infant utilizes his nourishment, body-water content decreases and mineral content increases to bring about calcification of bones.

The fact that both human and cow's milk is low in iron is no cause for concern. The iron obtained transplacentally is sufficient for the full-term infant's needs during this early period (p. 262).

### Water requirement

The newborn infant's water requirement is met if he receives a formula calculated at 20 calories per ounce (breast milk yields 20 calories to the ounce). Supplementary feedings of water may be ordered during the summer months or if the infant is febrile.

The newborn requires a simplified form of nourishment and nature provides this directly from the mother's body.

## Introduction to breast feeding[4]

There is no finer introduction for the newborn to extrauterine life than to be placed at his mother's breast. To be well-cared for, the neonate needs this emotional warmth. Woman's physiology prepares her to reestablish just such a symbiosis. The skin to skin contact reunites mother and infant; she again becomes his source of protection, security, and nourishment. Then, too, she needs to feel the infant's dependence on her, although she may not be aware of this.

The decision to breast feed must be the mother's, but the nurse's attitude has a tremendous influence on the mother who did not decide during her pregnancy how she wished to nourish her infant or who is still undecided after delivery. The nurse who understands the nutritional value of human milk and the psychological value to both mother and infant will take time to visit with the mother before the initial feeding, will discuss the art of breast feeding with her, and, thus, will help her get off to a happy start.

She will explain that the infant's behavior is not well organized at birth and that the demand for nourishment during the first few days of life is irregular; in some infants it is frequent, in others it is infrequent. He will take what he needs for nourishment and satisfy his need to suck. When lactation is fully established, the milk supply will be regulated by her infant's demands. The nurse will further explain that the first few days of nursing are for initiating the sucking stimulus primary to the flow of milk and, of course, that nursing provides the best possible way for both mother and child to become acquainted with each other. This sucking prepares her nipples for the task of vigorous nursing to follow. The mother may experience discomfort in her nipples if the infant nurses vigorously, but this will subside within a short time.

The success in initiating breast feeding depends on the mother's attitude toward this physiological process. Factors involved are (1) genetic makeup of the mother, (2) adequate understanding of the physiology of lactation, and (3) encouraging support of her husband, family, doctor, and nurses.

## Value of colostrum

During the first few days of life, if the infant is fed solely from the breast, one could say it goes through a period of physiological starvation as far as milk intake is concerned. If the infant has a good sucking reflex, it receives "small" amounts of colostrum at each nursing. Nature has a plan in that this unique preparation is adequate for the newborn until the flow of milk is established. Colostrum is yellow in color and rich in protein and minerals; it has less fat and slightly less sugar than mature human milk. The fluid portion is primarily serum albumin. Then, too, its laxative effect helps the infant get rid of meconium.

Many women are unaware of colostrum, and when they see the watery consistency of the secretions from the breasts, they assume their "milk" to be weak and arrive at the decision to abandon breast feeding before secretion of milk has even started.

It is known that antibodies are transferred to the fetus via the transplacental route, but whether human colostrum is a means of transferring passive immunity is still questionable. There is scientific proof indicating that antibodies against polio are present in human milk.[3,7]

Some pediatricians believe that it is important to give a carbohydrate substrate to the infant to avoid severe jaundice (bilirubinemia) and start the infant on glucose water 6 to 8 hours after birth; other pediatricians practice an initial starvation period.[2,6] Excess pregnanediol (excretion product of progesterone) in breast milk is said to inhibit the activity of glucuronyl transferase and contribute to bilirubinemia. This is only a temporary phenomenon and stimulation of lactation should be continued. On p. 64 you learned that the lactogenic hormone acted directly on the alveolar epithelium. As the milk is secreted, it is stored in the ampulla of the duct. The lactiferous ducts that serve as a reservoir terminate in the nipple and excrete the milk through minute openings in the nipple. For 1 or 2 weeks the mother secretes "transition" milk; it is not until near the end of the neonatal period that she secretes "mature" milk.

### Nutritive composition of breast milk

Women of different genetic makeup secrete milk of different nutritive composition. Women in what we rate as undernourished countries of the world are able to maintain satisfactory lactation periods far beyond what the majority of American mothers are able to maintain. "Studies of poor Indian women showed that increase in protein content of the mother's diet from 60 to 79 grams resulted in no change in the protein content of the milk."*

---

*From Guthrie, Helen Andrews: Introductory nutrition, St. Louis, 1967, The C. V. Mosby Co., p. 328.

When the mother is severely malnourished, the milk will be of inferior quality, but a satisfactory amount can be maintained, however, at the expense of further depleting her own health. The health of the lactating mother can only be ensured if her nutrition is satisfactory.

Even though living standards rise, prenatal education improves, and the value of breast feeding is emphasized, all of this means little to the American woman personally in her "midst of plenty." Those from the lower economic and educational groups nurse their infants less frequently than women of the higher income groups. Although cow's milk is modified to resemble human milk, it is a "substitute" nourishment for the infant; nevertheless, it is the preferred feeding of most American women. It is in areas of the world where

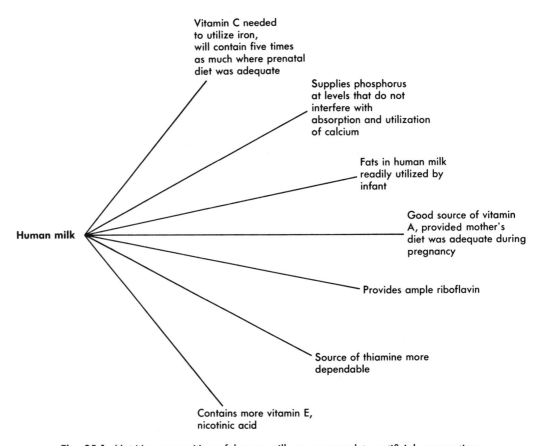

**Fig. 25-1.** Nutritive composition of human milk as compared to artificial preparations.

malnutrition is a threat that breast feeding is very important. (See Table 25-1 and Figs. 25-1 and 25-2.)

In looking at Table 25-2 you will see that human milk contains only half as much protein as cow's milk. This is compensated for in that the protein in human milk is predominately lactalbumin. Lactalbumin forms a soft curd in the infant's stomach and, thus, facilitates action of the digestive enzymes.

The advantage of the high lactose content in breast milk (twice that in cow's milk) over the other carbohydrates is that it facilitates amino acid, calcium, phosphorus, and magnesium absorption and nitrogen retention. Therefore mineral content of bones is increased. Lactose is also favorably acted on by *Lactobacillus bifidus* in the lower gastrointestinal tract, which converts it into lactic acid. Such an acid medium hinders growth of pathogens and thus decreases the likelihood of infection. Intestinal production of riboflavin and pyridoxine is favored when lactose is the principal carbohydrate in milk.

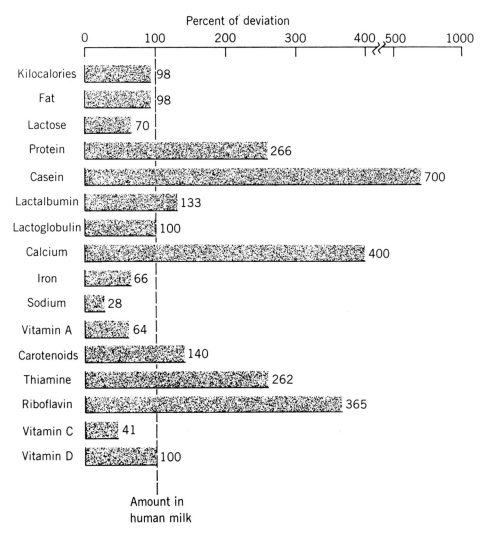

**Fig. 25-2.** Relative amounts of various nutrients in human and cow's milk. (From Guthrie, Helen Andrews: Introductory nutrition, St. Louis, 1967, The C. V. Mosby Co.)

Table 25-1. Substances excreted in breast milk

| Substance | Exceptions | Effect on infant |
|---|---|---|
| Alcohol | Not excreted unless intake is excessive; is eliminated rapidly from mother's body | None |
| Atropine* | Excreted in milk; diminishes milk flow | May affect infant |
| Barbiturates | Generally in small amounts | Acts as sedative if amount excreted is excessive |
| Bromides | | May cause occasional skin eruptions; produces symptoms of drowsiness |
| Caffeine | Excreted in small amounts | None |
| Dilantin | Little, if any, excreted | None |
| Hyoscine | | None |
| Morphine | | When mother is known drug addict, withdrawal symptoms will be noted in infant when mother attempts to wean infant |
| Penicillin | | None |
| Purgatives such as senna and cascara | | Does affect infant |
| Quinine | | None |
| Sodium salicylate | | None |
| Sulfonamides | | None |
| Nicotine | | Believed by some investigators to diminish flow of milk |

*Not excreted according to some investigators.

## Factors influencing secretion and flow of milk
### Problems of the new mother

While in the hospital, mothers have the problem of keeping the infant awake to nurse. This so often happens when infants are on a rigid hospital schedule. What the mother does not know is that the infant may have been crying for a long period of time in the nursery; his demands to be fed were not met, and when he is finally brought to the mother, he is exhausted, nurses for 1 or 2 minutes, and then falls asleep. He is contented for the time with the emotional warmth of the mother's breast. When the infant is taken from the comfort of its mother's arms and placed in the crib, he invariably awakens and starts the cycle all over again. The nurse not interested in breast feeding is all too ready to give him a supplementary feeding of artificial nourishment and notates on the infant's chart, "infant refused breast!" The nurse with little practical experience in breast feeding and inhibitions as to its psychological value will advocate bottle feeding to this troubled mother, and since the early puerperium is a period of instability, mothers are sensitive and easily persuaded. It is a fact that many new mothers desire and look forward to nursing their infant, but give up because of this

**Table 25-2.** The composition of colostrum; immature and mature human milk and cow's milk per 100 ml. of milk*

| Nutrient | Human Colostrum (1 to 5 days) | Human Transitional (6 to 10 days) | Human Mature | Mature cow's milk |
|---|---|---|---|---|
| Energy, kilocalories | 58.0 | 74.0 | 71.0 | 69.0 |
| Fat, grams | 2.9 | 3.6 | 3.8 | 3.7 |
| Lactose, grams | 5.3 | 6.6 | 7.0 | 4.8 |
| Protein, grams | 2.7 | 1.6 | 1.2 | 3.3 |
| Casein, grams | 1.2 | 0.7 | 0.4 | 2.8 |
| Lactalbumin, grams | | 0.8 | 0.3 | 0.4 |
| Calcium, mg. | 31.0 | 34.0 | 33.0 | 125.0 |
| Phosphorus, mg. | 14.0 | 17.0 | 15.0 | 96.0 |
| Iron, mg. | 0.09 | 0.04 | 0.15 | 0.10 |
| Vitamins | | | | |
| A, I.U. | 296 | 283 | 176 | 113 |
| Carotene, I.U. | 186 | 63 | 45 | 63 |
| D, I.U. | | | 0.42 | 2.36 |
| E, mg. | 1.28 | 1.32 | 0.56 | 0.06 |
| Ascorbic acid, mg. | 4.4 | 5.4 | 4.3 | 1.6 |
| Folic acid, μg. | 0.05 | 0.02 | 0.18 | 0.23 |
| Niacin, mg. | 0.075 | 0.175 | 0.172 | 0.085 |
| Pantothenic acid, mg. | 0.183 | 0.288 | 0.196 | 0.350 |
| Pyridoxine, mg. | | | 0.011 | 0.048 |
| Riboflavin, mg. | 0.029 | 0.033 | 0.042 | 0.157 |
| Thiamine, mg. | 0.015 | 0.006 | 0.016 | 0.042 |

*Based on Food and Nutrition Board, National Academy of Sciences: The composition of milks, National Research Council Publication no. 254, Washington, D. C., 1953, National Research Council; from Guthrie, Helen Andrews: Introductory nutrition, St. Louis, 1967, The C. V. Mosby Co.

early discouragement; some even think the infant rejects them. *Inept instructions and the supplementary bottle are the best ways to discourage breast feeding,* and by so doing the nurse encourages the mother to accept negative attitudes toward this biological function. There is certainly no doubt that it is less time consuming to give the mother medication to suppress lactation than to help her learn this art.

### Attitudes of nurses

The nurse with positive attitudes toward breast feeding has a tremendous influence and can derive deep satisfaction in promoting a secure mother-infant relationship. She does not take a sleeping infant to place at the mother's breast because she knows the infant will not nurse and the mother will become discouraged. She takes the infant to the mother when he demands nourishment. He must be fed when he wants to be fed.

It is true that the infant must nurse for a brief period of time to bring the colostrum through the ducts; the sleepy infant will not do this. The nurse can encourage sucking by showing the mother how to manually express a small amount of colostrum from the nipple after it is well inserted into his mouth. If the mother is relaxed, the colostrum will come through the ducts easily.

Even though milk is more easily obtained through a rubber nipple and certainly satisfies the demand for food, it is a poor substitute for the soft, warm contact with the breast nipple.

### Effect of analgesics and anesthetics

Infants born to mothers who had little or no sedation during labor and no inhalation anesthesia for delivery will instinctively take the breast readily immediately after birth.

Infants born to mothers who were heavily sedated during labor and under deep anesthesia for delivery are certainly not ready to nurse until some time after birth. It may be days before they work vigorously at the breast in search of nourishment. When the mother has had a long labor, it is wise to allow her a good rest before initiating nursing. Another factor to be considered is if the infant is ready to nurse. A large amount of mucus stimulates the gag reflex; this interferes with their sucking and interest in nursing. Therefore the decision as to when to start the initial feeding at the breast should be individualized and based on both the mother's and the infant's readiness. A rigid, fixed schedule may do for the artificially fed infant, but certainly this is not conducive to initiating the flow of milk.

### Self-regulatory feeding

The mother needs to understand that her baby's demand for food varies; that the early morning feeding may always be longer; and that at any one feeding the baby may nurse twice as long as at another. There are the quiet, sleepy infants and the restless, active infants; each has its own variations in metabolism. Each is a unique individual and his demands for nourishment cannot be compared with the needs of any other infant.

The nurse needs to explain to the mother that when she takes the infant home, she will be free to nurse him when he is hungry, and that his irregular demands are normal, but cannot be met in a hospital setting where a rigid feeding schedule exists. Also at home she can relax and cuddle up with her baby as he drinks his fill of the food Mother Nature so aptly provided.

The mother should be acquainted with self-regulatory feeding. Whether to feed the infant on schedule or when he demands feeding has many pros and cons. If we teach the mother concerning self-regulatory feeding and acquaint her with the variability of her infant's needs, both she and the infant can derive satisfaction from this plan. The method of feeding must suit the mother's temperament and the needs of "her" infant. They both will develop a satisfactory feeding pattern within a few weeks.

### Manual expression

If at any one feeding the infant does not empty the breast, the mother should be instructed how to manually express the remaining milk from the breasts (Fig. 25-3, *B*). This is essential to maintain an optimum supply; that is, the amount secreted is directly proportional to the amount released. When the mother finds that she is

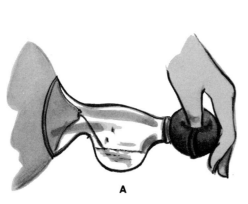
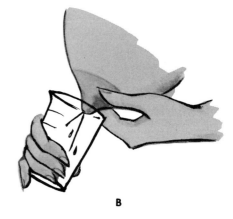

**Fig. 25-3. A,** Expression of milk with hand pump. **B,** Manual expression with compression of milk pocket at anterior and posterior margins of areola.

secreting more than her infant needs, she may express what remains in the breasts (after nursing) into a sterile bottle and place it in her freezer. This can be given to the infant if the mother chooses to be away from home at a feeding time.

### Length of time for nursing

Some infants grasp the nipple vigorously from the start and nurse steadily, whereas others suck less vigorously and tend to nurse more slowly. A 3- to 5-minute period of nursing seems a good guide for the first 24 hours, when the infant is on a 3- to 4-hour hospital schedule.

The turgor of the mother's nipples must be taken into consideration. If this is her first baby and if she is red haired and has fair skin, it is wise to limit time of nursing. We want to avoid fissured nipples, since this invites infection and discomfort for the mother. This need not happen if she is instructed properly. Room for flexibility should be the rule.

Whether to nurse the infant from both breasts at a feeding or on one breast at alternate feedings is a controversial subject. The patient may have her own prefer-

ence or abide by her doctor's or nurse's recommendation.

### Position of mother and infant for feeding

An infant does not normally fight the breast unless his air supply is interfered with. It is so important that the nurse assist the mother in establishing good patterns of nursing; otherwise if the infant is not comfortable, he will object and the mother will feel that he rejects her. (See Fig. 25-4.)

If the mother is lying down, have her raise her arm and place the baby close to her with her arm encircling the infant's head. A pillow at her back for support adds to her comfort. If she is sitting up, see that her feet are propped on a stool. A pillow on her lap helps raise the baby closer to the breast. The mother holds the infant so that his cheek comes in contact with the nipple; he will "naturally" turn his head in search of the nipple. The infant awake and hungry will root and find his source of nourishment.

It is not an infrequent incident that an infant suffers burns as the result of the mother smoking while the infant is nurs-

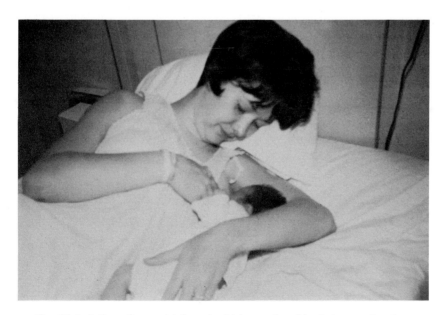

**Fig. 25-4.** Both mother and infant should be comfortable during nursing time.

ing. She needs to be cautioned about this. She also needs to be shown how to support her breasts while the infant is nursing and how to remove the infant from the breast when the infant is satisfied. Show the mother how to press her finger gently into her breast away from the corner of the baby's mouth to release suction. Gentle pressure on the lower chin will also cause him to release the nipple. Removing him forcibly invites fissured nipples.

After feeding hold the baby in the erect position or at a 45-degree angle to favor eructation of air bubbles; although it is believed by some that nursing babies do not swallow air, the gas formed is caused by action of dilute hydrochloric acid in the milk.

The mother who was delivered by cesarean section and wants to breast feed should certainly be permitted to do so. Although she may not feel as agile as her roommate for a few days, breast feeding will be restful and relaxing for her during her convalescence.

The most effective galactagogue for any nursing mother is that she *derive pleasure in the thought and contentment in the process*. There is an inherent longing in a woman to physically nurture her child. This cannot be realized by artificial feeding!

**Clinical advantages of breast feeding**

1. Mother experiences affectionate interaction with her baby that sets pattern for natural intimacy.
2. Breast feeding gives not only security to the infant but also to the mother, for it increases her sense of competence in meeting this most important need of her newborn.
3. Mother reaches the maturation point of maternal development.
4. Infant regulates his intake more readily.
5. Breast feeding favors involution of the uterus

**Clinical advantages of mother's milk**

1. Lowered mortality and morbidity rate
2. Infant given added protection against gastrointestinal and respiratory infections
3. Contains a poliomyelitis neutralizing agent.
4. Better utilization of proteins
5. Less water loss through renal excretion
6. Eliminates milk allergies
7. Less incidence of infantile eczema
8. Calcium and phosphorus from mother's milk apparently more efficiently utilized (even though cow's milk contains more of these minerals)
9. Rich in lysozyme (antibacterial substance)

**Contraindication to breast feeding**

Any debilitating disease such as severe anemia, kidney disease, epilepsy, heart disease, psychoses, or presence of a high fever.
**Exception:** Blood incompatibility between mother and infant is **not** a contraindication to breast feeding.[5]

## Instructions for the mother
*Concerning the milk ejection or let-down reflex[1]*

If you will study Fig. 25-5, *A*, you will see that sensory impulses evolved from the infant's sucking are transmitted to the posterior pituitary gland (neurohypophysis), which in turn discharges oxytocin via the blood back to the breasts. This oxytocin causes contraction of smooth muscles around the alveoli and as the infant nurses, milk flows through the ducts into the lactiferous sinuses.

This milk ejection, or let-down reflex, is conditioned by many factors such as (1) while the infant is nursing on one breast, milk will flow from the other breast; (2) when the mother hears her infant cry, she will experience a tingling sensation in the breasts;(3) when the mother is away from her infant she will feel the release of the milk while thinking about the infant or when it is near feeding time; and (4) other sensory contact between mother and in-

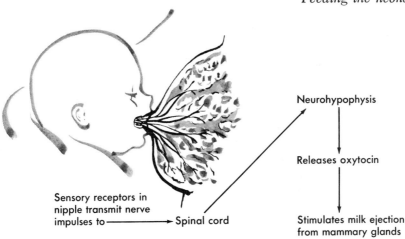

**Neurohypophysis**

**Releases oxytocin**

Sensory receptors in
nipple transmit nerve
impulses to ──────→ Spinal cord

**Stimulates milk ejection
from mammary glands**

**Fig. 25-5.** Neurogenic-hormonal milk ejection reflex. Regular stimulation releases oxytocin, which in turn is responsible for milk ejection reflex.

fant, such as infant's stroking the breast while nursing.

This let-down reflex can be inhibited by any distraction that affects the mother, such as tension or emotional stress. Under stress, adrenaline, a vasoconstrictor, is released into the blood and inhibits oxytocin from stimulating breast tissues.

These psychosomatic factors are the main reason why the American metropolitan environment, with its constant disruption of "family unity," undermines satisfactory lactation. Women in rural areas, where there is a more relaxed environment with less subjection to modern cultural tensions, are more successful at this art. Studies show that breast feeding is continued longer in a sedentary atmosphere, such as a farm community.

Synthetic oxytocin (Syntocinon) is now available to assist in the initial let-down of the milk. This oxytocic acts specifically on the myoepithelium surrounding the alveoli of the breasts by causing them to contract and release the milk into the ducts. It may be used transbuccally (lozenge) or as an intranasal application (spray solution). Administration of thyroid hormone also helps restore a declining milk flow.

The mother should know that the return of her menses has no influence on the quality or quantity of milk, unless it is caused by nervous reaction of the mother.

Smoking is not contraindicated, since the amount of nicotine transmitted is not sufficient to harm the infant. However, the mother should be cautioned about smoking while the infant is nursing (p. 273).

*Concerning successful lactation*

As you have no doubt learned by this time, teaching and instructing mothers is a very important function of the student during her clinical experience in the maternity department. The aid of a competent nurse is invaluable to the new mother.

The mother who is breast feeding needs to be instructed on continued care of her infant, and the nurse should plan to spend sometime with her prior to or on the day of discharge. She needs to understand both the physiological and psychological changes that will continue to occur during the puerperium. The emotional excitement involved in going home may diminish the flow of milk temporarily, but she need only be reassured that this is a normal response.

Ten days to 2 weeks after delivery the estrogen level in the blood rises and may inhibit the flow of sufficient prolactin hormone necessary for continued production of milk. Instruct the mother to allow the infant to empty the breasts during this time. The stimulation will counteract the effect of the inhibitory action of the estrogen. In 1 or 2 days the mother will again have adequate secretion and flow. Too often mothers stop nursing during this time because they become discouraged and frustrated by thinking that they are losing their milk.

The continued success at breast feeding depends on (1) how secure and content she feels in her ability to nurse and (2) a suitable diet and adequate rest.

### Concerning artificial feeding

The nurse needs to instruct the mother who is feeding her infant from the bottle. The following is an outline of such instructions:

1. The infant should not be allowed to take formula too rapidly.
2. Overfeeding should be avoided; it induces digestive disturbances, especially diarrhea, and is one of the main causes of functional vomiting.
3. Position the bottle at an angle so that the nipple is always filled with the formula.
4. Perforations in the nipple should not be too large, but if too small the infant tends to suck in quantities of air that result in abdominal discomfort.
5. Formula should be at room temperature before feeding.
6. Position of infant for eructing of air bubbles should be demonstrated.
7. Placing the infant on his right side after feeding allows formula to drain through the pyloric end to intestines more easily.

### STUDY QUESTIONS
*Multiple choice*

1. Mrs. B complains of pain and sensitivity in the nipple of her right breast. She asks if lactation will be interferred with if she nurses the infant from only the one breast for 1 or 2 days. The nurse knows that:
   (a) lactation will continue even though she nurses from the one breast only.
   (b) both breasts must be stimulated if she expects to lactate successfully.

(c) since lactation is hormonal it really does not matter.

2. Later on in the day when you are collecting babies to return to the central nursery, Mrs. B shows you a drop of blood on the disposable pad inside her nursing brassiere. Your response will be:
   (a) give Mrs. B a breast shield and tell her to use it at the next feeding.
   (b) apply sterile gauze to the nipple and tell Mrs. B not to nurse the infant on that breast until the doctor makes rounds the next day.
   (c) tell Mrs. B she had better take the infant off the breast and start artificial feeding.
   (d) call the doctor immediately and tell him about Mrs. B.

3. Mrs. A's baby is awake when you put him to the breast but he does not seem interested in grasping the nipple. Which of the following would you include in your response:
   (a) your baby is not hungry now. We must not force him because force causes frustration.
   (b) show the mother how to express the colostrum while the nipple is in the infant's mouth.
   (c) stroke masseter muscle of the jaw.
   (d) I will give you a bottle of water for the baby. We will try the breast at the next feeding.
   1. a and d      2. b and c      3. c only

4. It is important that the infant compress the base of the nipple when nursing and not the tip because:
   (a) compression on the base of the nipple will release milk from the ampulla.
   (b) sucking on the tip of the nipple causes fissures, cracks, and excoriations.
   (c) compression on the acini will release milk from the lactiferous lobules.
   1. a only      2. a and b      3. b and c

5. If a new mother shows an interest in breast feeding, the nurse should explain that:
   (a) the newborn's behavior is not well organized at birth and that it takes time for him to adjust to his postnatal environment.
   (b) the newborn's demand for nourishment tends to be irregular the first few days of life.
   (c) the infant must be conditioned to feed when nourishment is offered to him. This is the only way he can be regulated.
   1. a only      2. a and b      3. c only

6. When a lactating mother is severely malnourished:
   (a) her milk will be of inferior quality.

(b) satisfactory quantity can still be maintained.
(c) her own health will be further depleted.
1. a and b    2. a and c    3. all the above
7. If the infant is awake and hungry but "fights the breast" it is most likely because:
(a) the infant has pain.
(b) the infant does not like the taste of colostrum.
(c) the infant is not positioned at the breast properly.
(d) the infant rejects his mother.
8. Mrs. X questions you about the hypertrophy of her baby's breasts. You will tell her:
(a) it will recede by the end of the neonatal period.
(b) it will recede within a few days.
(c) to rub camphorated oil on the breasts several times a day.
9. Between 10 days to 2 weeks of life the full-term newborn's caloric requirement is:
(a) 50 to 55 calories per pound of body weight.
(b) 30 to 40 calories per pound of body weight.
(c) 80 to 100 calories per pound of body weight.
10. The fact that both human and cow's milk is low in iron:
(a) is always a great concern of the pediatrician.
(b) is supplemented in the formula at about 3 days after birth.
(c) is no cause for concern because the infant has reserve stores of this mineral in his liver.

*True or false*

(T) (F) 1. When lactation is fully established, the milk supply will be regulated by the infant's demands.
(T) (F) 2. The need for iron in the lactating mother's diet does not increase above that for pregnancy.
(T) (F) 3. Breast milk contains a poliomyelitis neutralizing agent.
(T) (F) 4. Breast feeding need not be contraindicated where there are known rhesus incompatibilities.
(T) (F) 5. Lactalbumin is an enzyme in human milk.
(T) (F) 6. The infant's demand for nourishment is well established at birth.
(T) (F) 7. Emptying time of the stomach is longer when the infant is on artificial feeding rather than breast feeding.
(T) (F) 8. Breast milk yields 40 calories to the ounce.
(T) (F) 9. Lactose is the principal carbohydrate in human milk.
(T) (F) 10. Syntocinon stimulates the milk-ejection reflex.

**REFERENCES**

1. The womanly art of breast feeding, Franklin Park, Ill., 1958, LaLeche League of Franklin Park, Inc., p. 50.
2. Breast-milk jaundice, J.A.M.A. **121**:1024, March 22, 1965.
3. Athreya, B. H., Coriell, L. L., and Charney, J.: Poliomyelitis antibodies in human colostrum and milk, J. Pediat. **64**:79, Jan., 1964.
4. Eppink, Henrietta: Time of initial breast feeding surveyed in Michigan hospital, Hosp. Top. **46**:116, June, 1968.
5. Meyer, Herman: Infant foods and feeding, Springfield, Ill., 1960, Charles C Thomas, Publisher, p. 56.
6. Smith, Carl: Blood diseases of infancy and childhood, ed. 2, St. Louis, 1966, The C. V. Mosby Co., p. 103.
7. Smith, Clement: Human milk and breast feeding, Pediat. Pract. **29**:44, March, 1965.

**SELECTED READINGS**

Andelman, M. B., and Sered, B. R.: Utilization of dietary iron by term infants, Amer. J. Dis. Child. **111**:45, Jan., 1966.
Bakwin, Harry, and Bakwin, Ruth: Clinical management of behavior disorders in children, ed. 3, Philadelphia, 1966, W. B. Saunders Co., chap. 11.
Beal, Virginia A.: Breast and formula feeding of infants, J. Amer. Diet. Ass. **55**:31, July, 1969.
Beal, Virginia: Calcium and phosphorus in infancy, J. Amer. Diet. Ass. **53**:450, Nov., 1968.
Blake, Florence, and Wright, F. Howell: Essentials of pediatric nursing, ed. 7, Philadelphia, 1963, J. B. Lippincott Co., chap. 3.
Fomon, Samuel: Infant nutrition, Philadelphia, 1967, W. B. Saunders Co.
Gross, Samuel: The relationship between milk protein and iron content on hematologic values in infancy, J. Pediat. **73**:521, Oct., 1968.
Hill, Lee F.: Infant feeding: historic and current. Pediat. Clin. N. Amer. **14**:255-263, Feb., 1967.
Meyer, Herman F.: Current feeding practices in hospital maternity nurseries, Clin. Pediat. **8**:69, Feb., 1969.
O'Connor, Patricia, and de Castro, Fernando: Maternal knowledge of nutritional anemia, Public Health Rep. **84**:527, June, 1969.
Rose, H. E., and Mayer, J.: Activity, caloric intake, fat storage, and the energy balance of infants, Pediatrics **41**:18, Jan., 1968.
Rubin, Reva: Food and feeding, Nurs. Forum **6**:195, Spring, 1967.
Schaffer, Alexander: Diseases of the newborn,

Philadelphia, 1965, W. B. Saunders Co., chaps. 96 and 97.

Watson, E. H., and Lowrey, G. H.: Growth and development of children, ed. 5, Chicago, 1967, Year Book Medical Publishers, Inc., chap. 11.

*Artificial feeding*

Bakwin, Harry, and Bakwin, Ruth: Clinical management of behavior disorders in children, ed. 3, Philadelphia, 1966, W. B. Saunders Co., p. 65.

Liley, H. M. I.: Modern motherhood, New York, 1966, Random House, Inc., chap. 13.

Meyer, Herman: Infant foods and feeding, Springfield, Ill., 1960, Charles C Thomas, Publisher, chaps. 4 to 7.

*Breast feeding*

Bogert, L. Jean, Briggs, George M., and Calloway, Doris: Nutrition and physical fitness, Philadelphia, 1966, W. B. Saunders Co., chap. 21.

De Castro, F. J.: Decline of breast feeding, Clin. Pediat. 7:703, Dec., 1968.

Evans, Ramona T., Thigpen, Lorna W., and Hamrick, Mabel: Exploration of factors involved in maternal physiological adaptation to breast feeding, Nurs. Res. 18:28, Jan.-Feb., 1969.

Guyton, Arthur: Textbook of medical physiology, Philadelphia, 1966, W. B. Saunders Co., chap. 79.

Hazlett, Wm.: The curious problem of breast feeding, Child Family 5:3, Fall, 1966.

Iffrig, Sister Mary Charitas: Nursing care and success in breast feeding, Nurs. Clin. N. Amer. 3:345-354, June, 1968.

Jelliffee, Derick B.: Breast milk and world protein gap, Clin. Pediat. 7:96, Feb., 1968.

Meyer, Herman: Infant foods and feeding, Springfield, Ill., 1960, Charles C Thomas, Publisher, chap. 3.

Meyer, Herman F.: Breast feeding in the United States, Clin. Pediat. 7:708, Dec., 1968.

Montagu, M. F. Ashley: Life before Birth, New York, 1964, New American Library, Inc., chap. 15.

Newton, Michael: Nine questions mothers ask about breast feeding, Consultant 7:27, Feb., 1967.

Newton, Michael, and Newton, Niles: The normal course and management of lactation. In Lytle, Nancy, editor: Maternal health nursing Philadelphia, 1967, W. B. Saunders Co., pp. 108-125.

Newton, Niles: Maternal emotions, New York, 1955, Paul E. Hoeber, Inc., chap. 6.

Newton, Niles: Decline of breast feeding: psychological implications, Nurs. Times 63:1267, Sept. 22, 1967.

Newton, Niles: Decline in breast feeding: social aspects of breast feeding, Nurs. Times 63:1310, Sept. 29, 1967.

Newton, Niles: Decline of breast feeding: psychophysical regulating mechanism, Nurs. Times 53:1346, Oct. 6, 1967.

Newton, Niles, and Newton, Michael: Psychological aspects of lactation, New Eng. J. Med. 277:1179, Nov., 1967.

Richardson, Frank Howard: The technic of breast feeding, Child Family 6:5, Spring, 1967.

Whipple, Dorothy: Breastfeeding in today's world, Child Family, 6:3, Spring, 1967.

The womanly art of breast feeding, Franklin Park, Ill., 1958, LaLeche League of Franklin Park, Inc.

Woody, N. C., and Woody, H. B.: Management of breast feeding, J. Pediat. 68:344, March, 1966.

**For student's quick notes:**

# Chapter 26

# The high-risk neonate—I

If all newborns were born healthy and strong with a fair chance to adjust to this life, much heartache would be prevented. That some infants are not, you will learn in this chapter.

It is the nurse who observes the newborn during the adjustment to extrauterine life and she is the one most likely to detect the first clue that all is not well with the infant. She knows what the infant's response to stimuli should be. She knows if the mother has been oversedated and recognizes when the infant's drowsiness persists beyond normal time. She distinguishes between the loud, lusty cry of the healthy newborn, and the weak, intermittent cry, the shrill cry, the whimpering cry of the infant who is ill.

Although the full-term newborn nursery caters only to the care of the healthy infant, the disorders and structural aberrations most likely to be recognized during the neonatal period are discussed here briefly to acquaint you with various deviations and to prepare you to assist the parents to accept the fact that their infant does have an anomaly.

History reveals that ancient feelings toward congenital anomalies are associated with symbolic meanings, but such myths are being replaced with facts presented to us by scientists and specialists. Each day means a step forward with new hope for the prevention and treatment of hereditary and congenital anomalies. For example, research has made possible the early detection and treatment of certain chemical defects such as phenylketonuria and galactosemia by which the mental retardation they cause may be prevented. Surgery, too, contributes hope, as evidenced by such remarkable results with the congenital heart anomalies. With these modern approaches the infant can be salvaged and the child directed and taught to make a satisfactory contribution to the society in which he lives.

When the mother learns that her infant suffers an anomaly, her emotional reaction may be resentment toward the infant, overprotection, a feeling of fright or guilt, and then self-blame and self-pity. One thing is certain— her attitudes will be unstable and confused. Both parents are bound to be apprehensive about the outcome. They need the support of their family, doctor, and nurse. By observing the mother's behavior and attitudes, the nurse is given a clue regarding how she should respond. First, the nurse must know just what information was given to the mother, if it was given by the father or the doctor, and if she has seen the infant. Second, she must determine if the patient wants to talk or prefers to be alone. She may want an interpretation of the doctor's explanation about the medical terms or possible treatments not quite clear to her. The nurse must at all times be tactful in the information she gives; she must know where her authority begins and ends. The patient must not be led to build false hopes about what is said to her.

## Respiratory disorders

There are a number of reasons why the newborn infant is not able to make adequate respiratory efforts: (1) infections acquired in utero, (2) oversedation from analgesics and anesthetics given to the mother, (3) weakness of respiratory muscles, such as in premature infants, (4) intrauterine anoxia, (5) intracranial hemorrhage, (6) diaphragmatic hernia, (7) congenital malformations of the heart, and (8) aspiration of amniotic fluid and meconium.

### Atelectasis

Atelectasis is defined as incomplete expansion of the lungs. Atelectasis may be *primary,* failure of alveoli to expand, or *secondary,* initial expansion and then collapse because entrance of air is inhibited by some obstruction such as formation of hyaline membrane.

Clinically, with primary atelectasis the infant may have intermittent cyanosis with irregular respirations and periods of apnea, or he may have persistent cyanosis with feeble respiratory efforts. With secondary atelectasis the infant may or may not show any distress at birth; then, within 12 to 24 hours, cyanosis and dyspnea are noted. The infant makes vigorous respiratory efforts. The nurse will notice retraction on inspiration and expiratory grunts with flaring of the alae nasi. Her responsibility is to detect early symptoms of distress, to aspirate infant's respiratory tract as needed

to keep the airway clear, and to make every effort to prevent infection.

The treatment is oxygen as needed to control cyanosis. The value of an environment with high humidity is questioned by some doctors, except when the atelectasis is due to obstruction by mucus. Since the infant with atelectasis is subject to secondary infection, the doctor usually orders prophylactic antibiotic therapy.

### Hyaline membrane syndrome

Hyaline membrane syndrome is the result of a membrane deposited along the walls of the bronchioles, alveoli, and alveolar ducts. The most likely victims are (1) low birth weight infants, (2) those delivered by cesarean section (especially if hemorrhage prompted the section; studies show a correlation of hyaline membrane with maternal hemorrhage), and (3) those born of diabetic mothers. It has been stated that the cesarean section in itself (elective) should not increase the risk of hyaline membrane.

The membrane is rarely present in the lungs of infants who die within a few hours of birth although they have the clinical signs of the disease.

Some years ago the theory was presented that pathogenesis of the membrane might be the result of the fetus swallowing and aspirating amniotic fluid, which is more likely when the infant is delivered by cesarean section. For this reason aspiration of gastric contents to prevent regurgitation into the lungs at the time of birth was the rule and probably still is in many hospitals. This procedure, unfortunately, has not decreased the incidence of this disease.

A later hypothesis (1963) stated that delayed clamping of the cord allowed placental blood to transfuse into the infant and thus provided adequate oxygenation of the pulmonary vascular bed.

For normal expansion of the lungs and prevention of alveolar collapse, a lipoprotein substance called *surfactant* must be secreted by the alveolar epithelium. The lungs of newborns who die of hyaline membrane disease do not have this surfactant in their lungs.

*Clinical course of the disease.* Some infants who develop this mysterious disease show a history of a poor or fair Apgar score in the delivery room; then, within a few hours they manifest increased respiratory rate with sternal retraction. Other infants have a good Apgar score at birth but within the hour show tachypnea, sternal retraction, and expiratory grunting. Cyanosis and dyspnea are apparent a little later. The respiratory rate rises to as much as 120 per minute. Periods of apnea followed by very rapid breathing and progressive cyanosis are grave prognostic signs. The infant usually lies with mouth open and body flaccid. He is edematous, with shiny palms and puffy eyelids, and has a whimpering cry. He gives the appearance of an overinflated chest with protruding abdomen during inspiration.

*Treatment.* To counteract the metabolic acidosis so prevalent in the infant with hyaline membrane disease, the doctor may order 65 ml. per kilogram per day of Na-HCO$_3$ in 10% glucose over a 24-hour period, and 60 ml. per kilogram per day of 5% glucose in 0.45% saline solution for infants born to diabetic mothers. This improves cardiac action and lung blood flow. Pneumonia develops secondarily in many of the affected infants. Therefore antimicrobial drugs such as kanamycin are usually ordered.

*Nursing responsibilities.* Of initial importance is providing an environmental temperature sufficient to maintain skin temperature at 97° F. This may require increasing Isolette temperature to 95° or 96° F. Infants seem to breathe better in an environment of high humidity. Such an environment does control fluid loss through the skin, but its value in dissolution of the membrane is highly doubtful. Increased humidity promotes maceration in the skin creases and favors growth of microorganisms, that is, *Pseudomonas aeruginosa.*[3]

The oxygen level is regulated to relieve cyanosis. The nurse's accurate monitoring of infant's clinical status and respiratory rate and her observation of the nature of distress, such as retraction and grunting (evidence of hypoxia), provide the pediatrician with clues for instituting therapy. Cyanosis, which is a late sign, is recorded as mild, moderate, or extreme. The infant should be handled minimally, but his position changed for comfort.

Infants born of mothers who had complications predisposing to intrauterine asphyxia need special watching and should be scrutinized for developing signs and symptoms. Prolonged fetal distress may be a factor, but this has yet to be proved.

## Digestive disorders

The usual symptoms of digestive disorders are vomiting and diarrhea. Both may be the mere result of feeding problems or they may be due to actual pathology. *Vomiting* differs from regurgitation only in degree. The former implies emptying of the stomach, whereas regurgitation implies returning small amounts of feeding.

### Functional vomiting

Functional vomiting may be due to gastric distention brought about by improper methods of feeding such as (1) propping the bottle, (2) openings in nipple may be too large, (3) feeding the infant too rapidly, (4) formula may be too dilute, (5) formula may be too high in fat content, and (6) failure in taking time to "bubble" the infant so that swallowed air may be eructated.

**NURSING DIAGNOSIS OF VOMITING**

| Observation | Possible causative factors |
|---|---|
| 1. Vomits frequent, small amounts of un-coagulated milk | 1. Chalasia—abnormally relaxed esophageal muscles |
| 2. Vomits uncurdled milk on starting or during the feeding; also ejects through nose | 2. Esophageal atresia |
| 3. Curdled vomitus | 3. Proof that formula did enter the stomach |
| 4. Hematemesis | 4. May be of maternal origin; use Downey-Apt test for diagnosis |
| 5. Bile-stained vomitus | 5. Suspicious of intestinal obstruction below bile duct; observe for abdominal distention and passage of meconium |
| 6. Projectile vomiting | 6. Observed during or immediately after feeding; seen with pyloric stenosis; accompanied by observable peristaltic waves over the stomach |
| 7. Persistent vomiting | 7. Pylorospasms; urinary tract or other infections |
| 8. Mucus or mucus and saliva (neutral reaction) | 8. Esophageal atresia or stenosis |

**Pylorospasms**

*Definition:* Involuntary contraction of pyloric muscle.

*Etiology:* Pylorospasms have been known to be associated with unfavorable environmental conditions such as a tense mother.

*Symptoms:* Onset of vomiting is not common during the first 2 weeks, but may occur occasionally during the first few days of life. Pylorospasms occur during or after feeding.

Vomiting may be intermittent or after every attempt to feed; it is seldom projectile.

Pyloric mass is usually not felt.

Constipation is less severe.

*Treatment:* Antispasmodic and antihistaminic drugs. Thickened formula.

**Pyloric stenosis**

*Definition:* Hypertrophic obstruction, usually congenital.

*Etiology:* Pyloric stenosis is more frequent in Caucasian than in Negro infants. A large number of those affected are firstborns and males. It has been stated that there is the possibility of a genetic factor.

*Symptoms:* Onset of vomiting is usually not until third or fourth week after birth, but may occur at any time.

Pylorospasms usually precede the hypertrophy of the pylorus.

Vomiting may be intermittent at first, then increases in frequency and projectility; occurs during or shortly after a feeding and never contains bile.

Pyloric mass can be felt, and peristaltic waves observed.

Constipation is pronounced.

*Treatment:* Medical—antispasmodic drugs, parenteral fluids to control dehydration. Surgical—Rammstedt operation.

Vomiting the first day usually indicates an obstruction in the gastrointestinal tract, although intracranial pressure commonly produces vomiting. Onset of vomiting 2 or more weeks after birth is usually due to narrowing of pyloric lumen (p. 283).

It is the nurse's responsibility to give the doctor an accurate report on the following: (1) frequency of vomiting; (2) amount of vomitus and whether it is green (bile) or contains flecks of blood; (3) the time of vomiting in relation to the time of feeding; (4) whether there is evidence of dehydration; (5) condition of the infant after a vomiting episode; and (6) whether it is simple regurgitation or projectile. This gives the pediatrician useful information as to the etiology or to possibility and location of obstruction.

If the infant is fed the thickened formula with a spoon, the nurse must use care to see that it is placed well back in the mouth because of the extrusion reflex. These infants seem more content if allowed to suck; putting a large hole in the nipple to facilitate release of thick feeding satisfies this need. Feed the infant slowly, with care, and bubble frequently.

### Diarrhea

Diarrhea may be due to (1) overfeeding or too rapid filling of the stomach, (2) adjustment to formula, (3) allergies to certain proteins in cow's milk, and (4) infections.

A great variety of pathogens are responsible for outbreaks of diarrhea in the newborn nursery. The pathogenic strains of *Escherichia coli* (normal inhabitant of adult intestinal tract) have a high degree of virulence for the newborn and are the greatest offenders.

Since infectious diarrhea is highly contagious, the infant should be removed from the nursery on the least suspicion, and feedings withheld until seen by the pediatrician. Newborns can become extremely ill from rapid loss of fluids and electrolytes, which result in dehydration and acidosis. Infants so afflicted should be transferred to the pediatric isolation unit. For nursing care and treatment, see a pediatric text.

The nurse may observe the following signs and symptoms preceding the loose bowel movements: (1) failure to feed well, (2) loss of weight, (3) lethargy, and (4) possible elevation of temperature. Diarrheal stools are usually green, liquid, and frothy. A diarrheal stool passes through the intestines so rapidly that normal chemical changes are interfered with; hence the green color.

## Birth injuries
### Intracranial hemorrhage

As you learned in Chapter 14, birth is a traumatic experience; the passenger is subjected to a hazardous ordeal on passage through the birth canal. His head is the most likely part of the body to be subjected to trauma.

In a normal labor of average length the shape of the head adjusts to the contour of the birth canal, but *sudden* or *extreme* force increases tension of the dura with subsequent hemorrhage. When the hemorrhage causes pressure on the medulla, all vital body functions are at stake.

Nature provides for some of this pressure by allowing for the overlapping of the skull bones, but when labor is prolonged and difficult, the pressure may be too great. Premature infants are especially subject to brain injury from such pressure, since their brain tissue is not so well protected as the full-term infants. The two main etiological factors are (1) trauma and (2) anoxia.

*Subdural hemorrhage.* Subdural hemorrhage is invariably the result of trauma. Predisposing factors to subdural hemorrhage are (1) application of forceps other than low, (2) breech or footling presentation with difficult extraction, (3) a large baby, and (4) the mother is a primigravida or older multigravida.

*Intraventricular hemorrhage.* Intraventricular hemorrhage affects smaller rather than larger babies and affects prematures rather than full-term infants; it usually occurs in a spontaneous delivery. Asphyxia is the outstanding contributory factor. Prematurity, preeclampsia, and eclampsia predispose to this type of hemorrhage.

*Subarachnoid hemorrhage.* Subarachnoid hemorrhage is more common, but usually mild. It, too, appears to be the result of asphyxia rather than mechanical injury and is more likely to occur in the premature infant and in infants born of mothers who had a history of preeclampsia. These infants seldom have a tense anterior fontanel or convulsion.

A number of clinical signs of brain damage that make their appearance within 24 hours of delivery are as follows: (1) weak and intermittent or shrill and high-pitched cry; (2) thrashing movements of the extremities; (3) anxious facies with eyes staring; (4) clonic and tonic convulsions; (5) periods of apnea and cyanosis; (6) poor reflexes; (7) rhythmic protrusion of the tongue; (8) trismus; (9) subnormal or elevated temperature; (10) jaundice (destruction of blood cells increases serum bilirubin); and (11) tense fontanels.

The Isolette is preferable for care of these infants because it facilitates observation, regulation of oxygen, and temperature stabilization. The doctor may order the head of the bed elevated to reduce cerebral venous pressure.

The prognosis for intracranial hemorrhage depends on extent of the injury. Those who do survive are subject to behavior disorders, epilepsy, and mental retardation.

*Cephalhematoma.* A cephalhematoma is compared with a caput succedaneum on p. 286 and in Fig. 26-1.

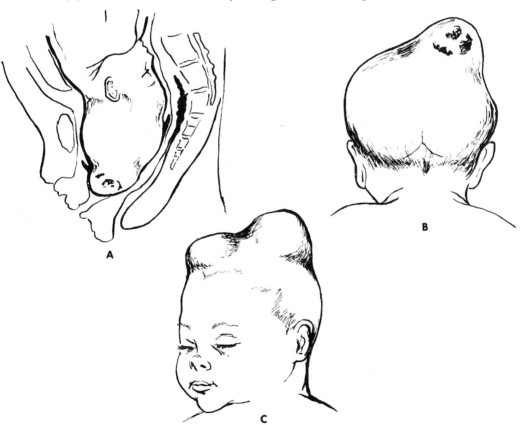

**Fig. 26-1. A,** Formation of caput succedaneum. **B,** Appearance of caput succedaneum. **C,** Cephalhematoma.

**Caput succedaneum**

1. A swelling of soft tissues of the scalp is formed by effusion of serum as the result of pressure on part of the scalp during labor and delivery; it lies over sutures.

2. The condition is present at birth.

3. The swelling is largest at birth, and then recedes.

4. The swelling is soft, boggy, and pits on pressure.

**Cephalhematoma**

1. Blood accumulates between the bone and periosteum, usually over one parietal bone. The location has much to do with position of the head during labor. This does not extend over suture line or fontanel and occurs twice as often in male infants.

2. The bleeding is slow and the condition is not noticeable until several hours after birth. Clinical jaundice due to resorption may be recognizable.

3. The bleeding increases in size for 2 or 3 days and takes 4 to 6 weeks for resorption; it may be accompanied by underlying skull fracture.

4. The hematoma may be soft or tense.

### Neonatal facial nerve palsy

A nerve paralysis causing distortion of the face is not necessarily related to birth trauma. This may be the result of intrauterine pressure, especially when the infant was in an abnormal posture. The nurse will observe movement of only one side of the face. When the infant cries, the mouth will be drawn toward the unaffected side. The eye usually remains open on the affected side.

### Brachial palsy (Erb-Duchenne palsy)

Brachial palsy is a paralysis resulting from injury to the fifth and sixth cervical nerve roots. This may occur when traction is exerted on the head to facilitate delivery of the shoulders. The arm lies limp at the side and when lifted is flaccid. Wrist and hand are normal; grasp reflex is good. Recovery depends on regeneration of the nerves, and whether they were merely stretched or severed. The doctor usually instructs the mother in massaging muscles to prevent formation of contractures.

### Klumpke's paralysis

Klumpke's paralysis is a form of brachial palsy involving the wrist and hand that are innervated from eighth cervical and first thoracic nerve roots. The hand and wrist are relaxed and the grasp reflex is poor or absent. Prognosis depends on extent of injury and whether the nerve is injured or torn. When the damage is not extensive, function may return in a few months. Treatment is partial immobilization, which may be accomplished by pinning the wrist portion of the shirt sleeve to the mattress sheet or by using a sling binder.

## Infections of the neonate

The following discussions give only a brief review of some of the illnesses of the newborn. The care of the sick infant is part of pediatric experience and thoroughly covered in pediatric textbooks.

During pregnancy many gamma globulins containing antibodies are transferred to the fetus through the placenta and amniotic fluid. Thus the newborn has some inner resources of protection (passive immunity) to some of the diseases.

A strong, healthy body at birth offers a good resistance to disease. The infant's ability to form gamma globulin is limited, and he needs immunization against childhood diseases, including diphtheria, poliomyelitis, smallpox, measles, and pertussis.

It is the nurse's responsibility to use protective measures to protect the newborn from infection and to be alert to signs indicating the onset of infection.

The neonate's reaction to virulent organisms differs from that of the older infant. He does not manifest signs and symptoms of infection as the adult does, and fever is often absent. This makes it extremely difficult for the nurse to recognize that he is ill. The earliest sign is failure to feed well and this should be reported to the doctor so that he may determine its significance.

Infections may be acquired during fetal existence, during the birth process, or after delivery. The *Staphylococcus,* water trap organisms, and *Escherichia coli* are the chief scourges; the latter is responsible for approximately 10% of neonatal infections.

### Impetigo neonatorum

The etiology of impetigo neonatorum may be *Staphylococcus* or *Streptococcus.* It is a superficial skin infection characterized by vesicles containing fluid. The characteristic blebs are most likely to develop in folds, creases, and moist surfaces of the skin, although any part of the body may be affected because autoinoculation favors the spread.

The epidermis should be removed with cotton applicators moistened with alcohol and the denuded area exposed to dry heat. Local application of preparations such as sulfadiazine, bacitracin, and neomycin may be ordered by the doctor. Since it is a highly contagious infection, strict isolation should be enforced.

### Thrush (oral moniliasis)

*Etiology.* The etiology of thrush is *Candida (Monilia) albicans,* a fungus infection. The principal source of this infection is the maternal vaginal secretions. The infant is usually infected on passage through the birth canal, although he may be secondarily infected by nursery personnel.

Moisture favors the growth, and lesions (white plaques mistaken for milk) are most likely to be observed in the mouth and genital and anal areas. The lesions appear as white elevated areas and resemble milk curds.

Clinically it goes unrecognized in our newborn nurseries, since the incubation period is 5 days and infants are discharged on the third or fourth day.

*Treatment.* Areas should be swabbed with cotton applicators dipped in soda-bicarbonate solution, 1 teaspoon to 4 ounces of water (destroys acid media in which *Candida* thrives), aqueous solution of nystatin (200,000 units into 1 ml. water) applied locally three to four times a day with soft cotton applicator, and Zephiran 1:1000 aqueous dilution or 1% gentian violet, applied once a day.

### Bacterial conjunctivitis (ophthalmia neonatorum)

The etiology may be *Staphylococcus, E. coli,* a virus, or the gonococcus; the latter will result in blindness if not treated. The infection is acquired on passage through the birth canal. Today it is rare due to the prophylaxis introduced in 1884 by Carl Credé.

### Omphalitis

When the umbilical cord is not cared for properly, it becomes soft and moist and provides a good medium for the growth of saprophytic bacteria. The result is a purulent discharge with fetid odor.

A more serious condition is the development of cellulitis of the skin around the area of the umbilicus. If not treated, bacteria may invade the umbilical vessels.

## The postmature infant

A *postmature* infant is one who is live born after 42 weeks' gestation, but is not necessarily a victim of placental dysfunction.

A *dysmature* infant is one who exhibits severe malnutrition, regardless of gestational age.

Not all postmature infants suffer from placental insufficiency; some infants continue to develop normally after term. Occasionally the nurse will admit a postmature infant to the nursery and she should be familiar with the clinical manifestations.

The postmature infant *not* subjected to placental insufficiency has a characteristic appearance: (1) skin is pale, dry, and cracked, with no protective vernix, (2) fingernails are long, (3) no lanugo is present, and (4) the facial expression is alert.

When the fetus has been exposed to placental dysfunction syndrome plus postmaturity, he appears to have lost weight, that is, the skin is loose. Passage of meconium is characteristic in fetal distress (intrauterine anoxia). This causes a green or yellow staining of the skin and cord that may be noted in these infants. They are victims of respiratory distress syndrome.

## Hemolytic disorders
### Hyperbilirubinemia

The full-term infant is said to have hyperbilirubinemia when the level of bilirubin reaches 12 mg. per 100 ml.; the low birth weight infant is described as such when the bilirubin level is 15 mg. per 100 ml.

*Etiology.* The most important cause is when an incompatibility in blood group of the mother and infant exists. With this hemolytic anemia the jaundice is noticeable in the first 24 hours after birth for the full-term and in the first 36 hours for the low birth weight infant. Other contributory factors are (1) dehydration, (2) pyloric stenosis, (3) anoxia, (4) intestinal obstruction, (5) infections, (6) hyaline membrane syndrome, and (7) certain drugs such as excess of synthetic vitamin K and sulfisoxazole (Gantrisin).

It has been stated that there is a relation between lack of carbohydrates and the increased incidence of jaundice. The carbohydrate starvation delays functioning of enzyme systems such as glucuronyl transferase and may be a contributory factor in the increased jaundice of low birth weight infants. It has also been observed that infants born of diabetic mothers, if fed before the usual 24- to 48-hour fasting, had less jaundice. Excess pregnanediol in breast milk is also said to inhibit the activity of the glucuronyl transferase (p. 267). When the hyperbilirubinemia is unrelated to erythroblastosis, the jaundice develops more slowly.

There have been reports on the effectiveness of ultraviolet phototherapy in preventing dangerous levels of bilirubin. The ultraviolet light breaks down pigment as it passes through skin capillaries.[1,4,5,7-9]

Activated charcoal has also been used to prevent reabsorption of bile into the circulation.

### Rh blood incompatibilities

In Chapter 4 you read about the transfer of incompatible erythrocytes that result in a destructive hemolytic process in the newborn. If this destruction is severe, the fetus may die in utero from anemia and heart failure, or if born alive, he is likely to have hydrops fetalis (severe anemia and edema).

Sometimes it is only after birth that destructive effects appear, but 90% of the babies afflicted can be saved by an exchange transfusion—withdrawal of the baby's blood and replacement with Rh-negative blood.[6,11]

Not all Rh-positive infants born to Rh-negative sensitized women are afflicted (15% to 20%), nor is the extent of hemolysis always so severe that an exchange transfusion is required. When the disease is severe, the infant may be jaundiced at birth with yellow discoloration of the cord and pallor of the mucous membranes. In such cases the exchange transfusion will remove the antibody-coated red blood cells and reduce the risk of kernicterus.

When a woman has a history of a rising titer in her serum, a history of a previous delivery of an erythroblastotic infant, or confirmation of bilirubin in the amniotic fluid, the doctor may induce labor.

In anticipation of an affected infant the recovery nursery personnel should be notified in advance, and preparation made for the exchange. When the infant is delivered, the cord is left rather long to facilitate use of the umbilical vein if an exchange transfusion is necessary. The nurse should keep the cord moist by application of gauze soaked in saline solution, and the cord should be kept in place with an abdominal band. At birth, cord blood is sent to the laboratory to determine presence of Rh antibodies attached to the erythrocytes (direct Coombs' test).

The purposes of the exchange transfusion are to (1) prevent kernicterus and (2) prevent death from heart failure after severe anemia and edema.

Criteria for the exchange varies, but the exchange is usually performed at birth when one of the following conditions is found: (1) positive direct Coombs' with cord blood hemoglobin is less than 11 grams per 100 ml. for the full-term infant; (2) positive direct Coombs' with cord blood hemoglobin is less than 14 grams per 100 ml. for the low birth weight infant; (3) cord bilirubin content is over 4 mg. per 100 ml.; (4) jaundice develops during first 6 hours; and (5) if within 6 to 8 hours the serum bilirubin reaches 18 to 20 mg. per 100 ml., hemoglobin is below 12 grams per 100 ml., hematocrit is less than 35%.

The doctor may administer albumin because of its ability to bind free bilirubin and thus prevent deposition of bilirubin in the tissues.

### Nursing responsibilities for exchange transfusion

1. Provide environmental warmth for the infant.
2. Careful monitoring of heart rate during the procedure.
3. Have oxygen and resuscitative equipment at hand.
4. Careful monitoring of intake and output.
5. Have 2 to 5 mEq. sodium bicarbonate available for immediate use in cases of bradycardia or cardiac arrest.
6. Calcium gluconate 0.5 ml. should be at hand to counteract hypocalcemia. (Some doctors give 1 ml. of 10% calcium gluconate after each 100 ml. of blood exchanged.)
7. Allow donor blood to reach room temperature gradually. Rapid temperature change such as from the refrigerator to a water bath affects the erythrocytes.
8. Check donor's Rh type (should be that of the mother's, that is, Rh negative).

The amount of blood exchanged approximates 80 ml. whole blood per pound of body weight for the full-term infant, taking into consideration the condition of the infant. Individual replacement exchange is 20 ml., again depending on weight and condition of the infant.

### Risks associated with exchange transfusion[6,10]

1. Overloading infant's circulation by giving more than is withdrawn
2. High concentration of potassium in stored blood, which results in hyperkalemia (this may cause cardiac arrest)
3. Hypocalcemia from depletion of calcium from infant's plasma
4. Acidosis resulting in bradycardia or cardiac arrest
5. Hypothermia
6. Air embolism

After the procedure is completed, the nurse continues to furnish environmental warmth and gives oxygen as needed. Observe the infant for symptoms of central nervous system disorders. This may occur 24 to 48 hours after the transfusion. Keep cord moist for second replacement.

### Kernicterus[12,13]

Kernicterus is defined as jaundice of nuclear masses and ganglia on the medulla. There is no one level of serum bilirubin at which the infant is certain to develop kernicterus. However, toxic action of the *indirect* (unconjugated) bilirubin (deposits of bile pigment in nerve cells) is believed to reach dangerous levels about 20 mg. per 100 ml. Kernicterus can develop with low levels of bilirubin, such as in intrauterine hypoxia, hypoglycemia, or infections. It is the "tissue" bilirubin, not serum bilirubin, that is dangerous to nerve cells. The difference between these two levels depends

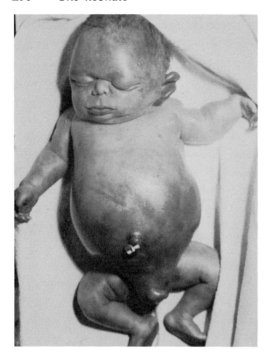

**Fig. 26-2.** Severely edematous infant—hydrops fetalis.

on albumin available to bind the bilirubin.

Kernicterus usually develops during the first 5 days of life; it strikes the full-term infant on the third or fourth day and the low birth weight infant between the fourth and tenth day. It never develops in utero because bilirubin is transferred to the mother's blood by the placenta.

The severely affected infant shows signs of developing brain damage, such as poor response to the Moro reflex, shrill cry, or failure to feed well. He may become flaccid or rigid. There is a tendency for the eyes to roll downward (setting-sun sign). When the hyperbilirubinemia is severe during pregnancy, the infant, if live-born, is severely edematous and anemic (hydrops fetalis), or the severity of the anemia leads to cardiac failure and the infant dies in utero (Fig. 26-2). If the infant does survive, the sequelae are deafness, mental defects, and athetosis (slow, involuntary, sinuous, writhing movements, especially of hands). The mortality rates are approximately 50% for the full-term infant and 75% for the low birth weight infant.

## Metabolic disorders
### Infants born of diabetic mothers

With good prenatal care (management of the pregnant diabetic woman), chances for survival of the infant are very good.

These infants are characteristically large at birth. Their size is so characteristic that all oversized infants born to an otherwise normal mother indicate a further check for diabetes. These infants are also heavier at birth and longer than average length, even though they are delivered some weeks before term. They are plethoric and have a plump, puffy appearance, with rather round face. The excess weight is attributed more to fat than to edema and belies their true condition.

The majority of infants appear well at birth and continue to progress satisfactorily. For other newborns, the Apgar score may be favorable at birth but clinical signs of respiratory distress syndrome appear within 24 hours. This is the most common complication afflicting these infants, although intracranial hemorrhage (generally caused by placental insufficiency or asphyxia), congenital anomalies, and congestive heart failure contribute to the mortality. The majority of deaths are associated with their immaturity and the outcome for many of them depends a great deal on how mature the infant is when born. Mortality is higher among those infants who are overweight (12 to 14 pounds) than those weighing 6 to 8 pounds.

The conscientious nurse will watch over these infants with special care to detect early signs of respiratory distress or hypoglycemia. The nursing care does not differ from any other infant with respiratory distress syndrome. Clinical signs include (1) twitching of the extremities, (2) irritability, (3) pallor, intermittent cyanosis, and convulsions, (4) jaundice, (5) hypothermia, and (6) atonia.

Because some doctors believe that aspiration of amniotic fluid contributes to the development of hyaline membrane disease, they order gastric lavage on these infants.

Since there is marked hypertrophy of islet tissue, some of these infants have a fall in true blood glucose below 20 mg. per 100 ml. This occurs during the first few hours after birth, the result of temporary hyperinsulinism, but returns to normal level in about 8 hours. The doctor may give the infant glucose solution to support blood glucose levels.

Oral or gavage feedings, 75 ml. per kilogram per day of 5% glucose solution, are started 3 to 4 hours after birth. If the infant is asymptomatic at 24 hours, formula is started. These infants also tend to have hypocalcemia, hyperbilirubinemia, and increased adrenal corticosteroids.

It has been stated that some infants who are abnormally large at birth tend to develop diabetes at a later time in life.

### Phenylketonuria

Phenylketonuria (PKU) is the result of an inborn metabolism error whereby the infant is unable to metabolize the amino acid phenylalanine because of deficiency of phenylalanine hydroxylase normally made by the liver. Most of the infants afflicted are the offspring of two heterozygous carriers of the pathological gene. The incidence is approximately one in 10,000. It is less frequent in Negroes than in Caucasians and equally frequent in males and females. The abnormality is not present at birth, since the placenta removes the phenylalanine.

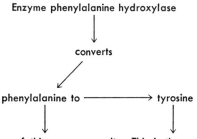

Enzyme phenylalanine hydroxylase
↓
converts
phenylalanine to ⟶ tyrosine

Absence of this enzyme results in phenylalanine accumulating in the blood and in phenylketone bodies being excreted in the urine. Infants afflicted are blond and have fair skin and blue eyes.

This is the precursor of melanin compounds that pigment eyes, skin, and hair.

With the lack of the enzyme, phenylalanine and its metabolites accumulate in the blood 2 to 4 days after the infant is started on feeding. The Guthrie B subtilis inhibition assay test (filter paper blood test), done on 4-day-old infants, will provide earliest reliable indication of PKU. The normal phenylalanine level in the blood does not normally exceed 2 to 3 mg. per 100 ml. Where the blood exhibits 4 mg. per 100 ml. or higher, a follow-up examination is recommended. Definite diagnosis is established when blood plasma or serum phenylalanine levels reach 10 mg. or more per 100 ml. The view is that this high level of blood phenylalanine arrests normal brain development.

Urinary excretion of phenylpyruvic acid will be detected when serum phenylalanine level exceeds 15 mg. per 100 ml., usually 10 to 14 days after birth. Filter paper urine specimens may be obtained from the baby at 3 weeks of age.

Phenylketonuria, if detected early enough, is treatable by special diet. For management and prognosis, see a pediatric textbook.

## Congenital anomalies
### Central nervous system

Congenital anomalies of the central nervous system include the absence or abnormal size of the head and defects in closure of the bony spine. The three most common are (1) anencephalus, (2) hydrocephalus, and (3) spina bifida.

***Etiology.*** Excessive secretion of fluid or obstruction of the circulating fluid may result from prenatal infections, anomalous development of the brain or cord, or the result of trauma such as subdural hematoma.

***Types***

*Internal hydrocephalus.* Cerebrospinal fluid accumulates in the ventricles.

*External hydrocephalus.* Excessive fluid accumulates outside the cerebrum (between brain and dura mater).

***Clinical manifestations.*** The head is usually normal or slightly enlarged in size at

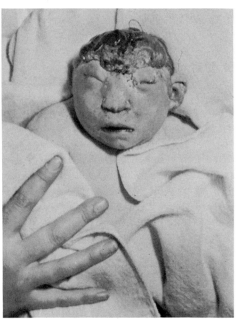

**Fig. 26-3.** Anencephalus—absence of cranial vault of the skull. Cerebral hemisphere is a mass of dark, red tissue attached to base of skull.

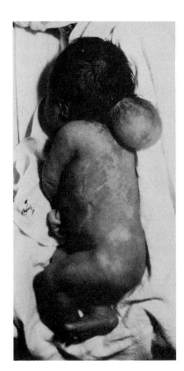

**Fig. 26-5.** Meningomyelocele—meninges, spinal cord, or nerve roots protrude through a defect in vertebral column and form a sac.

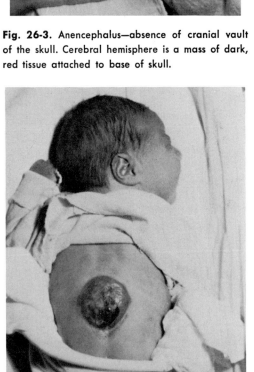

**Fig. 26-4.** Meningocele—meninges protrude through spina bifida and form a sac; no neurological deficit involved.

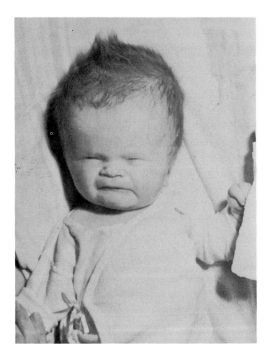

**Fig. 26-6.** Hydrocephalus—abnormal increase in cerebrospinal fluid volume within intracranial cavity.

birth. The suture lines are widened and fontanels are tense. In some cases one may recognize a downward displacement of the eyes (setting-sun sign) and abnormal bulging of the forehead in the area of the anterior fontanel. The infant has a high-pitched cry and is subject to vomiting and convulsions. A number of cases are known to be familial and do not become symptomatic until after the neonatal period. Some cases develop in utero and cannot be delivered without a craniotomy. The condition is associated with encephalocele.

### Alimentary tract

The nurse is expected to develop skill in early recognition of alimentary tract obstruction. The more alert she is, the more quickly diagnosis and treatment can be instituted. Delay in diagnosis is a factor contributing to mortality of those afflicted.

Suspect alimentary tract obstruction when (1) excessive mucus accumulates in the infant's mouth and he has constant drooling and (2) vomiting occurs, especially on the first day of life. The type and character of the vomitus provide the following guide to location of obstruction: (1) the abdomen is distended and more pronounced if the obstruction is in the lower tract with visible peristaltic waves; (2) stools are scanty with graying or gray-green meconium when obstruction is located high; and (3) there is an absence of stools. Normally, the newborn passes meconium within 24 hours.

#### Tracheoesophageal fistula.
There are different types of tracheoesophageal fistulas, but the most common variety is the one in which the lower portion of the esophagus opens into the trachea and the upper part ends in a small saclike pouch (Fig. 26-7).

The first clue is observation of excessive amounts of mucus coming from the infant's mouth—almost "constant drooling." This should be recognized before the first feeding because once fluid is taken, it fills the pouch and is immediately regurgitated through both nose and mouth. The infant

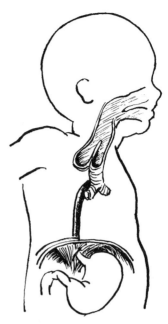

**Fig. 26-7.** Tracheoesophageal fistula, with upper esophagus ending in a blind pouch—the most common form.

coughs, gags, and aspirates contents into the lungs with subsequent pneumonitis. The infant may also have intermittent periods of cyanosis.

The doctor may order a catheter passed into the esophagus to determine the site of obstruction, but this may be misleading since the tube may actually coil in the pouch. Giving the infant a few milliliters of Lipiodol via an esophageal catheter under a fluoroscope will confirm doctor's suspicion. Treatment is immediate surgery, unless the infant shows sign of pneumonitis.

The infant should be kept in an upright position to minimize aspiration of drainage. Gentle esophageal suction to remove excess mucus and humidified oxygen to reduce viscosity of oral secretions are usually ordered.

It is becoming routine practice in many hospitals to pass a soft catheter through each nostril and into the stomach immediately after birth for removal of contents and to determine (without delay) if there is any congenital obstruction of the upper gastrointestinal tract.

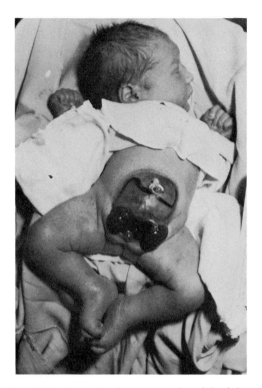

**Fig. 26-8.** Omphalocele—congenital umbilical hernia. Abdominal contents protrude through defect in anterior abdominal wall. A thin transparent membrane covers protruding viscera.

*Meconium ileus.* A segment of the bowel is blocked with thick, mucilaginous, putty-like meconium. This abnormal consistency of the meconium is due to lack of pancreatic secretions. Meconium ileus is the earliest manifestation of cystic fibrosis of the pancreas. A laboratory method of diagnosis is analysis of pancreatic juice for pancreatic enzymes. Diagnosis is made on the absence of trypsin and an increase of sodium chloride in the sweat. The history of intestinal obstruction in siblings is also helpful.

The nurse should be aware of the clinical signs and symptoms such as (1) failure to pass stool, or scanty, thick meconium, (2) abdominal distention (this outstanding symptom is seen as early as 3 to 12 hours after birth), and (3) vomiting may be bile stained at times. If the infant does survive surgery (ileotomy), it usually develops pulmonary disease.

*Imperforate anus.* The absence of a normal anal opening is called an imperforate anus. Initial attempt to take rectal temperature will reveal imperforate anus or patent anus with shallow blind pouch. Later signs of abnormality of lower bowel are (1) failure to pass meconium and (2) progressive distention of the abdomen.

### Respiratory system

*Choanal atresia.* Choanal atresia is an obstruction of the posterior nares. The infant becomes quite disturbed when the nurse attempts to feed him because infants do not accommodate to mouth breathing and cannot suck and breathe at the same time. They develop dyspnea during attempts to feed. If one forcibly closes the mouth, the infant will become dyspneic and cyanotic.

These infants are usually gavage fed, but must be observed between feedings, for the tongue may drop backward, obstruct the airway (glossoptosis), and cause cyanosis. It is the nurse's responsibility to keep the nostrils clean and to use utmost care in feeding to prevent aspiration of formula. If the obstruction is membranous, it may be dilated by threading a catheter through the membrane; if the obstruction is bony, operative intervention is the treatment of choice.

*Congenital laryngeal stridor.* An abnormal collapse of the larynx with inspiration is called congenital laryngeal stridor. The infant starts with noisy respirations at birth or shortly thereafter. The nurse will hear a crowing sound on inspiration that is intensified when the infant is lying supine or is crying. This does not interfere with sucking and the color remains good. Depending on severity of the stridor, the infant may become dyspneic with periods of cyanosis. Nursing responsibility is the same as with choanal atresia. The mild form usually subsides within 6 months to 1 year. For a severe stridor, surgery may be necessary.

*Diaphragmatic hernia.* Diaphragmatic hernia is a protrusion of the abdominal viscera into the thoracic cavity through a defect in the diaphragm. It tends to occur more on the left side. (See Fig. 26-9.)

The infant may manifest severe respiratory difficulties at birth, such as dyspnea and cyanosis; in other instances an infant shows no problems until hours or even days later. Early recognition by the nurse is very important; asymmetry of the chest and an underdeveloped, smaller than normal abdomen are early signs. After the doctor examines the infant and a roentgenogram confirms his diagnosis, no time is lost in surgical intervention.

### Miscellaneous anomalies

*Cleft palate and cleft lip.* Cleft palate is the incomplete fusion of intermaxillary process that may be unilateral or bilateral. Maldevelopment of the palate is often associated with cleft lip. Approximately one in 2,500 have the cleft palate but normal development of the lip. Cleft lip is the failure of fusion of upper lip. Seventy percent of these are afflicted with cleft palate and the condition occurs more often in males. Heredity is a factor with these anomalies, but environmental factors may also play a part. (See Fig. 26-10.)

The mother needs instructions and practice in feeding the infant. The infant has difficulty creating suction and tends to become irritable during feeding. The Lamb's or Ducky nipple is longer, softer, and more practical than the regular type nipple. These infants tend to swallow excessive air and need to be fed slowly and bubbled frequently.

*Gentiourinary system.* Congenital anomalies of the genitourinary system are more frequent than any other system. They account for 20% of the stillbirths and neonatal deaths. (See Fig. 26-11.)

*Bilateral renal agenesis.* The characteristics of this abnormality are (1) bowing of the legs, attributed to fixed position in the uterus, as the result of oligohydramnios, (2) mature expression of the face with recession of the chin, (3) ears are large and set "low" on sides of the head, and (4) occurs more often in males.

*Sex anomalies.* Infants born with gonadal tissue of both sexes are called hermaphrodites. In the male infant the presence of testes but undetermined external genitalia is called pseudohermaphroditism. The external genitalia may resemble

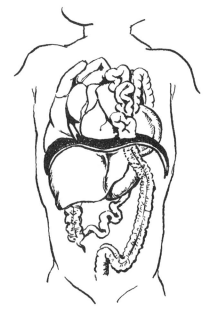

**Fig. 26-9.** Diaphragmatic hernia showing abdominal viscera herniated into the thoracic cavity.

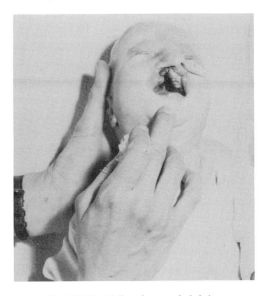

**Fig. 26-10.** Cleft palate and cleft lip.

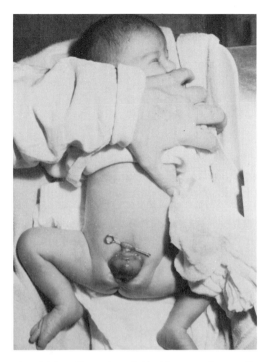

**Fig. 26-11.** Exstrophy of bladder—an abnormality in union of lower abdominal wall, exposing bladder. This abnormality involves the genital organs.

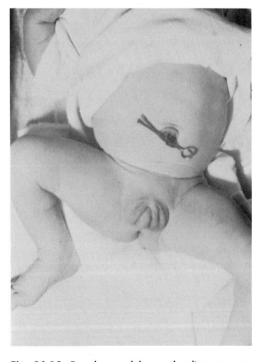

**Fig. 26-12.** Female pseudohermaphrodite—two ovaries present but external genitalia ambiguous.

that of the female. Masculinization of female fetus is often produced by the administration of progestational hormones to the mother. This type is not progressive. (See Fig. 26-12.)

A more common cause is the congenital adrenal hyperplasia (adrenogenital syndrome). Female genitalia deviate from the normal due to excessive excretion of androgens or cortical adrenal hormones. This type is progressive after birth.

**Down's syndrome.** Through the research of geneticists it has been determined that a genetic error in the number or in the construction of the chromosome may result in various anomalies in the newborn. Down's syndrome is the name given to just such a chromosomal abnormality.

Normally within each body cell there are 23 *pairs* of chromosomes for a total of 46. When the chromosome appears in triplicate instead of in pairs of two, it is called *trisomy.* In Down's syndrome the chromosome number is 47 instead of 46. It seems to be the two chromosomes of pair 21 that fail to separate during gametogenesis; hence the name "trisomy 21." This extra chromosome causes physical, sexual, and mental retardation. It would appear that this aberration has a tendency to increase with advanced maternal age.

Not all infants with Down's syndrome have the defect in pair 21 of their chromosomes. In fact, the chromosome count may be normal, but it has been postulated that a chromosome of one pair may separate and attach itself to another chromosome or there may be an exchange of portions of different chromosomes. This form of the disorder is called *translocation* and may be transmitted through many generations, usually the offspring of young mothers who are more likely to give birth to siblings with Down's syndrome.

Infants with Down's syndrome have the following characteristics:

1. Infants are small for their gestational age.
2. Eyes slant upward and a prominent

epicanthal fold of skin involves the inner aspect of upper eyelid.

3. Tongue protrudes and infant breathes through his mouth.
4. Hand has simian crease pattern, with short fingers, and absence of middle phalanx of fifth finger.
5. Face has characteristic expression and grimace.
6. White flecks can be seen in the iris.
7. The entire body is hypotonic.

*Fixed posture anomalies.* Some congenital anomalies originate from fixed posture of the fetus in utero. Examples are congenital clubfoot, congenital torticollis, and distortion of the mandible. It is believed these are associated with oligohydramnios.

## The circumcision[2,14,15]

Initially, God gave the rite of circumcision to Abraham and commanded him to circumcise his son and any male servants at least 8 days of age. Genesis 17:10-13, "This is my covenant, which you shall keep, between me and you and your descendants after you: Every male among you shall be circumcised. You shall be circumcised in the flesh of your foreskins, and it shall be a sign of the covenant between me and you. He that is eight days old among you shall be circumcised; every male throughout your generations, whether born in your house, or bought with your money from any foreigner who is not of your offspring, both he that is born in your house and he that is bought with your money, shall be circumcised." In Exodus: 4:25, Zipporah, wife of Moses, performed circumcision upon her son with a sharp stone.

The rite of circumcision has subsisted in the Jewish religion to the present day; it was instituted by God as a physical reminder of the covenant established between God and the Israelites. Bris milah, as circumcision is officially called, represents the Jewish parents' love and devotion for their child by dedicating him to God. Interestingly enough, the rite takes place on the eighth day, the time when the pro-

thrombin level is again normal. Since it is a religious ceremony, the circumcision is performed by the mohel (the Rabbi) and commemorates God's choosing the Jews to be his own people.

There are many pros and cons regarding the necessity of circumcision, but interestingly enough the rate of penile cancer has been negligible among the Jews. Doctors attribute this asset to the scrupulous hygiene the Jewish people maintain.

Nurses may be led to believe by medical and lay writers that the infant suffers no pain during the circumcision, but this is not true. The prepuce contains a network of nerve endings and his sensitivity to pain increases day by day.

Whether or not the infant should be circumcised is a matter to be decided by the parents. Some male infants have a fully retractable prepuce, others do not. The important factor is the time selected for the procedure. It is routine in many newborn nurseries to do a bleeding and coagulation time on all male infants prior to circumcision. The normal bleeding time at birth is 2 minutes and coagulation time is 3 minutes. The prothrombin time is highest at birth; it then declines until the eighth day when it again reaches normal levels.

The nurse needs to keep watch over the infant after circumcision, for infants die each year as the result of hemorrhage. Placing a red tag on the infant's unit serves as a good reminder that the infant needs to be checked frequently for bleeding.

Contraindications would be (1) abnormal bleeding and coagulation time, (2) clinical manifestations of jaundice, (3) vomiting, and (4) skin eruptions.

**STUDY QUESTIONS**

*Matching*

Match the terms in the first column with their appropriate definitions in the second column:
1. (a) Presence of __Ears set low on side of
    a respira-        head
    tory dis-
    order

(b) Vomiting and diarrhea    —Fontanels are depressed

(c) Calcium gluconate    —Intestinal obstruction below the bile duct

(d) Vomiting    —Fontanels become tense

(e) Regurgitation    —Clinical sign of brain damage

(f) Narrowing of pyloric lumen    —Vomiting usually starts second or third week of life

(g) Bile-stained vomitus    —Observation of infrequent and irregularly spaced respirations

(h) Rhythmic protrusion of the tongue    —Usual symptoms of digestive disturbance

(i) Brain damage    —Implies return of small amount of feeding

(j) Dehydration    —Implies emptying of stomach

(k) Bilateral renal agenesis    —To counteract hypocalcemia during transfusion

2. (a) Surfactant    —Contributes to hyperbilirubinemia

(b) Diarrhea    —Contagious skin infection

(c) Charcoal    —Injury to nerve fibers of brachial plexus

(d) Klumpke's paralysis    —Form of paralysis involving hand

(e) Soda bicarbonate    —Vomiting first day of life

(f) Gantrisin    —May be due to overfeeding infant

(g) Impetigo    —Prevents reabsorption of bile into circulation

(h) Pyloric stenosis    —Vomiting seldom projectile

(i) Esophageal atresia    —Ejects vomitus through the nose

(j) Erb-Duchenne palsy    —Projectile vomiting and peristaltic waves over stomach

(k) Gastrointestinal obstruction    —To counteract metabolic acidosis

(l) Pylorospasm    —Lipoprotein substance secreted by alveolar epithelium

## Multiple choice

1. A cephalhematoma:
   (a) is noticeable at birth.
   (b) may contribute to clinical jaundice.
   (c) disappears soon after birth.
   (d) Is a blood tumor between skull and periosteum.
   (e) is a blood tumor between the periosteum and brain substance.
   1. a, c, and e    2. b and d    3. a, c, and d

2. An infant has bile-stained vomitus on the second day after birth. You will observe the infant for:
   (a) abdominal distention.
   (b) passage of clay-colored stools.
   (c) passage of meconium.
   1. a and b    2. a and c    3. a only

3. Mrs. A is concerned because her infant is severely jaundiced. The doctor told her of the possibility of the need for an exchange transfusion and she questions you about the danger involved in the procedure. The most appropriate answer would be:
   (a) there is always danger but if not transfused, the infant will surely die.
   (b) transfusion is a wonderful advance in medical science. The infant not transfused or transfused too late is usually the victim of brain damage.
   (c) the blood your baby is to receive will replace the blood cells that are causing the jaundice. Today's methods of exchange transfusion are most effective.

4. An infant is admitted to the nursery with yellow discoloration of the cord. The nurse knows this might be due to:
   (a) hyperbilirubinemia.
   (b) fetal anoxia.
   (c) breech presentation.
   (d) all of these.
   1. d    2. a and b    3. a and c

5. Mrs. B is admitted in active labor with a history of having made one prenatal visit to the clinic. When the infant is admitted to the nursery, there is a notation to the effect that the mother is a known drug addict. The nurse will expect Mrs. B's infant to exhibit the following symptoms of withdrawal:
   (a) twitching of the extremities.
   (b) shrill cry.
   (c) diarrhea and vomiting.
   (d) infant to be listless with episodes of cyanosis.
   1. a, b, c    2. c and d    3. a and d

6. Mrs. D, a known diabetic, delivered a 9-pound boy with a diaphragmatic hernia. In addition to congenital anomalies, other conditions contribute to the mortality of infants born to diabetic mothers such as:
   (a) congestive heart failure.
   (b) hyaline membrane disease.
   (c) intracranial hemorrhage.
   (d) all of these.

7. If the nurse observes edema and discoloration of the external genitalia on a newborn infant, she would check to see what the presentation was because this is rather common with:

(a) breech.
(b) posterior.
(c) compound.

8. The nurse would expect a newborn infant to keep his lower extremities in the same attitude as in utero if the presentation was:
(a) footling.
(b) frank breech.
(c) complete breech.

*True or false*

(T) (F) 1. There is a correlation of hyaline membrane disease with maternal hemorrhage.

(T) (F) 2. Intracranial pressure commonly produces vomiting.

(T) (F) 3. Infants with hyaline membrane disease always have a poor Apgar score at birth.

(T) (F) 4. Failure to feed well is an early sign that the infant is ill.

(T) (F) 5. Soda bicarbonate solution is a treatment for impetigo neonatorum.

(T) (F) 6. When hyperbilirubinemia is unrelated to erythroblastosis fetalis, the jaundice develops more slowly.

(T) (F) 7. With Klumpke's paralysis, nerve roots of the brachial plexus are affected.

(T) (F) 8. Two main etiological factors predisposing to intracranial hemorrhage are trauma and anoxia.

(T) (F) 9. It is not uncommon for an infant to have a wryneck if delivered in breech presentation.

(T) (F) 10. Fever is the first sign of infection in the newborn.

(T) (F) 11. The postmature infant has a great deal of lanugo.

(T) (F) 12. Postmature infants are usually victims of respiratory distress syndrome.

(T) (F) 13. Grunting is evidence of hypoxia.

## REFERENCES

1. New light on neonatal jaundice, New Eng. J. Med. **280**:779, April, 1969.
2. The medical controversy over circumcision, Good Housekeeping **167**:179, 1968.
3. Babson, Gorham S., and Benson, Ralph C.: Primer on prematurity and high-risk pregnancy, St. Louis, 1966, The C. V. Mosby Co., p. 97.
4. Behrman, R. E.: Phototherapy and hyperbilirubinemia, J. Pediat. **74**:989, June, 1969.
5. Behrman, R. E.: Summary of a symposium on phototherapy for hyperbilirubinemia, J. Pediat. **75**:718, Oct., 1969.
6. Britten, Anthony F.: Neonatal exchange transfusion, Clin. Pediat. **7**:125, March, 1968.
7. Lucey, Jerold F.: Light on jaundice, New Eng. J. Med. **280**:1076, May, 1969.
8. Lucey, Jerold F.: Benefits of phototherapy outweighs theoretical risks, Hosp. Top. **48**:69, Jan., 1970.
9. Lucey, J., Ferreiro, M., and Hewitt, J.: Prevention of hyperbilirubinemia of prematurity by phototherapy, Pediatrics **41**:1047, June, 1968.
10. Pangopoulos, G., Valaes, T., and Doxiodis, S. A.: Morbidity and mortality related to exchange transfusion, J. Pediat. **74**:247, Feb., 1969.
11. Pochedly, Carl: The exchange transfusion, Clin. Pediat. **7**:383, July, 1968.
12. Potter, Edith L.: Pathology of fetus and infant, Chicago, 1962, Year Book Medical Publishers, Inc., pp. 477-478.
13. Schaffer, Alexander: Diseases of the newborn, Philadelphia, 1965, W. B. Saunders Co., p. 629.
14. Schaffer, Alexander: Diseases of the newborn, Philadelphia, 1965, W. B. Saunders Co., p. 442.
15. Weiss, Charles: Does circumcision of newborn require an anesthetic? Clin. Pediat. **7**:128, March, 1968.

## SELECTED READINGS
*Respiratory distress*

Avery, Mary Ellen: The lung and its disorders in the newborn infant, Philadelphia, 1964, W. B. Saunders Co., chaps. 10 and 11.

Babson, Gorham S., and Benson, Ralph C.: Primer on prematurity and high-risk pregnancy, St. Louis, 1966, The C. V. Mosby Co., pp. 129-133.

Desmond, Murdina, Rudolph, Arnold, and Pineda, Rebecca: Clinical diagnosis of respiratory difficulties in the newborn, Pediat. Clin. N. Amer. **13**:669, 1966.

Fate of survivors of hyaline membrane disease, New Eng. J. Med. **279**:1111, Nov., 1968.

Graw, Robert G.: Respiratory distress syndrome, Clin. Pediat. **7**:510, Sept., 1968.

Hargrove, Cecilia: Hyaline membrane disease, RN **30**:78, Feb., 1967.

Harrison, V. C., Heese, H. de V., and Klein, M.: The significance of grunting in hyaline membrane disease, Pediatrics **41**:548, Sept., 1968.

Hodson, W. Alan, and Chernick, Victor: Respiratory emergencies in the infant, Hosp. Med. **5**:18, Feb., 1969.

Hull, David: Lung expansion and ventilation during resuscitation of asphyxiated newborn infants, J. Pediat. **75**:47, July, 1969.

Kendig, Edwin, editor: Disorders of the respiratory tract in children, Philadelphia, 1967, W. B. Saunders Co., sect. 3.

Mitchell, Ross G.: Apnoeic attacks in the newborn infant, Nurs. Times 62:101, Jan., 1966.

Nelson, Nicholas, and Scully, Robert: Respiratory distress and cyanosis in the newborn infant, New Eng. J. Med. 278:496, Feb., 1968.

Pringle, Janet: Respiratory distress unit, Amer. J. Nurs. 68:2370, Nov., 1968.

Schaffer, Alexander: Diseases of the newborn, Philadelphia, 1965, W. B. Saunders Co., chap. 10.

Shanklin, Douglas R.: An approach to prevention of hyaline membrane disease, Hosp. Top. 47:59, Aug., 1969.

Shaklin, Douglas R., and Wolfson, S. L.: Oxygen as a cause of pulmonary hemorrhage in infants, New Eng. J. Med. 277:833, Oct., 1967.

Shepard, Frank M.: Residual pulmonary findings in clinical hyaline membrane disease, New Eng. J. Med. 279:1063, Nov. 14, 1968.

Sinclair, John C.: Prevention and treatment of respiratory distress syndrome, Pediat. Clin. N. Amer. 13:711, Aug., 1966.

Smith, Clement: Respiratory distress syndrome. In Gellis, Sydney, and Kagan, Benjamin, editors: Current pediatric therapy, Philadelphia, 1967, W. B. Saunders Co., pp. 846-848.

*High-risk neonate*

Behrman, Richard: Care of high-risk infant. In Varga, Charles: Handbook of pediatric medical emergencies, ed. 4, St. Louis, 1968, The C. V. Mosby Co., p. 73.

Duffy, Edw. A.: Foci of high infant mortality, Clin. Pediat. 7:63, Feb., 1968.

Hardy, Janet: Birth injuries. In Gellis, Sydney, and Kagan, Benjamin, editors: Current pediatric therapy, Philadelphia, 1967, W. B. Saunders Co., pp. 840-844.

Hart, E. W.: Hemorrhagic states in the newborn infant, Nurs. Mirror 127:28, Oct. 25, 1968.

Kendig, Edwin: The place of BCG vaccine in the management of infants born of tuberculous mothers, New Eng. J. Med. 281:520, Sept., 1969.

Langworth, J., and Steele, R.: Sudden unexpected death in infancy, Canad. Nurse 62:42, Sept., 1966.

Lees, Martin H.: Heart failure in newborn infant, J. Pediat. 75:139, July, 1969.

Northway, W., Jr., and Rosan, R.: Oxygen therapy hazards in the neonate, Hosp. Pract. 4:59, Jan., 1969.

Prosser, Robert: Recent advances in knowledge of the newborn, Nurs. Times 63:1708, Dec., 1967.

Pryor, Helen, and Thelander, Hulda: Abnormally small head size and intellect in children, J. Pediat. 73:593, Oct., 1968.

Rickham, Peter: The ethics of surgery in newborn infants, Clin. Pediat. 8:251, May, 1969.

Windle, Wm. F.: Brain damage at birth, J.A.M.A. 206:1967, Nov., 1968.

*Hyperbilirubinemia*

Bentley, Herschel P., Jr.: Hyperbilirubinemia of the newborn infant. In Shirkey, Harry C., editor: Pediatric therapy, ed. 3, St. Louis, 1968, The C. V. Mosby Co., chap. 89.

Bowman, John M., and Frisen, Rhinehart: Hemolytic disease of the newborn. In Gellis, Sydney S., and Kagan, Benjamin M., editors: Current pediatric therapy, Philadelphia, 1967, W. B. Saunders Co., pp. 330-334.

Oski, Frank A., and Naiman, J. Lawrence: Hematologic problems in the newborn, Philadelphia, 1966, W. B. Saunders Co., chap. 6.

Reiquam, C. W., Beatty, E. C., and Connell, John R.: Erythroblastosis fetalis, Clin. Pediat. 6:411, July, 1967.

Schaffer, Alexander: Diseases of the newborn, Philadelphia, 1965, W. B. Saunders Co., chap. 72.

Smith, Carl: Blood diseases of infancy and childhood, ed. 2, St. Louis, 1966, The C. V. Mosby Co., chaps. 9 and 10.

*Birth defects*

Alexopoulos, K. A.: Choanal atresia, Clin. Pediat. 6:579, Oct., 1967.

Apgar, Virginia: Birth defects, J.A.M.A. 204:371, April, 1968.

Avery, Mary Ellen: The lung and its disorders in the newborn infant, Philadelphia, 1964, W. B. Saunders Co., chap. 8.

Betson, Carol, Valoon, Patricia, and Soika, Cynthia: Cardiac surgery in neonates: a chance for life, Amer. J. Nurs. 69:69, Jan., 1969.

Blake, Florence, and Wright, F. Howell: Essentials of pediatric nursing, ed. 7, Philadelphia, 1963, J. B. Lippincott Co., chap. 11.

Broadribb, Violet: Foundations of pediatric nursing, Philadelphia, 1967, J. B. Lippincott Co., chap. 8.

Bryden, June, and Tyndale, Anne: When a handicapped child is born, Nurs. Times 64:1516, Nov., 1968.

Eckstein, H. B.: Complications of ventriculoatrial drainage for hydrocephalus, Nurs. Mirror 126:29, May, 1968.

Goldman, Allen S.: Congenital malformations and a world survey, Clin. Pediat. 6:675, Dec., 1967.

Hillsman, Gladys: Genetics and the nurse, Nurs. Outlook 14:34, Jan., 1966.

Holmes, Lewis, and Atkins, Leonard: An abnormal C-group chromosome in a child with severe growth retardation, J. Pediat. 73:119, July, 1968.

Ingalls, Theodore H., and Henry, Thomas A.:

Trisomy and D/G translocation mongolism in brothers, New Eng. J. Med. **278**:10, Jan., 1968.

Ingraham, Franc D., and Matson, Donald D.: Neurosurgery in infancy and childhood, Springfield, Ill., 1954, Charles C Thomas, Publisher, chap. 1.

Juberg, Richard C.: Heredity counseling, Nurs. Outlook **14**:28, Jan., 1966.

Lagos, Jorge, and Siekert, Robert: Intracranial hemorrhage in infancy and childhood, Clin. Pediat. **8**:90, Feb., 1969.

Larsen, Grace I.: What every nurse should know about congenital syphilis, Nurs. Outlook **13**:52, March, 1965.

Laurence, K. M.: Spina bifida cystica, Nurs. Times **63**:620, May, 1967.

Lorber, John: Children with spina bifida, Nurs. Mirror **127**:19, Sept., 1968.

Lorber, John: Neurologic assessment of neonates with spina bifida, Clin. Pediat. **7**:676, Nov., 1968.

Milunsky, Aubrey, Graef, J. W., and Gaynor, M. F., Jr.: Methotrexate-induced congenital malformations, J. Pediat. **72**:790, June, 1967.

Montagu, M. F. Ashley: Prenatal influences, Springfield, Ill., 1962, Charles C Thomas, Publisher, pp. 113-116.

Naggan, Lechaim, and MacMahon, Breau: Ethnic differences in the prevalence of anencephaly and spina bifida, New Eng. J. Med. **277**:1119, Nov., 1967.

Rosen, Mortimer G.: Studies of brain damage in the fetus and the newborn, Hosp. Top. **47**:91, March, 1969.

Rudolph, Jerome: A tip-off congenital anomalies in the newborn, Consultant **6**:10, 1966.

Saxoni, Fotini, Lapaanis, P., and Pantelakis, S. N.: Congenital syphilis, Clin. Pediat. **6**:687, Dec., 1967.

Schaffer, Alexander: Diseases of the newborn, Philadelphia, 1965, W. B. Saunders Co., chap. 104.

Stern, Curt: Some general aspects of human genetics, Amer. J. Obstet. Gynec. **99**:604, Nov., 1968.

Stimson, Cyrus: Understanding the mongoloid child, Today's Health, **46**:56, Nov., 1968.

Thompson, Marg.: Genetic counseling in clinical pediatrics, Clin. Pediat. **6**:199, April, 1967.

Touloukian, Robert and Pickett, Lawrence: Management of the newborn with imperforate anus, Clin. Pediat. **8**:389, July, 1969.

Townes, Philip: Mongolism in a child with 48 chromosomes, J. Pediat. **73**:97, July, 1968.

Valenti, Carl, Schutta, E. J., and Kehaty, T.: Cystogenic diagnosis of Down's syndrome in utero, J.A.M.A. **207**:1513, Feb., 1969.

Valentine, G. H.: The chromosome disorders, Philadelphia, 1966, J. B. Lippincott Co., chap. 5.

Watkins, Arthur G.: Spina bifida cystica, Nurs. Times **64**:316, March, 1968.

Winick, Myron: Birth defects: what is being done about them, Nurs. Outlook **14**:43, Jan., 1966.

Wright, Stanley: Down's syndrome. In Gellis, Sydney, and Kagan, Benjamin, editors: Current pediatric therapy, 1967, W. B. Saunders Co., p. 21.

*Abnormalities in sexual development*

Bakwin, Harry, and Bakwin, Ruth: Clinical management of behavior disorders in children, ed. 3, Philadelphia, 1966, W. B. Saunders Co., p. 436.

Beas, Francisco, Vargas, Luis, Spada, Raúl P., and Merchak, Norman: Pseudoprecocious puberty in infants caused by a dermal ointment containing estrogens, J. Pediat. **75**:127, July, 1969.

Crigler, John: Hermaphroditism. In Gellis, Sydney, and Kagan, Benjamin, editors: Current pediatric therapy, Philadelphia, 1967, W. B. Saunders Co., p. 392.

Grollman, Arthur: Clinical endocrinology and its physiologic basis, Philadelphia, 1964, J. B. Lippincott Co., chap. 11.

Hughes, James G.: Synopsis of pediatrics, St. Louis, 1967, The C. V. Mosby Co., pp. 562-569.

Montagu, M. F. Ashley: Prenatal influences, Springfield, Ill., 1962, Charles C Thomas, Publisher, pp. 349-354.

Schaffer, Alexander: Diseases of the newborn, Philadelphia, 1965, W. B. Saunders Co., p. 524.

Valentine, G. H.: The chromosome disorders, Philadelphia, 1966, J. B. Lippincott Co., p. 122.

Voorhess, Mary L.: Masculinization of female fetus associated with norethindrone-mestranol therapy during pregnancy, J. Pediat. **71**:128, July, 1967.

*Postmaturity*

Clifford, Stewart H.: Postmaturity and dysmaturity. In Gellis, Sydney, and Kagan, Benjamin, editors: Current pediatric therapy, Philadelphia, 1967, W. B. Saunders Co., p. 840.

Miller, James: Dermal ridge patterns; technique for their study in human fetuses, J. Pediat. **73**:614, Oct., 1968.

Montagu, M. F. Ashley: Life before birth, New York, 1964, New American Library, Inc., p. 181.

Montagu, M. F. Ashley: Prenatal influences, Springfield, Ill., 1962, Charles C Thomas, Publisher, p. 413.

Potter, Edith L.: Pathology of fetus and infant, Chicago, 1962, Year Book Medical Publishers, Inc., pp. 30-31.

Schaffer, Alexander: Diseases of the newborn, Philadelphia, 1965, W. B. Saunders Co., p. 30.

*Phenylketonuria*

Davis, Louis: Practical points in PKU testing, Nurs. Outlook **14**:46, Jan., 1966.

Desper, Mary: PKU symptoms, diagnosis, treatment and prognosis, RN **30**:63, March, 1967.

Epps, Roselyn Payne: Phenylketonuria in an American Negro infant, Clin. Pediat. **7**:607, Oct., 1968.

Fisch, Robert O.: Down's syndrome with phenylketonuria, Clin. Pediat. **7**:226, April, 1968.

Forbes, Nancy, Shaw, Kenneth N., Koch, Richard, Coffelt, R. Wendell, and Straus, Reuben: Maternal phenylketonuria, Nurs. Outlook **14**:40, Jan., 1966.

Frankenburg, Wm.: Maternal phenylketonuria: implications for growth and development, J. Pediat. **73**:560, Oct., 1968.

Hughes, James G.: Synopsis of pediatrics, St. Louis, 1967, The C. V. Mosby Co., pp. 662-666.

Keleski, Lorelei, Solomons, G., and Opitz, E.: Parental reactions to PKU in the family, J. Pediat. **70**:793, May, 1967.

Koch, Richard, and Dobson, James: Hospital screening programs aid identification of PKU, Hosp. Top. **46**:111, June, 1968.

Lyman, Frank L., editor: Phenylketonuria, Springfield, Ill., 1963, Charles C Thomas, Publisher.

O'Flynn, Margaret: Some observations on the dietary treatment of PKU, J. Pediat. **72**:260, Feb., 1968.

Pineda, G.: Variability in the manifestations of phenylketonuria, J. Pediat. **72**:528, April, 1968.

Schaffer, Alexander: Diseases of the newborn, Philadelphia, 1965, W. B. Saunders Co., p. 918.

Warkany, Josef, and Fraser, F. Clark: Defect in metabolism and amino acids. In Nelson, Waldo E., editor: Textbook of pediatrics, ed. 8, Philadelphia, 1964, W. B. Saunders Co., p. 290.

*Infants born of diabetic mothers*

Behrman, Richard: Infant of diabetic. In Vargo, Charles: Handbook of pediatric medical emergencies, ed. 4, St. Louis, 1968, The C. V. Mosby Co., pp. 66-67.

Farquhar, James: Infants born to diabetic mothers: In Gellis, Sydney, and Kagan, Benjamin, editors: Current pediatric therapy, Philadelphia, 1967, W. B. Saunders Co., p. 398.

Fischer, Alfred E.: Management of newborn infants born to diabetic mothers. In Rovinsky, Joseph, editor: Medical, surgical and gynecologic complications of pregnancy, Baltimore, 1965, The Williams & Wilkins Co., pp. 613-617.

Greenhill, J. P., editor: Obstetrics, ed. 13, Philadelphia, 1965, W. B. Saunders Co., p. 1002.

Hagbard, Lars: Pregnancy and diabetes mellitus, Springfield, Ill., 1966, Charles C Thomas, Publisher, pp. 80-85.

Halldorson, Salvar, editor: Hypoglycemia in infants, Clin. Pediat. **6**:94, 1967.

Kahn, Charles B.: Clinical and chemical diabetes in offspring of diabetic couples, New Eng. J. Med. **281**:343, Aug., 1969.

McKay, R. J., Jr., and Smith, Clement A.: Infants of diabetic mothers. In Nelson, Waldo, editor: Textbook of pediatrics, ed. 8, Philadelphia, 1964, W. B. Saunders Co., p. 392.

Schaffer, Alexander: Diseases of the newborn, Philadelphia, 1965, W. B. Saunders Co., p. 41.

**For student's quick notes:**

Chapter 27

# The high-risk neonate—II

How does the transition to extrauterine life differ for the tiny infant exposed before completion of the gestational period? What are his limitations and the problems he must surmount if he is to survive? This you will learn about in Chapter 27. In addition, you will become aware of the tremendous responsibility the nurse assumes as she gives her undivided attention and care to this helpless creature of humanity.

## The low birth weight and premature infant

It has been customary to classify infants with a birth weight of less than 2,500 grams (5½ pounds) as "premature." Seven percent of the births in the United States come under this classification. Birth weight is not in itself a sufficient criterion for defining prematurity. The period of gestation is also an important adjunct to be considered.

The American Academy of Pediatrics has accepted a recommendation by the Expert Committee on Maternal and Child Health of the World Health Organization that classifies live-born infants with a birth weight of 2,500 grams or less as *low birth weight,* and live-born infants with gestational period of less than 37 weeks as *premature,* regardless of their weight. The inaccuracy of this definition is that many women do not or cannot give an accurate date as to the first day of their last menses, but it does emphasize the fact that low birth weight infants may or may not be premature and that a premature infant is not necessarily of low birth weight.

Many of the so-called low birth weight infants do have a gestational age of 37 weeks or more, in many instances because of some interference with intrauterine growth. A weight of 1,500 grams identifies "very small" infants.

Other criteria for determining prematurity are as follows: (1) head circumference less than 33 cm.; (2) head circumference 3 cm. or more over circumference of the thorax; and (3) crown-rump measurement less than 32 cm.

### Etiology

The incidence of prematurity and low birth weight infants is associated with a combination of factors. High-risk pregnancies predispose to early delivery. See premature labor, pp. 183 and 184.

### Incidence

The incidence is higher with the following: (1) age—youngest and oldest mothers (under 16 and primigravidas over 40), (2) plural births, (3) inadequate nutrition, (4) lack of or inadequate prenatal care, (5) history of previous early labors, abortions, and premature deliveries, and (6) cigarette smoking. The incidence of low birth weight infants is doubled when the mother is a heavy smoker because tobacco smoke robs the blood of oxygen.

There is a definite correlation between premature births and economic status. Among low income groups, the rate of prematurity is higher. "The prematurity rate is more related to the socioeconomic environment during the mother's childhood than to her social status in adult life."*

## Mortality

Prematurity accounts for 55% of neonatal deaths. Over one half of the deaths occur within the first 24 hours of life. These deaths are associated with (1) atelectasis, with or without hyaline membrane disease, (2) infections, (3) intracranial hemorrhage from anoxia or trauma, and (4) malformations.

## Clinical signs specifically pointing to "early exposure"

1. The skin is thin, reddish pink, translucent.
2. The infant is inactive and somnolent.
3. The fontanels are small and the sutures are narrow.
4. The cry is feeble.
5. All responses are readily fatigued.
6. Labia minora are prominent; in the male the scrotum is small and testes frequently undescended.
7. Reflexes are not well defined.
8. Subcutaneous fat is lacking (one reason why these infants are unable to maintain satisfactory body temperature).

Within a short time the nurse will observe:

1. Skin becomes pale (physiological drop in hemoglobin level).
2. Jaundice appears in 36 to 72 hours, continues in severity to about the seventh day, and persists for 2 weeks.
3. The infant will lose approximately 7 ounces within the first 4 to 6 days (10% to 20% of birth weight).
4. The infant will regain his birth weight within 2 to 3 weeks and dou-

ble it in 2 months, depending on maturity at birth.

## Limitations of premature infants

The premature infant requires intensive care by skilled nurses because his transition to extrauterine existence is indeed hazardous, especially during neonatal period.

Because the infant left the protection and security of the uterus long before his physical development was complete, he is born with many limitations. He has specific physical needs that must be met if he is to survive.

What are some of the life sustaining environmental conditions this infant was denied by his early exposure?

1. He lacks fat needed to insulate and conserve body heat.
2. He has poor reflex control of skin capillaries.
3. He cannot maintain adequate temperature to sustain life independently.
4. His respiratory system functions inadequately, which is attributed to immaturity of central nervous system, especially the centers in the brain regulating and maintaining constant rhythmic breathing. Maintaining respirations is a major factor in his fight for life.
5. Blood vascular system is fragile. Poor formation of prothrombin predisposes to bleeding.
6. Poor development of cardiac sphincter means poor defense against tracheal aspiration.
7. Since mineralization of bones occurs in the last month of gestation, the premature will have a small calcium deposit in his bones at birth. The bones of the skull, therefore, are not able to withstand pressure of the birth process. This leads to hemorrhages with irreversible brain damage.
8. Glomeruli and tubules are inefficient. This predisposes to electrolyte and water imbalance with edema and resulting acidosis.

*From Babson, Gorham S., and Benson, Ralph C.: Primer on prematurity and high-risk pregnancy, St. Louis, 1966, The C. V. Mosby Co., p. 16.

*Admission care and nursing responsibilities*

Tremendous indeed are the nursing responsibilities as the nurse strives to maintain and stabilize adequate body temperature, to conserve heat and energy, and to support the infant's feeble respiratory efforts. Supportive measures include the following:

1. Place infant in Isolette or incubator. If environmental temperature is not 90° F., leave infant wrapped in receiving blankets. The doctor may require the weight immediately for determining solutions or medications he may wish to order. If so, weigh with coverings left on infant. Remove and weigh blankets after infant is transferred to Isolette and subtract this weight. In other instances, weighing the infant can be postponed until hours later. Omit sponging with pHisoHex and cord care. *Rest* is most important after the hazardous ordeal of birth.
2. Aspirate nasal secretions gently with bulb syringe.

*Oxygen needs*

1. Observe skin color for pallor, jaundice, or cyanosis.
2. Give oxygen only in sufficient amount to relieve cyanosis and dyspnea; administer oxygen by funnel only in an emergency.
3. Check and record oxygen concentration every 2 hours with oxymeter.

*Temperature*[2,3]

1. Maintain adequate environmental warmth (90° to 97° F.) and maintain controlled body temperature at 97° F.
2. Take axillary temperature every 2 hours until stabilized (not necessary with skin thermistor control).
3. Ideal incubator temperature of 90° F. maintains axillary temperature of 97° F. for infants over 1,000 grams.
4. Make every effort to maintain temperature at 97° F.
5. Report temperature under 96° F. or over 99° F. (decrease in temperature increases infant's oxygen requirement).

*Humidity.* Humidity within neutral range (40% to 70%) aids in stabilization of body temperature and prevents drying effect on the membrane lining the respiratory tract. Humidity may also decrease the irritating effect oxygen might have on tissues.

*Respirations.* Observe the respiratory rate, sternal retraction, and expiratory grunting. Periodic breathing with episodes of apnea is characteristic of the very low birth weight infants (usually observed after 12 hours) as the result of disturbance in acid-base balance. The infant may need gentle stimulation during these intervals. Prolonged apnea is a sign of central nervous system disturbance or infection.

*Positioning infant*

1. Place infant on his right side with blanket roll at back for support, or on his back with slight elevation of head and shoulders (especially with respiratory distress). Placing the small premature infant on his abdomen interferes with his breathing since, in this position, the liver will push against the diaphragm.
2. Change position at feeding time.

*Infant clothing*

1. No clothing should be put on infants under 3½ pounds.
2. Diaper only those 3½ to 4 pounds.
3. At 4½ pounds dress infant and open portholes on Isolette. Infant is ready to be placed in open crib when he can maintain his own temperature in nursery environment.

*Other factors*

1. Observe for variations in behavior or appearance. (May be an early indication of infection.)
2. Protect infant from infection.
3. The nurse must be alert at all times to recognize deviations from the normal and know how to cope with emergency situations.
4. Keep Isolettes and incubators scrupulously clean. Change water in Iso-

lette or incubators daily, or add 1.5 ml. of silver nitrate solution (1:1000) per liter of water and change every third day.

### Silverman-Andersen score

"This method, which was developed for scoring the breathing performance of premature infants, is based on signs of respiratory retraction. . . . Recorded as important signs of distress are (1) retraction of the chest as compared with abdominal respiration during inspiration, (2) retraction of lower intercostal muscles, (3) retraction of the xyphoid, (4) chin-tug with inspiration, and (5) expiratory grunt. A score of 0 indicates good ventilation. When scored by this method the prognosis of infants, particularly as applied to those born prematurely, shows a high degree of clinical significance.

It should be noted that contrary to the scoring procedure of Apgar, which applies a rating of 10 points to an infant in good condition and 0 to an infant in bad condition the ratings of the Silverman-Andersen scale are the reverse. A score of 0 indicates an infant with good ventilation, whereas a score of 10 denotes an infant in severe respiratory distress."[*]

### Nutrition and feeding

When to start feedings on these small infants should be an individualized decision. The 24- to 48-hour starvation period has given way to *early* feeding because

[*]From Abramson, Harold, editor: Resuscitation of the newborn infant, St. Louis, 1960, The C. V. Mosby Co., p. 137.

doctors now believe this prevents nutritive depletion and avoids hypoglycemia and hyperbilirubinemia. "Malnourished infants require glucose and water soon after birth to support brain metabolism, due to deficient glycogen stores in liver."[*]

Infants with respiratory distress, cyanosis, and apnea are fed parenterally. Meeting nutritional and fluid requirements by this method is an important facet in the care of these tiny infants. Important electrolytes can be furnished by solutions of glucose in saline solution and, in cases of metabolic acidosis, in sodium bicarbonate.

Gavage feeding is the choice when the infant is under 1,500 grams, since he has poor sucking and swallowing reflexes. If urged to suck before these reflexes are active, there is danger of aspiration. When the infant starts sucking on the gavage tube, he should be tried on a soft nipple. The premature in good condition is started on 5% or 10% glucose water within 6 to 12 hours after birth. (See Fig. 27-1.)

Energy needs and rapid growth call for added carbohydrates, protein, and calories. His caloric requirements are 30% to 50% greater per pound of body weight than for full-term infants. Even so the immaturity of his digestive system and the small capacity he can tolerate complicate meeting his requirements. He requires small, frequent feedings.

Birth stores of iron are not adequate as they are in the full-term infant. Since his

[*]From Babson, Gorham S., and Benson, Ralph C.: Primer on prematurity and high-risk pregnancy, St. Louis, 1966, The C. V. Mosby Co., p. 107.

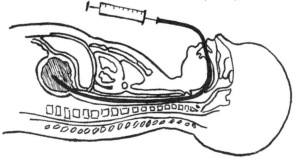

**Fig. 27-1.** Schematic drawing that shows tube in place for gavage feeding.

early entrance predisposes him to hypochromic anemia during the first year, iron supplements should be provided (0.5 to 0.8 mg. per kilogram per day, usually started the third or fourth week). Vitamins C and D are supplemented about the second week. Vitamin C aids in metabolism of phenylalanine and tyrosine.

Within 1 week, when progress is normal, the infant is usually ready for 2½ ounces of formula per pound of body weight over a 24-hour period, or 60 to 70 ml. A gain in weight is not the only controlling criterion for determining nutritional needs. The infant should (1) retain all feedings, (2) sleep between feedings, (3) show hunger directly prior to feeding time, and (4) have approximately six semisolid stools in a 24-hour period.

Do not urge the infant to take more than he accepts with ease. Overfeeding invites diarrhea and aspiration of vomitus. If the infant shows reluctance to feed on two successive attempts, it should be reported to the doctor. Always discontinue or withhold feeding if the infant shows abdominal distention, cyanosis, vomiting, or loose bowel movements. A change in feeding pattern is often the first indication that the infant is ill. Turn the infant on his right side when feeding is completed.

### Anomalies peculiar to the premature infant

*Retrolental fibrosplasia.*[1] Retrolental fibroplasia was first recognized in 1942. *Prolonged* exposure to *high* concentrations of oxygen produces spasms of fine arterioles. This restriction of blood flow in the retina leads to fibrosis and retinal detachment, with likelihood of blindness. Since vascular maturity is attained during the eighth month of gestation, the disease specifically attacks the premature and more so those who weigh less than 1,800 grams at birth. It seldom strikes the infant weighing more than 4 pounds.

*Wilson-Mikity syndrome.* The Wilson-Mikity syndrome is a respiratory disorder attacking premature newborns. The etiology of the disease is obscure. The lungs show areas of cystic emphysema. Clinical signs are respiratory distress, sternal, retraction, and persistent cyanosis.

### The mother, the premature, and the nurse

The nurse, in addition to understanding the physical hazards to which the premature infant is exposed, also needs to know something about the emotional impact experienced by the parents and the problems associated with psychological effects of maternal deprivation.

The first crisis to be faced by the mother is accepting the fact that she did deliver a premature infant; then she must accept the trauma she suffers wondering if he will live and about the possibility of abnormalities.

The mother needs to know about her infant's daily progress. The nurse should use tact in avoiding false promises. One or two visits with the nurse each day while in the hospital gives the mother opportunity to convey her concerns about the infant.

Some mothers are disturbed and feel hostility when they observe nurses caring for their infant. This in itself creates negative attitudes toward her feeling of competence. The mother needs direction in assuming responsibilities involved in the infant's care.

The rigid hospital barrier of separating the mother from her premature infant is slowly being broken down. There is no reason why the mother, free from infection and given proper instructions in hand washing and gowning, should not be permitted to hold, love, and feed her baby before she goes home. Arrangements may also be made whereby she visits and cares for the infant during the interval before his discharge. This prepares her to cope with days and weeks of waiting to take her baby home.

Criteria for discharge are usually based on (1) adequate home environment determined by report from the public health nurse, (2) evidence of freedom from infectious diseases in the home, (3) infant's vigorous cry, (4) infant's desire to feed, and (5) hematocrit over 25%.

## STUDY QUESTIONS
*Multiple choice*
1. You are assigned to the high-risk nursery and when checking one of the low birth weight infant's temperature, you find it to be 99.4° F. You should:
   (a) report this immediately.
   (b) check environmental temperature of the incubator before reporting.
   (c) check environmental temperature of the incubator, then check infant's temperature again in 20 minutes and report findings.
2. Later on in the day you observe overactivity in one of the low birth weight infants. One of the likely causes of this is:
   (a) decrease in temperature.
   (b) increase in temperature.
   (c) excessive sensory stimulation.
3. The environmental temperature for the low birth weight infant should be:
   (a) stabilized at 90° F. at all times.
   (b) adjusted according to each infant's metabolic needs.
   (c) adjusted according to infant's weight.
4. In caring for these low birth weight infants you would report a temperature:
   (a) below 96° or over 99° F.
   (b) below 97.6° or over 98.6° F.
   (c) below 98.6° F.
5. A humidity within neutral range aids in stabilization of body temperature. For the premature this neutral range is:
   (a) 40% to 70%.
   (b) 70% to 80%.
   (c) 50% to 70%.
6. Taking into consideraion the maturity and hydration of the premature infant at birth, they usually regain their birth weight in about:
   (a) 2 to 3 weeks.
   (b) 10 days.
   (c) 4 to 6 weeks.

*True or false*
(T) (F) 1. Most premature infants manifest physiological jaundice.
(T) (F) 2. The premature infant does not store proteins well.
(T) (F) 3. Respiratory distress should be considered present whenever a premature infant shows a respiratory rate over 60 per minute.
(T) (F) 4. A change in feeding pattern may be the first sign of illness.

## REFERENCES
1. Adler, Frances: Textbook of ophthalmology, ed. 7, Philadelphia, 1963, W. B. Saunders Co., p. 400.
2. Torrance, Jane: Temperature readings of premature infants, Nurs. Res. **17**:312, July-Aug., 1968.
3. Neal, Mary V., and Nauer, Claire: Ability of premature infant to maintain his own body temperature, Nurs. Res. **17**:396, Sept.-Oct., 1968.

## SELECTED READINGS
*Classification of low birth weight and premature infants*

Bartsch, Violette: Standardization of terminology, reporting of live births, fetal deaths, Hosp. Top. **46**:97, Oct., 1968.
Battaglia, Frederick, and Lubchenco, Lulu: A practical classification of newborn infants by weight and gestational age, J. Pediat. **71**:159, Aug., 1967.
Creery, R. D. G.: The infant of low birth-weight, Nurs. Mirror **10**:12, Oct., 1967.
Ghosh, Shanti, and Daga, Sarla: Comparison of gestational age and weight as standards of prematurity, J. Pediat. **71**:173, Aug., 1967.
Robinson, R. J.: Low birth weight babies: premature and small-for-dates, Nurs. Mirror **127**:32, 1968.
Wolman, Irving J., and Freedman, Alan R., editors: Clinical estimation of gestational age. In Clinical pediatrics handbook **8**:179, March, Sept., 1969.
Yerushalmy, J.: The classification of newborn infants by birth weight and gestational age, J. Pediat. **71**:164, Aug., 1967.

*Wilson-Mikity syndrome*

Avery, Mary Ellen: The lung and its disorders in the newborn infant, Philadelphia, 1964, W. B. Saunders Co., p. 158.
Light, G., and Parkhurst, R.: Wilson-Mikity syndrome, Clin. Pediat. **7**:742, Dec., 1968.
Schaffer, Alexander: Diseases of the newborn, Philadelphia, 1965, W. B. Saunders Co., p. 113.

*Retrolental fibroplasia*

Greenhill, J. P., editor: Obstetrics, ed. 13, Philadelphia, 1965, W. B. Saunders Co., p. 1003.
Hughes, James G.: Synopsis of pediatrics, St. Louis, 1967, The C. V. Mosby Co., pp. 236, 237, and 904.
Illingworth, R. S.: The development of the infant and young child, ed. 3, Baltimore, 1966, The Williams & Wilkins Co., p. 41.
Isler, Charlotte Help for victims of retrolental fibroplasia, RN **30**:37, Aug., 1967.

Klaus, Marshall, and Meyer, Belton: Oxygen therapy for the newborn, Pediat. Clin. N. Amer. 13:731, Aug., 1966.

McKay, R. J., Jr., and Smith, Clement A.: In Nelson, Waldo E., editor: Textbook of pediatrics, ed. 8, Philadelphia, 1964, W. B. Saunders Co., pp. 353 and 1497.

Vaughan, Daniel, Cook, Robert, and Asbury, Taylor: General ophthalmology, Los Altos, Calif., 1965, Lange Medical Publishers, pp. 132 and 332.

*High-risk neonate*

Abramowicz, Mark, and Kass, Edward: Pathogenesis and prognosis of prematurity, New Eng. J. Med. 275:878, Oct., 1966; 275:1053, Nov., 1966.

Bakwin, Harry, and Bakwin, Ruth: Clinical management of behavior disorders in children, ed. 3, Philadelphia, 1966, W. B. Saunders Co., pp. 56-58.

Blake, Florence, and Wright, F. Howell: Essentials of pediatric nursing, ed. 7, Philadelphia, 1963, J. B. Lippincott Co., chap. 9.

Broadribb, Violet: Foundations of pediatric nursing, Philadelphia, 1967, J. B. Lippincott Co., chap. 8.

Chase, Helen: Ranking countries by infant mortality rates, Public Health Rep. 84:19, Jan., 1969.

Fierer, Joshua, and others: Contaminated resuscitators: fatal threat to newborns, Hosp. Top. 46: 77, Oct., 1968.

Gluck, Louis: Treatment of premature infant. In Shirkey, Harry C., editor: Pediatric therapy, ed. 3, St. Louis, 1968, The C. V. Mosby Co.

Green, G. H.: Multiple pregnancy, Nurs. Mirror 126:13, Feb., 1968.

Hayes, Wayland, and Gazaway, Rena: Human relations in nursing, Philadelphia, 1964, W. B. Saunders Co., chap. 17.

Hurlock, Elizabeth B.: Child development, New York, 1964, McGraw-Hill Book Co., chap. 3.

Illingworth, R. S.: The development of the infant and young child, ed. 3, Baltimore, 1966, The Williams & Wilkins Co., p. 131.

Latham, Helen C., and Heckel, Robert V.: Pediatric nursing, St. Louis, 1967, The C. V. Mosby Co., chap. 20.

McKay, R. J., Jr., and Smith, Clement A.: Premature. In Nelson, Waldo E., editor: Textbook of pediatrics, ed. 8, Philadelphia, 1964, W. B. Saunders Co., pp. 352-357.

Montagu, M. F. Ashley: Prenatal influences, Springfield, Ill., 1962, Charles C Thomas, Publisher, p. 398.

Polk, Lewis D.: No more preemies, Clin. Pediat. 7:247, May, 1968.

Richardson, Stephen, and Guttmacher, Alan, editors: Childbearing: its social and psychological aspects, Baltimore, 1967, The Williams & Wilkins Co., p. 10.

Richie, Joshua, and others: Edema and hemolytic anemia in premature infants, New Eng. J. Med. 279:1185, Nov., 1968.

Schaffer, Alexander: Diseases of the newborn, Philadelphia, 1965, W. B. Saunders Co., chap. 2.

Watson, E. H., and Lowrey, G. H.: Growth and Development of children, ed. 5, Chicago, 1967, Year Book Medical Publishers, Inc., chap. 5.

**For student's quick notes:**

Chapter 28

# Epilogue

It will be to the advantage of the student if the instructor directs her in planning a postnatal home visit. This will be the student's opportunity to continue supportive relationships during the last phase of the childbearing cycle.

In such a setting the student will not be likely to have the equipment at hand to care for the infant, as she did in the hospital setting. Both will learn how to improvise with whatever facilities may be available. In the home setting the mother's natural attitudes can be encouraged. The nurse is a supportive figure while the mother organizes her plan of care for her newborn. The mother feels more relaxed and can verbalize her feelings without feeling inadequate, while at the same time the student learns to recognize the mother's specific concerns and anxieties as she observes the mother caring for the infant.

Both will benefit from a second visit. The student will evaluate the mother's progress and her own role as a student-teacher. She again discusses the mother's own needs, emphasizing adequate rest, and reminds her of the importance of the 6-week visit to the doctor.

Such home visits complete the student's learning experience while on her maternity nursing assignment. She certainly will derive satisfaction that comes from knowing that she, as a nurse, contributed in her own unique way to the well-being of the childbearing family.

# Appendixes

# Obstetrics and obstetrical nursing through the ages

## History of obstetrics

Let us wander back through the ages and read the story of progress in obstetrics —of woman's fortitude in bringing forth a new life.

### Among primitive peoples

Primitive obstetrics can be traced back for centuries. It is still being practiced today among some Indian and Eskimo tribes. Family and friends still participate in the sacred rituals while the woman labors. Their practices of mythology, sacred songs, and dances are still of psychotherapeutic value to the woman in labor. History relates that labor and delivery among primitive women was a relatively simple process (providing the fetus presented in a normal position). Partly because the daily life of these women involved much physical labor and partly because they toiled long hours of the day, their babies were small. Then, too, since women accepted childbirth as a natural process, they were not predisposed to psychological fears. There was little intermingling of races and therefore, anatomically, little incidence of pelvic disproportion. Women in primitive times cared for themselves during childbirth; occasionally other women assisted them and from this develops the midwife. When labor was difficult, it could usually be attributed to the abnormal presentation of the fetus, and no matter how crude practices might have been, persons were willing to give aid. Primitive women knew

nothing of childbed fever; no one contaminated the birth canal with repeated examinations, nor was she placed on filthy linens and exposed to cross infection, as you will read about later in our story. With the refinement of civilization came infection and social diseases, and as women moved into this environment, they were introduced to infection and exposed to the evils of the time; rarely was the mortality from childbirth attributed to infection.

### Obstetrics and civilization— from superstition to science

The Greeks were the first to separate medicine from magic, religion, and superstition. About the period of 500 B.C. to A.D. 500, there was the emergence of scientific rationale among Greek physicians, but the temples of healing were still in the hands of the priests and all of their procedures were tinted with superstitious and religious dogma. The Greek physicians were apprentice trained and at least willing to listen to scientific explanations, inaccurate as they might have been. They were bound to oaths of high ethical standards. It was the Greek physicians who placed so much importance on clinical observations and examinations.

Here history introduces us to Hippocrates, the "father of medicine" and the "prince of physicians." It was this great man who paved the way toward the development of scientific medicine and led the Greeks in organizing their knowledge. Despite this progress, pregnant women about to go into labor were not permitted in Greek temples of healing. Labor was woman's lot, to be borne as best she could with the aid of the midwife. They did have a law regarding the practices of midwives, but the Greeks still sang to the gods to deliver her in her travail.

Greek medicine and teachings migrated to Rome about 146 B.C. and were eventually accepted. However, they were still mixed with the "spirits" of superstition. Soranus of Ephesus lived in Rome during the second century A.D. and wrote about the practices of midwifery. He worked toward relieving some of the sufferings of women during childbirth. He reintroduced the podalic version. His philosophy, like Hippocrates, was based on knowledge, not superstition. He deserves the title "father of obstetrics" because he devoted his services to alleviate the sufferings of childbirth. He was known as a humble man, since he would "stoop so low" as to concern himself with childbearing women. You will learn more about this great man when you read about his interest in midwifery.

### During the medieval period

With the decline of the Roman Empire, the Greek philosophy of medicine deteriorated and the Christian religion was again in full reign. Under the power and influence of the church, the medical knowledge of the Greeks was crushed. It was the age of filth and faith forced upon ignorant, innocent people. The power of the church held sway over these people, and its religious rites spread ascetic practices. The woman in labor not only had to endure crude methods of aid, but she was open to barbarism, torture, and infection.

Primitive women had one way out of their dilemma—they resorted to abortion; but the Roman Catholic Church forbad this practice. Cesarean sections were advocated, no matter how crude the method might have been. The Roman law required that in the event of a woman's death, the fetus be removed by operation. This law

was known as Caesarean law; hence, Caesarean operation. The belief of the church was that because of the sin of woman's flesh, the salvation of her soul was in damnation. The church had one concern relating to childbirth—baptism of the infant or fetus—and attempts at intrauterine baptism were done with a baptismal syringe. There was little concern for fetal or maternal mortality. The physicians of this era did not perform surgery, so if the woman was delivered by cesarean section, it was left to the barber-surgeon.

For the primitive woman, suffering in childbirth was attributed to neglect; for women of the medieval period, suffering in childbirth was the price of sin.

The hospitals of this period were called hotels and meant "houses of hospitality" and "place of God's hospitality." These hospitals were established in the great cities of France. Hôtel-Dieu of Beaune, France, was established in 1443 and is still serving the poor and sick.

### During the Renaissance

Although quackery, superstition, and herb-doctoring still flourished through the early Renaissance, this period did mark some advances in medicine. Unfortunately, progress in maternal and infant care was much slower than in other branches of medicine. The latter part of this period could be called the beginning of the conquest of death among childbearing women.

Here history introduces us to Ambroise Paré, a great medical leader of the sixteenth century. He received early training in surgery at the only public hospital in Paris, the Hôtel-Dieu. Paré was a man of gentleness as was Soranus. The "age of filth" was still with these people. The "houses of hospitality" were open to anyone and gave shelter to all of the poor. Persons crowded together and when there were no beds, they were placed on floors covered with vermin and filth. A woman in labor could have shared a bed with a typhus patient or a beggar, for beggars made a practice of imposing upon the charities. These shelters became hotbeds of infection and it is easy to see how cross-infection became a scourge. It was during Paré's experiences in these "houses of hospitality" that he was led to depart from ancient established practices and fight for what he believed in. Soranus's interests were in the welfare of childbearing women; Paré's interests were in the welfare of the infant to be delivered. Paré described the podalic version and made the procedure more practicable. The mortality of the cesarean section was so very high that the podalic version was a tremendous advance.

Glory be to the few men of this era who were frontline soldiers in the beginning battle for a safe period of childbirth for the mother and for a fair chance of life for the new infant. Today, women benefit to the fullest by the victories of these men. During the Renaissance of European civilization there was a revival of practices of Greek physicians such as Hippocrates. The progress was slow, but obstetrics finally became an independent field of medicine. Physicians gradually eased their way into practicing this art and science.

History relates that in 1588 two brothers by the name of Chamberlen invented the obstetrical forceps, but they kept their invention a family secret for nearly a century. In 1720 Jean Palfyn, a Belgian, also invented obstretrical forceps and presented them at the Academy of Medicine in Paris. Thus we have been introduced to podalic version, cesarean sections, and forceps, each having its particular province.

### During the seventeenth and eighteenth century

François Mauriceau of France was an outstanding leader in knowledge of obstetrics during the seventeenth century. He contributed his views on epidemic puerperal fever and pelvic anatomy. He also dispensed with the use of the obstetrical chair for deliveries and started using the bed.

Hendrik van Deventer of Holland earned the title of "father of modern midwifery." His book gave the first accurate description of the pelvis and how pelvic deformities complicated labor. He also wrote on the mechanism of labor about 1701.

William Smellie of London gave us the foundation of modern knowledge of the placenta. He also introduced the steel-lock forceps in 1744. His book on midwifery in 1752 stressed safe rules for using forceps.

During this period there was a marked transference of care of women in labor from midwives to trained male obstetricians.

### During the nineteenth century

In the nineteenth century obstetrics was recognized as a part of medical practice, and many outstanding contributions were made. In the midst of this progress was the growing prevalence of puerperal fever, then called childbed fever. That puerperal fever was contagious and fatal was noted in a treatise by Pierre-Jacques Malouin at Hôtel-Dieu in 1746, and other references were made to it during the seventeenth and eighteenth centuries. Edward Strother described puerperal fever in 1716; Charles White of Manchester, England, wrote about the importance of scrupulous cleanliness as a preventive of the fever in 1773. This infection was greatest in the lying-in hospitals of Europe. Hygienic conditions had not improved and entering these hospitals was a "sentence of death" for every woman in labor.

About this time history introduces us to Ignaz Philipp Semmelweis and Oliver Wendell Holmes. Both of these men made outstanding contributions to progress in obstetrics. Semmelweis devoted his life's work to discovery of how puerperal fever was transferred from patient to patient, and Holmes, through word and pen, tried to awaken indifferent, stubborn physicians to the nature of the disease.

In 1843 Oliver Holmes prepared two papers on the contagiousness of puerperal fever. He presented these to the Boston Society for Medical Improvement. In his essay he spoke of the work of Ignaz Philipp Semmelweis and related how Semmelweis's clinical observations had decreased the mortality of puerperal infection by disinfection of the hands. He tried to show the physicans of America that the infection may be carried on the hands by doctors, midwives, or students from one patient to another, through lack of cleanliness. His paper was received with opposition and condemnation. Holmes was not an obstetrician, but a man filled with compassion for the many women victims of this fever. To Semmelweis goes the credit for discovering the means of preventing puerperal fever; to Holmes goes the credit for his determination to voice his belief in Semmelweis's theories.

Semmelweis received his degree in midwifery in 1844 in Vienna. He then worked as an assistant in Vienna's General Hospital. This was a charity institution and was divided into two clinics, one for the training of physicians and the other for training of midwives. In the ward used for training of physicians the mortality from this fever was tremendous. Women on entering the hospital begged not to be sent to this ward, and many would have preferred to deliver their infants in the streets because they knew when entering that they would probably die. In the ward devoted to the midwives the mortality was lower than in the other ward. This was the problem Semmelweis worked on with determination. His answer came when a friend of his, Dr. Jakob Kolletschka, died after acquiring a scalpel wound in his finger during an autopsy on a victim of puerperal fever. After a postmortem examination, it was revealed that the pathological changes were identical with those of women who died of the fever. His answer: the students were carrying the infection to the patients on their hands. He proved his theory by requesting that every student or physician wishing to examine a woman in labor scrub his hands in chlorinated lime solution. The results were dramatic—mortality dropped considerably.

This was proof of his theory, but he was laughed at, persecuted, and his suggestions ignored. He was depressed by the ingratitude of the people. In 1865, after much oppression and ridicule, he became infected and died a victim of the infection he worked so desperately to eradicate, so that women need not die during childbirth.

Semmelweis had little recognition in the history of the world, even though a statue of him was unveiled in Budapest in 1906. Louis Pasteur furthered the work of Semmelweis when he discovered the streptococci in 1860 as the etiology of the fever.

Thus you have been introduced to the outstanding early leaders in the conquest of maternal and fetal mortality: Soranus, Paré, Holmes, Semmelweis, Palfyn, and Pasteur.

### Introduction of anesthesia

Anesthesia was introduced into obstetrics in the middle of the nineteenth century, but not without stormy protest. The pangs of childbearing were women's heritage, and it was wrong to interfere! So went the tongues of many men. Biblical misinterpretation formed the basis for objections to the use of anesthesia. "How could women cry to God for help, if they were asleep?"

Dr. James Y. Simpson, professor of obstetrics at the University of Glasgow, was one of the first to use ether to alleviate the pain of childbirth, and he contributed much toward its acceptance. In 1847 he published his findings on the use of chloroform; he was also ridiculed and his work denounced by pen and spoken word. Simpson experienced the same opposition to his ideas as Semmelweis, except that he lived to enjoy the success of his work. Dr. C. D. Meigs of Philadelphia was one of the physicians so reluctant to accept Simpson's views and did all he could to thwart his work. The storm subsided when Dr. John Snow administered chloroform to Queen Victoria for delivery of Prince Leopold in 1853.

*Preventive phase of obstetrics*

The men who started the battle for improved care and consideration of the childbearing woman have had many dedicated followers through the ages. The practice of obstetrics, as we know it today, is the result of endeavors of doctors, scientists, and nurses to make pregnancy a healthy, emotionally satisfying experience for the woman, to make labor and delivery safe for her, and to give the infant a healthy start in life. Obstetrics today is in the preventive phase, with stress on antenatal care (puericulture). One of the early leaders in this concept was John William Ballantyne, who wrote about antenatal pathology and hygiene.

Thus in your reading of the history of obstetrics, you have been introduced to the early, outstanding leaders in the conquest of maternal and fetal mortality, you have followed the milestones of progress in an effort to make the mechanism of labor and the process of birth safe for the mother and to give the infant a just start in life.

## History of midwifery

Midwifery is defined as "the art and practice of assisting woman in childbirth." In ancient times this assistance was given exclusively by women because this was "woman's work." She may have been bounced, rolled, or trod upon; if all else failed the midwife called in the priest or medicine man to mumble his prayers and call forth the child. If need be, he removed the infant piecemeal. Fortunately, childbirth for most of these women was a natural, simple process, but for others it was a time of terror, torture, and tribulation.

The midwife was often referred to as "female healer" or "wise woman." Part of her duty was to sing sacred songs during labor and to show the child to the father after the child was born. If the father did not acknowledge the infant, she ofttimes placed it on a hilltop or in the market place where the infant's fate was determined, either to be adopted by a passerby or to die from exposure and starvation.

The midwife also performed abortions, since it was not illegal for her to do so.

The Bible (in the book of Exodus) makes reference to the midwife. From the writings of Soranus of Ephesus (A.D. 98 to 138), we read of his interest in midwifery. Soranus disapproved of the heartless manner in which some of the midwives attended the women in labor and of their means to hasten labor. If the woman did have a difficult labor, it was attributed to the disposition of the infant; therefore, the midwife had grounds for destroying the infant without an afterthought of the deed, since there was so little value placed on life.

Midwifery was practiced among the ancient Jews, but their prime concern was the hygiene of pregnancy. This was more important to them than the assistance of the midwife. To these people, cleanliness was a religious observation. Ancient Hebrews were referred to as the "founders of prophylaxis." Jewish women were delivered in the lap of the midwife or on an obstetrical chair. Reference is made to the obstetrical chair in Exodus and in Greek history. It is still in use today by some of the people of the Far East.

A Dominican monk, Albertus Magnus, wrote a book in the 1200s for the guidance of midwives, but its purpose was not to aid the childbearing woman nor the midwife, but to save the life of the infant until he was baptized. Early in the 1500s another manual was prepared by Eucharius Roesslin to direct midwives. It did revive some of the theories of the Greeks, but its pages were filled with superstitions and quackery.

In 1452 in Germany efforts were made to control the practices of midwives by establishing a guild for midwives. They also established a school in 1589.

About 1600, at the Hôtel-Dieu in Paris, a school was opened for the training of midwives. Louise Bourgeois was one of the first to graduate. This was one step forward in the interest of childbearing women. After centuries of neglect she was finally receiving consideration from physicians. However, they still did not participate, except when the midwife could not deliver the infant. The physician-barber may then have done a podalic version, or removed the infant as best he could. The physician could not "stoop so low" as to assist.

In 1670 Julian Clément delivered the Dauphin of France. This opened the way for male participation among the ladies of the court. He was given the title of accoucheur.

Van Deventer received the title of "father of midwifery." It was in the interest and determination of this man that brought about the beginning of male (physicians) participation in midwifery but not, however, without great opposition. Physicians who did attempt practicing midwifery were called "he-midwives" or "meddlesome midwives." Deliveries at this time by males were performed under cover because of the prevalance of prudery. It was not until the nineteenth century that physicians participated extensively in obstetrics.

In the eighteenth century a Dr. William Smellie established a school of midwifery. This Dr. Smellie published the first exact pelvic measurements, although it was Andreas Vesalius in 1543 who first showed the true relation of the pelvic bones.

A school of midwifery was started in 1762 by a Dr. Wm. Shippen, Jr., of Philadelphia. The first record of a male midwife in the United States was a Dr. Attwood of New York in 1745. In 1918 the Maternity Center Association was organized. The first American school for nurse-midwives opened in New York City in 1932 under direction of the Maternity Center Association. Credit is given to Bellevue Hospital for being the first hospital to give instructions in midwifery in the United States.

Today the nurse-midwife functions as part of the obstetrical team. She is a liaison between doctor, patient, and family.

She has advanced training in obstetrical nursing. Her program of preparation includes a master's degree, certification in a school of nurse-midwifery, and eligibility for membership in the American College of Nurse-Midwifery. She is then recognized as a practitioner of normal obstetrics. She assumes responsibility for the woman during the entire maternity cycle. Visiting with the woman at intervals during her pregnancy gives the nurse-midwife the opportunity to establish good rapport. This enables her to function with confidence and the mother in turn is relaxed because she too has learned to have faith and confidence in the nurse-midwife. She has every opportunity to teach the woman good health habits and assist her in preparation for the infant. She teaches the woman concerning the mechanism of labor and is present to assist the patient and reinforce what they discussed as she faces each stage of labor; she coaches her during the greatest of life's experiences. She has the basis for using good judgment by recognizing deviations from the normal and by knowing how to respond to an emergency situation. She offers not only physical but psychological support that every woman craves during labor. She is there to help the family during the "waiting hours" and to help them give the infant the best possible introduction into life. For the nurse who enjoys maternity nursing, nurse-midwifery offers a full, rich experience in human service.

### Calendar of contributions to progress in prenatal care

1900s First antenatal visits made to homes
1909 Association formed for the study and prevention of infant mortality; later became American Child Hygiene Association
1909 First White House Conference—recommended that a special bureau be established in the interest of the welfare of children
1911 Organization of baby health stations
1912 United States Children's Bureau established
1917 Three antenatal centers started in New York City

| | |
|---|---|
| 1918 | These centers incorporated as Maternity Center Association |
| 1919 | Second White House Conference on maternal and child welfare |
| 1921 | Shephard Towner Act—a national program for promotion of welfare and hygiene of mother and infant |
| 1925 | Joint Committee on Maternal Welfare was established |
| 1930 | Third White House Conference on child health and protection |
| 1935 | Title V of the Social Security Act provided grants to improve health and welfare of maternal and childcare |
| 1957 | American Association for Maternal and Infant Health |

## Obstetrical programs

The following universities offer courses to prepare graduate nurses for nurse-midwifery and to qualify for certification.

Catholic University
Department of Nursing
Washington, D. C.

Columbia University
Department of Nursing
New York, New York

Yale University
School of Nursing
New Haven, Connecticut

The following schools of nurse-midwifery offer programs leading to certification in nurse-midwifery.

Frontier Graduate School of Mid-wifery
Hyden, Kentucky

Catholic Maternity Institute
Santa Fe, New Mexico

Maternity Center Association
School of Nurse-midwifery
New York City, New York

**SELECTED READINGS**
*History of obstetrics and midwifery*

Chabon, Irwin: Awake and aware, New York, 1966, The Delacorte Press, chap. 3.

Clift, Margaret: Midwifery training in Uganda, Nurs. Mirror **127**:15, Aug. 9, 1968.

Grasby, E. Dudley: Epochs in obstetrics, Nurs. Times **63**:1207, Sept. 8, 1967.

Greene, John W.: The nurse midwife, Child Family **6**:12, Fall, 1967.

Hellman, Louis: Nurse midwifery in the United States, J. Obstet. Gynec. **30**:883, Dec., 1967.

Linder, E. M.: Childbirth practices in two primitive cultures, Nurs. Mirror **127**:29, July 19, 1968.

Loughlin, Bernice: Pregnancy in the Navajo culture, Nurs. Outlook **13**:55, March, 1965.

Malkin, H. J.: Wider horizons in midwifery, Nurs. Mirror **126**:19, May 31, 1938.

Mead, Margaret and Newton, Niles: Sensory stimulation and body mechanics, under cultural patterning of perinatal behavior. In Richardson, Stephen A., and Guttmacher, Alan F., editor: Childbearing: its social and psychological aspects, Baltimore, 1967, The Williams & Wilkins Co., pp. 205-222.

Perkes, R. C.: Training tomorrow's midwives, Nurs. Mirror **128**:36, June, 1969.

Ross, Evelyn: When an Indian baby is born, Nurs. Mirror **127**:30, Aug. 23, 1968.

Stallworthy, John: Changes in midwifery—progression or regression, Nurs. Mirror **128**:34, Feb. 7, 1969.

Thomas, Beryl: Midwives of tomorrow, Nurs. Times **65**:762, June, 1969.

Thompson, Barbara: Childbirth and infant care in a West African village, Nurs. Mirror **124**: 595, Sept. 29, 1967.

Thomson, L. C.: Midwifery in England, Canad. Nurse **64**:35, July, 1968.

Welsh, Dorothy M.: Old wives' tales about obstetrics, RN **30**:64, July, 1967.

# Pregnancy tests

## Table B-1

| Name of test | Test animal | Test positive | Factors involved |
|---|---|---|---|
| Aschheim-Zondek | Immature white mice | When ovaries enlarge 2 to 3 times normal size, corpus luteum present (95% to 98%) | 100 hours; 4 animals needed for test |
| Friedman | Rabbit 12 to 14 weeks old | Follicles are hemorrhagic; corpus luteum present (90% to 95%) | 24 to 48 hours; expensive |
| Kupperman | Female rat 3 to 6 weeks old | When ovary shows hyperemia | 2 to 24 hours |
| Galli Mainini | Male frog (*Ranapipiens*) or male toad (*Bufo Americanus*) | When frog or toad expells spermatozoa within 2 to 4 hours | Most suitable animal; easy to obtain and accurate and adequate |
| Hogben | Female toad | If animal ovulates within 24 hours after injection | Toads extremely sensitive to drugs; liable to kill toad |

# Appendix C

# Maternal and neonatal statistics

Table C-1. Maternal mortality by age, race, and cause of death—United States, 1963-1965 and 1953-1955*

| Age and cause of death | Average annual death rate per 100,000 live births | | | | Percent decline since 1953-1955 | |
| | White | | Nonwhite | | White | Nonwhite |
| | 1963-1965 | 1953-1955 | 1963-1965 | 1953-1955 | | |
|---|---|---|---|---|---|---|
| All ages† | 22.4 | 38.0 | 90.2 | 146.7 | 41 | 39 |
| Under 20 | 12.7 | 24.4 | 45.7 | 89.2 | 48 | 49 |
| 20 to 24 | 12.9 | 21.0 | 47.4 | 76.0 | 39 | 38 |
| 25 to 29 | 16.5 | 26.9 | 92.4 | 120.7 | 39 | 23 |
| 30 to 34 | 32.4 | 45.6 | 136.5 | 247.9 | 29 | 45 |
| 35 to 39 | 61.3 | 94.2 | 255.1 | 342.7 | 35 | 26 |
| 40 to 44 | 94.5 | 178.2 | 295.6 | 536.0 | 47 | 45 |
| All causes | 22.4 | 38.0 | 90.2 | 146.7 | 41 | 39 |
| Toxemia | 3.7 | 10.6 | 19.3 | 50.0 | 65 | 61 |
| Hemorrhage | 3.9 | 7.8 | 13.9 | 25.8 | 50 | 46 |
| Abortion | 3.9 | 4.5 | 18.9 | 22.2 | 13 | 15 |
| Sepsis | 2.7 | 4.5 | 10.2 | 11.2 | 40 | 9 |
| Ectopic pregnancy | 1.0 | 2.1 | 8.2 | 15.1 | 52 | 46 |
| Other complications | 7.3 | 8.5 | 19.7 | 22.4 | 14 | 12 |

*From Statistical Bulletin, vol. 49, Dec., 1968, New York, Metropolitan Life Insurance Co.
†Ages 45 and over included in all ages.

**Table C-2.** Maternal mortality in selected countries, 1963-1965 and 1953-1955*†

| Country | Average annual death rate per 100,000 live births | | Percent decline since 1953-1955 |
|---|---|---|---|
| | 1963-1965 | 1953-1955 | |
| United States‡ | | | |
| New England | 18.0 | 31.1 | 42 |
| Middle Atlantic | 35.5 | 45.4 | 22 |
| East North Central | 26.1 | 38.5 | 32 |
| West North Central | 22.9 | 43.6 | 47 |
| South Atlantic | 43.8 | 76.4 | 43 |
| East South Central | 54.7 | 102.7 | 47 |
| West South Central | 43.7 | 67.9 | 36 |
| Mountain | 30.1 | 45.6 | 34 |
| Pacific | 25.9 | 36.2 | 28 |
| Total United States | 33.6 | 53.5 | 37 |
| White | 22.4 | 38.0 | 41 |
| Nonwhite | 90.2 | 146.7 | 39 |
| Canada | 32.6 | 75.6 | 57 |
| Europe | | | |
| Sweden | 20.0 | 55.1 | 64 |
| Norway | 21.7 | 67.6 | 68 |
| Denmark§ | 20.6 | 65.6 | 69 |
| Finland | 39.3 | 114.9 | 66 |
| England and Wales | 26.6 | 71.3 | 63 |
| Scotland‖ | 32.9 | 72.3 | 54 |
| Belgium | 30.3 | 86.3 | 65 |
| Netherlands | 31.5 | 70.0 | 55 |
| France | 34.3 | 66.8 | 49 |
| Germany, Federal Republic | 76.0 | 158.7 | 52 |
| Switzerland | 43.8 | 111.5 | 61 |
| Spain¶ | 62.1 | 99.6 | 38 |
| Portugal | 85.5 | 155.8 | 45 |
| Italy# | 88.9 | 133.7 | 34 |
| Total—Selected European Countries | 51.7 | 103.2 | 50 |
| Other Countries | | | |
| Israel** | 31.8 | 67.8 | 53 |
| Japan | 96.0 | 181.2 | 47 |
| Australia‖ | 31.0 | 65.0 | 52 |
| New Zealand‖ | 31.3 | 44.6 | 30 |

*From Statistical Bulletin, vol. 49, Dec., 1968, New York, Metropolitan Life Insurance Co.
†Source of basic data: Reports of Division of Vital Statistics, National Center for Health Statistics, and *Demographic Yearbook*, Statistical Office of the United Nations, Department of Economic and Social Affairs.
‡United States: data by color for 1963 exclude New Jersey.
§Denmark: excludes Faroe Islands and Greenland.
‖Scotland, Australia (excluding aborigines) and New Zealand (excluding Maoris prior to 1962): data by year of registration rather than by year of occurrence.
¶Spain: based on data for 1952-1953 and 1961-1963.
#Italy: data for 1963-1965 not available; 1962-1964 figures used.
**Israel: data by year of registration in 1953-55 (Jewish population only).

**Table C-3.** Neonatal mortality in selected countries 1963-1964 and 1953-1954*†

| Country | Average annual death rate per 1,000 live births 1963-1964 | 1953-1954 | Percent decline |
|---|---|---|---|
| Italy‡ | 23.3 | 28.1 | 17 |
| West Germany§ | 19.4 | 29.5 | 34 |
| United States‖ | 18.1 | 19.4 | 7 |
| White | 16.5 | 18.1 | 9 |
| Nonwhite | 26.3 | 26.9 | 2 |
| Ireland¶ | 18.0 | 22.4 | 20 |
| Canada | 17.7 | 20.4 | 13 |
| Belgium‡ | 17.6 | 22.7 | 22 |
| Scotland¶ | 16.6 | 20.0 | 17 |
| France# | 16.4 | 21.9 | 25 |
| Israel** | 15.3 | 17.4 | 12 |
| Switzerland | 15.0 | 20.5 | 27 |
| Denmark†† | 14.5 | 18.3 | 21 |
| England and Wales | 14.1 | 17.8 | 21 |
| Australia¶ | 14.0 | 16.3 | 14 |
| Finland | 13.7 | 19.5 | 30 |
| New Zealand¶‡‡ | 12.4 | 14.3 | 13 |
| Sweden | 12.0 | 13.8 | 13 |
| Norway | 11.9 | 12.3 | 3 |
| Netherlands# | 11.8 | 16.4 | 28 |

*From Statistical Bulletin, vol. 48, Aug., 1967, New York, Metropolitan Life Insurance Co.
†Source of basic data: *Epidemiological and Vital Statistics Reports* and *World Health Statistics Annuals,* World Health Organization. *Demographic Yearbook 1957,* United Nations.
‡Italy and Belgium: data available for 1963 only.
§West Germany: data for 1953-1954 exclude Saarland.
‖United States: data by color for 1963 exclude New Jersey.
¶Australia, New Zealand, Scotland, and Ireland: data by year of registration rather than by year of occurrence.
#France and Netherlands: rates adjusted to include live births who died before registration.
**Israel: data by year of registration in 1953-1954. Jewish population only.
††Denmark: excludes Faroe Islands and Greenland.
‡‡New Zealand: excludes Maoris.

**Table C-4.** Neonatal mortality in the ten largest (1960 census) U. S. cities*†

| City | Average annual death rate per 1,000 live births, 1963-1964 Total | White | Nonwhite | Percent change since 1953-1954 Total | White | Nonwhite |
|---|---|---|---|---|---|---|
| New York, N. Y. | 19.7 | 16.2 | 29.7 | +7 | − 1 | + 3 |
| Chicago, Ill. | 20.4 | 16.2 | 27.6 | +5 | − 6 | + 7 |
| Los Angeles, Calif. | 17.8 | 16.1 | 22.9 | −5 | −11 | ‡ |
| Philadelphia, Pa. | 22.8 | 19.6 | 28.0 | −3 | + 1 | −17 |
| Detroit, Mich. | 21.6 | 16.9 | 28.9 | +4 | −10 | +13 |
| Baltimore, Md. | 21.7 | 17.8 | 25.6 | −5 | −12 | − 6 |
| Houston, Texas | 19.5 | 17.0 | 24.9 | −9 | −14 | − 6 |
| Cleveland, Ohio | 23.8 | 19.1 | 32.3 | +5 | − 3 | + 7 |
| Washington, D. C. | 25.0 | 18.8 | 27.3 | +6 | −14 | + 8 |
| St. Louis, Mo. | 22.8 | 18.9 | 27.9 | +2 | + 1 | −11 |

*From Statistical Bulletin, vol. 48, Aug., 1967, New York, Metropolitan Life Insurance Co.
†Source of basic data: Reports of the Division of Vital Statistics, National Center for Health Statistics.
‡Less than 0.5%.

# Appendix D

# Glossary

*abdominal* pertaining to the abdomen.
  *a. delivery* delivery of the fetus by cesarean section (see cesarean section).
  *a. pregnancy* pregnancy occurring in the abdominal cavity (see ectopic).
*ablatio placentae* see abruptio placentae.
*abortion* interruption of a pregnancy before the period of viability.
*abruptio placentae* premature separation of a normally situated placenta after viability, but before delivery.
*accouchement* delivery; childbirth.
*accoucheur* obstetrician; midwife.
*acrocyanosis* bluish discoloration of the digits.
*afibrinogenemia* decreased fibrinogen in the blood.
*afterbirth* see secundine.
*afterpains* pains resulting from contractions of uterine muscles after parturition.
*agalactia* failure or absence of secretion of milk.
*albuminuria* presence of serum albumin (protein) or serum globulin in the urine.
*amenorrhea* absence of menstruation.
*amnesia* loss of memory.
*amniocentesis* penetration of the uterus to withdraw fluid from the amniotic sac.
*amnion* inner membrane of the sac enclosing the fetus and amniotic fluid.
*amnionitis* inflammation of the amnion.
*amnioscope* instrument used to detect presence of meconium through intact fetal sac.
*amniotic* pertaining to the amnion.
  *a. embolism* if amniotic fluid is drawn into general circulation through gapping venous sinuses of the placenta and reaches pulmonary vessels, emboli may form.
  *a. fluid* fluid contained within the sac; also called liquor amnii.
  *a. sac* membranes enclosing fetus and amniotic fluid. Synonym: membranes or bag of waters.
*amniotome* instrument used to rupture the fetal membranes or sac.
*amniotomy* artificial rupture of the fetal membranes or sac.
*analgesia* loss or absence of sensibility to pain.

*android* resembling a man.
  *a. pelvis* male-type pelvis.
*anencephalia* monstrosity with absence of neural tissue in the cranium.
*anesthesia* absence of sensivity to stimuli, with or without loss of consciousness.
*anomaly* deviation from the normal.
*anoxia* absence or deficiency of oxygen.
*antenatal* before birth.
*antepartum* occurring before parturition or onset of labor.
*anteroposterior* direction from the front toward the back.
*anthropoid* apelike.
  *a. pelvis* pelvis contracted transversely.
*Apgar score* numerical rating of an infant's condition at 1 and 5 minutes after birth, based on heart rate, respiratory effort, muscle tone, reflex irritability, and color.
*apnea* temporary cessation of respirations.
*areola* pigmented area surrounding the nipple of the mammary glands.
*asphyxia* increased carbon dioxide tension in the blood and tissues; suffocation.
  *a. neonatorum* interference with exchange of gasses in the lungs of the newborn.
*ataractic* agent that tends to tranquilize.
*atelectasis* incomplete expansion or collapse of the lungs.
*atony* lack of normal tone.
  *uterine a.* muscles of the myometrium fail to contract and retract normally.
*atresia* absence of a normal anatomical opening.
  *choanal a.* obstruction of posterior nares.
  *esophageal a.* abnormal closure at some point along the esophagus.
*attitude* in obstetrics, relation of fetal extremities to its trunk.
*auscultation* in obstetrics, listening for certain sounds in the mother's abdomen such as the fetal heart and funic or uterine souffle.
*autosome* chromosome in man not concerned with sex determination.

*bag of waters* membranes (amnion and chorion) enclosing the fetus in the liquor amnii.

*ballottement* term used for rebound of the fetus when maneuvered by examining fingers through the abdominal wall or vaginal route.

*Bandl's ring* pathological uterine retraction ring, occurring in obstructed labors.

*Bartholin's glands* two small mucous glands, one on each side of the vaginal orifice, at the base of the labia majora.

*battledore placenta* insertion of umbilical cord into margin of the placenta instead of the center.

*Baudelocque's diameter* distance between the upper anterior aspect of the symphysis pubis and the depression below the spine of the fifth lumbar vertebra; same as external conjugate measurement.

*Bednar's aphthae* oval-shaped gray lesions at the posterior margin of the hard palate.

*bilirubin* red bile pigment formed from the hemoglobin of erythrocytes.

   *b. anemia* presence of bilirubin in the blood.

   *b. direct* bilirubin conjugated by the liver.

   *b. indirect* unconjugated or insoluble bilirubin.

*birth* act of being born or separation of infant from maternal body.

   *b. canal* that part of the genitalia comprising the cervix, vagina, and vulva.

   *b. mark* congenital blemish on the skin.

   *b. rate* number of births per 1,000 population in a given year.

*blastocyst* hollow ball of cells; modified blastula.

*blastoderm* germinal membrane of the ovum.

*blastodermic vesicle* one-layered vesicular structure of cells surrounding the fertilized ovum.

*blastula* stage of embryonic development following the morula stage.

*Brandt-Andrews' maneuver* method of expressing a separated placenta from the birth canal; one hand exerts gentle pressure over the abdomen between the fundus and symphysis, elevating the fundus, while traction is exerted on the cord with the other hand.

*Braun's physiological retraction ring* boundary between the upper and lower uterine segment brought about by retraction of muscle fibers (physiological retraction ring).

*Braxton Hicks's contractions* intermittent painless uterine contractions occurring throughout pregnancy.

*Braxton Hicks's version* combined external and internal manual maneuver whereby the position of the fetus is changed in the uterus.

*breech* the buttocks.

   *b. presentation* when the buttocks present for delivery in place of the head.

*bregma* junction of the coronal and sagittal sutures.

*brim* edge of the pelvic inlet or the superior strait.

*Calkins' sign* sign that the placenta has separated; uterus changes from a discoid shape before separation to a globular shape after separation.

*Candida* genus of yeastlike fungi.

   *c. albicans* species causing human infection.

*caput* head.

   *c. succedaneum* edema occurring under the fetal scalp during parturition.

*caudal* inferior end of the body.

   *c. anesthesia* a means of relief from pain of parturition by anatomical approach—caudal block.

*caul* portion of the amnion that sometimes envelops the fetal head and face at birth; called the veil by laity.

*cephalhematoma* localized effusion of blood beneath the periosteum of the skull of the newborn caused by disruption of blood vessels during the birth process.

*cephalic* pertains to the head.

*cerclage* encircling with ring or loop, such as encirclement of an incompetent cervical os.

*cervicitis* inflammation of the cervix of the uterus.

*cervix* neck of an organ.

   *c. uteri* lower, narrow portion of the uterus between the internal os and the external os.

   *dilatation of c.* opening of the cervical canal.

   *effacement of c.* thinning out of the cervical canal.

   *incompetent c.* one that is prone to dilate before normal period of gestation, usually between the sixteenth and twenty-eighth week.

*cesarean section* removal of the fetus by means of an incision through the abdominal and uterine wall.

*Chadwick's sign* bluish discoloration of the mucous membrane of the vagina; a presumptive sign of pregnancy that occurs after the fourth week.

*chalasia* relaxation of bodily opening. Example: esophageal gastric sphincter, a cause of vomiting in the neonate.

*childbirth* process of giving birth. Synonym: parturition.

   *cooperative c.* mother actively participates in the process of parturition.

*chloasma* hyperpigmentation of yellow-brown color occurring in circumscribed areas of the skin, generally the face and neck, during gestation.

*chorioepithelioma* uterine choriocarcinoma known to occur after a hydatidiform mole.

*chorion* outermost membrane of the developing embryo.

   *c. frondosum* villi in contact with the decidua basalis; that part forming the embryonic portion of the placenta.

   *c. laeve* smooth portion of the chorion or the villi extending toward the uterine cavity.

*chorionic* pertaining to the chorion.

*chromatin* portion of the cell nucleus; carrier of the genes in inheritance.

*sex c.* mass of chromatin bodies present in cell nucleus of females; not in normal males.

*chromosome* structure in the nucleus of cells that carries the genes or hereditary factors.

*cilium* hairlike process or fine projection from the surface of cells.

*circumcision, female* incision of fold of tissue over the glans clitoris.

*circumcision, male* excision of the foreskin of the penis.

*cleft lip* congenital fissure of the upper lip.

*cleft palate* congenital fissure in the roof of the mouth forming one cavity for nose and mouth.

*clitoris* structure of the female genitalia located where the labia minora unite anteriorly; homologous to the penis of the male.

*coitus* mating process in human beings.

*colostrum* yellowish fluid secreted by the female mammary glands during pregnancy and after parturition; serves as first nourishment for the newborn.

*colporrhaphy* operation of suturing the vagina or vaginal wall.

*conception* union of the ovum and sperm that marks the beginning of a new organism.

*confinement* term applied to the period of childbirth and puerperal period.

*congenital* present at the time of birth; a disease or abnormality occurring before birth.

*contraction* shortening in connection with muscles.

   *clonic c.* contraction of muscles alternating with periods of relaxation.

   *tonic c.* sustained contraction of muscles without alternating intervals of relaxation.

*Coombs' test* this test, as it applies to erythroblastosis, detects the presence of antibody globulin attached to the surface of red cells.

   *direct C.* usually done at birth, using cord blood to check for maternal antibodies that are attached to or coat the cells.

   *indirect C.* this test is done at intervals during pregnancy to detect presence of circulating anti-Rh antibodies in maternal serum or plasma.

*copulation* mating process; usually applied in reference to lower animals.

*corpus* body or principal part of an organ.

   *c. luteum* a yellow body formed in the cavity of the graafian follicle after the ovum has been expelled; persists during pregnancy.

   *c. uteri* body of the uterus.

*cotyledon* any lobe or subdivision on the maternal surface of the placenta.

*Couvelaire uterus* uterus overdistended with blood due to premature separation of the placenta; uterine musculature becomes infiltrated with blood, while the abdomen becomes boardlike.

*cradle cap* scaly crusts that form on the crown of the infant's head.

*craniotomy* decompression of the fetal skull to facilitate delivery.

*cranium* bones of the head; the skull.

*Credé's placenta expression* method of expressing a separated placenta from the birth canal.

*Credé's prophylaxis* treatment of the eyes of the newborn at birth using silver nitrate solution.

*crown rump* sitting height of the infant.

*crowning* said of the fetal head as it emerges from the vaginal orifice.

*cryptorchidism* condition in which one or both testes fail to descend into the scrotum.

*cul-de-sac* a pouch.

   *c. of Douglas* pouch or sac formed by peritoneum between the anterior wall of the rectum and the posterior wall of the uterus.

*Cullen's sign* a bluish tint noted around the area of the umbilicus; regarded as a sign of a ruptured ectopic pregnancy; the result of intraperitoneal bleeding over several days.

*cyesis* pregnancy.

*cystocele* protrusion of the urinary bladder into the vagina.

*cytolysis* dissolution of cells; trophoblasts or primary villi have the power of cytolysis to obtain nourishment for the developing embryo.

*cytotrophoblast* inner layer (Langhan's) of the trophoblasts.

*decidua* membranous lining of the uterus during gestation.

   *d. basalis* that portion directly underlying the implanted zygote.

   *d. capsularis* that portion directly overlying the implanted zygote.

   *d. vera (parietalis)* that lining the uterus other than the site of implantation of the zygote.

*delivery* expulsion or extraction of the fetus at birth.

   *abdominal d.* delivery of the fetus through incision of the abdominal wall into the uterus.

   *breech d.* delivery of the fetus in breech presentation.

   *instrumental d.* extraction of the fetus from the birth canal by application of forceps.

   *precipitate d.* very rapid, unattended delivery.

   *spontaneous d.* delivery completed without artificial aid, such as the use of forceps.

   *vaginal d.* delivery through the uterus and vagina.

*diaphoresis* profuse perspiration.

*diastasis recti* separation of the rectus muscles of the abdomen away from the midline.

*diuresis* increased secretion of urine.

*dizygotic* derived from two separate zygotes; twins from two ova.

*Döderlein's bacillus* gram-positive, nonpathogenic microorganism commonly found in normal vaginal secretions; believed to inhibit growth of pathogenic bacteria.

*Douglas' cul-de-sac* see cul-de-sac of Douglas.

*Downey-Apt test* used to differentiate maternal from fetal blood.

*Down's syndrome* chromosomal abnormality where the chromosome number is 47.

*dry labor* term used by laity when a pregnant woman's membranes rupture sometime before the onset of true labor.

*ductus* a duct.

   *d. arteriosus* blood vessel peculiar to fetal circulation between pulmonary artery and the aorta.

   *d. venosus* blood vessel peculiar to fetal circulation, connecting the umbilical vein and the inferior vena cava.

*Dührssen's incision* enlarging the cervical opening by means of three radial incisions corresponding to the numbers 10, 2, and 6 on a clock dial.

*Duncan's mechanism* method of expression of the placenta; placenta is folded upon itself with maternal side outermost as it approaches the vulva.

*dystocia* abnormal labor.

   *fetal d.* that caused by anomaly of the fetus or abnormal fetal position in utero.

   *maternal d.* that due to inadequate pelvic measurements, fetopelvic disproportion, or deficiency in power of uterine contractions.

*ecbolics* drugs to increase uterine contractions; oxytocics.

*eclampsia* convulsive attacks and coma.

   *e. of pregnancy* preceded by severe toxemia (high blood pressure, albuminuria, and proteinuria).

*ectoderm* outer layer of the three primitive germ layers of the embryo.

*ectopic* situated other than in the normal place; out of place.

   *e. pregnancy* nidation of the fertilized ovum outside the uterine cavity, such as in the tubes, ovaries, or abdomen.

*effacement* see cervix, effacement of.

*effleurage* gentle, stroking movements used in a massage.

*ejaculation* sudden, forcible act of expulsion, as of semen from the male urethra.

*embryo* stage of embryonic development from the second to the eighth week.

*encephalocele* defect in the skull with a herniation of neural tissue.

*endocrine* secreting internally; gland secretions enter directly into the blood or lymph and not through a duct.

*endometritis* inflammation of the endometrium.

*endometrium* mucous membrane lining of the uterine cavity.

*engagement* in obstetrics, largest plane of the presenting part has reached the level of the ischial spines of the pelvis.

*engorgement* in obstetrics, lymph and venous stasis occurring in the breasts prior to the flow of mother's milk.

*entoderm* innermost of the three primitive germ layers of the embryo.

*enzyme* complex colloidal substance with catalytic properties that brings about chemical changes in other substances without being changed in itself.

*epidural* external to the dura mater.

*episiotomy* incision of the vulva and perineum during delivery.

*epispadias* congenital defect of the male urethra; urethra opens on dorsum of the penis.

*epistaxis* hemorrhage from the nose.

*Epstein's pearls* white-yellow masses of epithelial cells over the posterior portion of the hard palate.

*Erb-Duchenne paralysis* injury to the brachial plexus; limited to fifth and sixth cervical nerve roots.

*ergot* fungus of rye; acts as a smooth muscle stimulant; an oxytocic.

*erythema* congestion of capillaries causing a redness of the skin.

*erythroblastosis* erythroblasts in the circulating blood.

   *e. fetalis* hemolytic anemia of the fetus or newborn caused by placenta transmission of antibodies from the mother; it is usually secondary to blood incompatibilities.

*escutcheon* pubic hair.

*estrogen* substance producing estrum; female sex hormone secreted by the ovaries and the placenta.

*eutocia* normal parturition.

*external os* junction of the cervix with the vagina.

*extraction* act of pulling out.

   *breech e.* extracting the fetus from the birth canal when the presenting part is breech.

*extraperitoneal* outside peritoneum.

*extrauterine* outside the uterus.

*fallopian tube* tube extending from the cornu of the uterus, one on each side, and terminating near the ovary; it conveys the ovum from the fimbriated end of the ovary to the uterus. Synonym: oviduct, salpinx.

*Farber's test* detects the presence of swallowed lanugo, hairs, and vernix caseosa in the meconium; used where intestinal obstruction is suspected.

*fecundation* act of impregnation; fertilization.

*fenestra* in obstetrics, opening in the blade of the forceps.

*fertilization* impregnation of an ovum with the spermatozoon.

*fetal* pertaining to a fetus.

   *f. death* when a fetus of 20 weeks or more by gestational age dies in utero. Synonym: stillbirth.

*f. mortality rate* number of fetal deaths per 1,000 live births within a given year.

*fetus* offspring from the eighth week of gestation until birth.

*fimbria* in obstetrics, fringelike end of the fallopian tube.

*follicle* secretory cavity or sac.

*atretic f.* graafian follicle that does not develop completely and undergoes degeneration.

*graafian f.* sac in the cortex of the ovary in which the ovum matures.

*primordial f.* graafian follicle before it ruptures.

*fontanel* membrane-covered space at junction of the cranial bones of the fetal skull.

*anterior f.* space between frontal and parietal bones; called the "soft spot."

*posterior f.* space between occipital and parietal bones.

*Foote's sign* rhythmic protrusion of the tongue; sometimes seen in an infant with intracranial hemorrhage.

*foramen* orifice or opening.

*f. ovale* in the fetus, opening between atria of the heart.

*forceps* obstetrical instruments used to make traction on the fetal skull to facilitate delivery.

*foreskin* fold of skin covering the glans penis; the prepuce.

*forewaters* fluid in front of the presenting part that escapes before or when the membranes rupture.

*fornix uteri* arch formed where the cervix converges with the vagina.

*fossa navicularis* shallow depression between the hymen and the fourchette.

*fourchette* area formed by junction of the labia majora and labia minora posteriorly.

*frenulum* fold of mucous membrane serving to support or restrain parts.

*f. linguae* fold of mucous membrane extending from the base of the mouth to the under surface of the tongue along the midline.

*fundus* larger part of a hollow organ.

*f. uteri* upper, rounded portion of the uterus.

*funic souffle* sound heard over the uterus, synchronous with fetal heart sounds.

*funis* cord connecting the embryo to the chorionic frondosum or fetal component of the placenta.

*galactagogue* any agent increasing the flow of milk.

*galactin* lactogenic hormone. Synonym: prolactin.

*galactocele* tumor of the mammary gland filled with milkylike fluid.

*galactopoiesis* maintenance of milk secretion.

*galactopoietic* agent that promotes the secretion of milk.

*galactorrhea* excessive secretion of milk.

*gamete* mature germ cell such as an ovum or sperm.

*gametogenesis* production of gametes.

*gavage* feeding by a stomach tube.

*gene* biological unit of heredity within the chromosome.

*genitalia* organs of the reproductive system.

*gestation* development of the fertilized ovum within the uterus; period of pregnancy, normally 40 weeks.

*abdominal g.* when the fertilized ovum develops in the abdominal cavity.

*ectopic g.* when the fertilized ovum develops outside the uterus. Synonym: ectopic pregnancy.

*gland(s)* secreting organ producing a specific product.

*Bartholin's g.* vulvovaginal gland, one on each side of the vaginal opening at the base of the labia majora.

*Cowper's g.* bulbourethral gland in the male; corresponds to Bartholin's gland.

*mammary g.* milk-secreting glands of female mammals.

*Montgomery's g.* sebaceous glands in the areola.

*nabothian g.* mucous glands in the cervix.

*Skene's g.* two tiny glands situated within the meatus of the female urethra.

*glans* small, glandlike body.

*g. clitoris* distal end of the clitoris.

*g. penis* head of the penis.

*glucuronyl transferase* liver enzyme that catalyzes bilirubin and favors its excretion.

*glycosuria* abnormally high sugar in the urine.

*gonad* a sex gland; an ovary or testis.

*gonadotropin* substance that stimulates the gonads, such as the hormone secreted by the anterior pituitary gland.

*chorionic g.* produced by chorionic villi of the placenta; found in urine and blood of pregnant women.

*Goodell's sign* softening of the cervix during pregnancy; an early or presumptive sign of pregnancy.

*graafian follicle* a mature follicle in the cortex of of the ovary containing an ovum.

*gravid* pregnancy.

*gravida* a pregnant woman.

*Guthrie test* blood test for presence of phenylketonuria.

*gynecoid* term applied to a normal female pelvis.

*gynecology* branch of medicine dealing specifically with diseases of the genital tract in women.

*halo sign* severely edematous fetus as seen on roentgenogram.

*Hegar's sign* softening of the lower uterine segment; a presumptive sign of pregnancy.

*hematoma* blood tumor.

*hematopoiesis* formation of blood.

*hemimelia* deformity or absence of distal half of a limb.

*hemorrhage* loss of over 500 ml. of blood during parturition.

*hemorrhoid* varicose dilatation of a vein in the anal region.

*hermaphrodite* congenital anomaly whereby an infant is born with gonadal tissue of both sexes.

    *pseudo h.* presence of ovaries or testes but undetermined external genitalia.

*homologous* similar in fundamental origin and structure. Example: Cowper's glands in the male are the homologues of Bartholin's glands in the female.

*hormone* chemical substance produced in an organ or gland that has a specific effect on the function of another organ or gland, such as stimulating it to increased activity.

*hyaline* glassylike, translucent.

    *h. membrane* in the newborn, a coating of the alveoli of the lungs with a hyaline-like material, interfering with normal exchange of gases.

*hydatid* cyst formed in the tissues; a cystlike structure.

*hydatidiform mole* degenerative process in the chorionic villi of the developing placenta that gives rise to multiple cysts.

*hydramnios* see polyhydramnios.

*hydrocele* serous tumor of the testes.

*hydrocephalus* increase in cerebrospinal fluid volume within the ventricles of the brain, accompanied by enlargement of the head.

*hydrops* edema; abnormal accumulation of fluid.

    *h. fetalis* in the newborn infant, this edema occurs in severe hemolytic disease due to blood discrepancy.

*hymen* fold of membrane wholly or partially occluding the vaginal orifice.

    *imperforate h.* absence of opening in the hymen.

*hymenotomy* incision of the hymen.

*hyperbilirubinemia* excess bilirubin in the blood; 12 mg. per 100 ml. for the full-term infant and 15 mg. per 100 ml. for the premature infant.

*hyperemesis* excessive vomiting.

    *h. gravidarum* pernicious vomiting during pregnancy.

*hyperinvolution* in obstetrics, the reduction in size of the uterus beyond normal during the puerperium.

*hypnosis* artificially induced trancelike condition in which there is increased responsiveness to commands and suggestions.

*hypocalcemia* deficiency of calcium in the blood.

*hypofibrinogenemia* deficiency of fibrinogen in the blood.

*hypogalactia* deficiency in milk secretion.

*hypoglycemia* deficiency of sugar in the blood.

*hypokalemia* deficiency of potassium in the blood.

*hypoprothrombinemia* deficiency of prothrombin in the blood.

*hypospadias* congenital defect of male urethra; opens on the undersurface of the penis.

*hypoxia* anoxia; lack of sufficient oxygen in inspired air.

*hysterectomy* excision of the uterus.

*icterus* yellow pigmentation of the tissues with bile. Synonym: jaundice.

    *i. neonatorum* type of hemolytic jaundice in the neonate.

*iliopectineal line* pertains to a ridge on inner surface of the ileum; separates the true from the false pelvis.

*illegitimate* born out of wedlock.

*imperforate anus* congenital absence of normal outlet of rectum.

*impetigo* bacterial skin disease characterized by vesicles containing fluid.

*impregnate* to fertilize an ovum.

*incompetent cervix* see under cervix.

*induction of labor* labor induced artificially; may be medical or surgical.

*inertia uteri* weak, ineffectual contractions of the muscular wall of the uterus.

*infant* human being from birth to the age of 2.

    *dysmature i.* one who exhibits severe malnutrition regardless of gestational age.

    *immature i.* a live-born, premature infant with a weight of 1,500 grams or less.

    *i. mortality* deaths of infants under 1 year of age.

    *i. mortality rate* number of deaths of live-born infants before the first birthday per 1,000 live births in a given year.

    *low birth weight i.* those live-born infants with a birth weight of 2,500 grams or less.

    *postmature i.* a live-born infant with a gestational period over 42 weeks.

    *premature i.* a live-born infant with a gestational period of less than 37 weeks, regardless of the weight at birth.

*inferior strait of pelvis* transverse diameter of the pelvic outlet.

*inlet* passage or route of entrance.

    *i. of pelvis* entrance into the pelvic cavity called the "brim" of the pelvis.

*insemination* deposit of sperm into the vaginal canal during coitus.

    *artificial i.* introduction of semen into the vaginal canal by artificial means.

*internal os* junction of the cervix with the corpus of the uterus.

*intertrigo* erythema showing diffused redness in the folds of the skin.

*introitus* in obstetrics, entrance of the vagina.

*inversion* turning inside out of an organ.

    *i. of uterus* a turning of the uterus inside out; fundus protrudes through the cervix or vagina.

*involution* in obstetrics, reduction in the size of the uterus during the puerperium.

*isthmus* narrow passage that connects two parts.

    *i. of uterus* transverse constriction between cervix and corpus of the uterus.

*jaundice* yellow appearance of the skin, white of the eyes, and mucous membranes due to deposition of bile pigments.

*jelly* thick, gelatinous mass.

 *Wharton's j.* mucoid substance covering umbilical vein and arteries.

*kernicterus* erythroblastosis fetalis with brain damage; high levels of bilirubin result in deposition of bile pigment within the tissues of the brain and spinal cord.

*Klippel-Feil syndrome* fusion or absence of one or more cervical vertebrae; head rests on shoulders.

*Klumpke's paralysis* form of branchial palsy involving wrist and hand.

*labia* (pl. of labium) liplike structures.

 *l. majora* folds of adipose tissue; forms anterior and posterior commissure.

 *l. minora* folds of mucous membrane within the labia majora (nymphae).

*labor* physiological mechanism by which the products of conception are expelled from the uterus to the outside world. Synonym: parturition.

 *dry l.* term used by laity when a pregnant woman's membranes rupture sometime before the onset of true labor.

 *false l.* uterine contractions misinterpreted for true labor; no cervical dilatation.

 *induced l.* that brought on by medical or surgical intervention.

 *precipitate l.* labor completed in less than 3 hours and usually unattended.

 *premature l.* labor occurring between the twenty-eighth and thirty-eighth week of gestation.

 *prolonged l.* labor extending beyond 16 hours.

 *spontaneous l.* labor completed without artificial aid such as with use of forceps.

*laceration* tearing of tissues.

*lactalbumin* albumin from milk.

*lactation* secretion of milk.

*lactogenesis* initiation of lactation.

*lactogenic* stimulating the secretion of milk.

 *l. hormone* prolactin or luteotrophin.

*lactoglobulin* protein in milk.

 *immune l.* antibodies occurring in colostrum of animals.

*lactose* milk sugar.

*lactosuria* lactose in the urine.

*Ladin's sign* soft spot felt anteriorly in the midline of the uterus; a presumptive sign of pregnancy.

*lambdoid suture* suture between the occipital and two parietal bones.

*Langhans' layer* inner layer of the trophoblastic cells, cytotrophoblasts; secretes chorionic gonadotrophins.

*lanugo* fine, downy hairs that are present on the body of some newborns, especially those born prematurely.

*laparotrachelotomy* cesarean section when the incision is made through the lower uterine segment.

*layette* clothing usually acquired during pregnancy in preparation for the newborn.

*legitimate* born of parents legally married.

*leukorrhea* whitish mucous discharge from the cervical canal.

*LH* abbreviation for luteinizing hormone; also called ICSH, or interstitial cell–stimulating hormone.

*lightening* descent of the uterus into the pelvic cavity prior to or during labor.

*linea* (pl. lineae) narrow ridge or streak.

 *l. alba* white line down middle of the abdomen.

 *l. nigra* pigmentation noted down middle of abdomen during pregnancy.

*liquor* liquid or fluid.

 *l. amnii* amniotic fluid surrounding the fetus.

 *l. folliculi* fluid in which the ova are suspended.

*lithopedion* a petrified fetus.

*live birth* delivery of a fetus, irrespective of duration of pregnancy, that shows evidence of life such as breathing, heart beat, and voluntary muscular movements.

*lochia* discharge of blood, tissue, and mucus from the uterus during the puerperium.

 *l. alba* the discharge when it becomes yellow to white, containing many microorganisms and degenerative cells; that of the final phase of the maternity cycle.

 *l. rubra* discharge immediately after birth, consisting mostly of blood from the vessels at the site of the placenta, lasting approximately 4 days.

 *l. serosa* discharge following rubra phase; pinkish to brown, decrease in red blood cells, increase in white blood cells and mucous cervical glands.

*lochiometra* retention of lochia.

*low birth weight infant* live-born infants with a birth weight of 2,500 grams or less.

*LTH* abbreviation for luteotropic hormone.

*lunar* pertaining to the moon; a full-term pregnancy is 10 lunar months.

*lutein* yellow pigment from serum; one source is from corpus luteum.

 *l. cells* ovarian cells containing yellow pigment involved in formation of corpus luteum.

*luteinizing hormone* (LH) (ICSH) stimulates production of progesterone by the ovary.

*luteotropic hormone* (LTH) promotes growth of breast tissue; maintains lactation and corpus luteum and stimulates secretion of progesterone.

*luteum* yellow.

 *corpus l.* yellow body formed in the graafian follicle after it ruptures; persists during gestation.

*lutin* hormone of corpus luteum. Synonym: progestin.

*lying-in* period of the puerperium.

*macrocephalous* having an excessively large head.

*malformation* deformity; defective in shape or structure.

*mammary* pertaining to the breast.

   *m. glands* glands of the female breast secreting milk.

   *m. papilla* nipple of the mammary gland.

*mask of pregnancy* see chloasma.

*mastitis* inflammation of the breast.

*maternal* pertaining to a mother.

*maternal mortality rate* number of deaths for every 10,000 live births in a given year.

*maternity* motherhood.

*matutinal* occurring early in the morning, as morning sickness.

*maturation* maturing as a graafian follicle; the process of cell division occurring in spermatogenesis or oogenesis, in which the number of chromosomes is reduced from diploid number to haploid number.

*meatus* opening or passage.

   *urinary m.* external urethral opening through which the urine is discharged.

*mechanism* combination of processes by which a result is obtained.

   *m. of labor* process by which the products of conception are expelled from the uterus and birth canal.

*meconium* first fecal matter discharged from intestines of newborn; it is greenish black in color and of mucilaginous consistency.

   *m. ileus* obstruction of small intestines by abnormal consistency of meconium; meconium is thick and puttylike.

   *m. plug* mass of meconium formed in terminal part of the rectum during fetal growth and development.

*menarche* beginning of the menstrual function.

*meningocele* congenital anomaly with protrusion of the meninges through a spina bifida to form a sac.

*menses* monthly flow of blood; menstruation.

*menstruation* periodic, physiological discharge of blood from the uterus.

*mentum* the chin.

*mesoderm* a primary germ layer of the embryo, between the ectoderm and entoderm.

*Methergine* trademark for preparations of methylergonovine; an ecbolic.

*metritis* inflammation of the uterus.

*metrorrhagia* bleeding from the uterus at a time other than during the menstrual period.

*microcephalus* pertains to an abnormally small head.

*midwife* woman who practices the art of assisting in the delivery of infants.

*midwifery* art of assisting in the delivery of infants.

*milia* pinpoint papules caused by overdistended sebaceous glands; prominent over the nose and chin of the neonate.

*milk leg* see phelgmasia alba dolens.

*miscarriage* synonym: abortion.

*mittelschmerz* cramplike pain and spotting of blood experienced midway between menstrual periods; associated with period of ovulation and rupture of graafian follicle.

*molding* shaping of the fetal head as it adapts to the pelvis and birth canal.

*mongolian spots* areas of dark blue pigmentation over the lumbar, sacral, and gluteal regions.

*mongolism* see Down's syndrome.

*moniliasis* infection of the mucous membranes or the skin; caused by yeastlike fungi.

*monozygotic* originating from one zygote; pertains to identical twins.

*mons* a prominence.

   *m. pubis* prominence over the symphysis pubis.

   *m. veneris* mons pubis in the female.

*Montgomery's tubercles or glands* small prominences scattered around the areola of the breast.

*morbid* sick; diseased.

*morbidity* state of being sick or diseased.

   *puerperal m.* includes all puerperal fevers.

*morula* mass of cells formed by cleavage of a fertilized ovum.

*multigravida* a woman during her second and subsequent pregnancies.

*multipara* a woman who has delivered two or more viable infants.

*myometrium* muscle coat of the uterus.

*nabothian glands* mucus-secreting glands of the cervix.

*Nägele's rule* calculation used to estimated date of delivery.

*natal* pertaining to birth.

*navel* the umbilicus.

*neonatal* pertaining to the neonate.

   *n. death* one occurring within the neonatal period, or the first 28 days of life.

   *n. mortality rate* the number of neonatal deaths per 1,000 live births in a given year.

   *n. period* the first 28 days of the infant's life.

*neonate* newborn infant during the first 28 days of life.

*nevus* birthmark; a congenital pigmented circumscribed area of the skin.

*nidation* implantation of the zygote in the endometrium of the uterus.

*Nitrazine paper test* tests the reaction of urine; if membranes are ruptured, the amniotic fluid will turn the paper a blue-green to deep blue color.

*nullipara* a woman who has not borne a child.

*nympha* labia minora.

*obstetrician* a physician who cares for the woman during her pregnancy, parturition, and puerperium.

*obstetrics* that branch of medicine dealing with pregnancy, parturition, and the puerperium.

*obstetrix* a midwife.

*occiput* back part of the skull.

*oligohydramnios* abnormally small amount of liquor amnii.

*omphalic* pertaining to the umbilicus.

*omphalitis* inflammation of the umbilicus.

*omphalocele* congenital umbilical hernia.

*oocyesis* an ectopic pregnancy in the ovary.

*oocyte* primitive ovum.

*oogenesis* development of female germ cells into mature ova.

*operculum* plug of mucus covering the external cervical os during pregnancy.

*ophthalmia* inflammation of the eye.

　*o. neonatorum* purulent conjunctivitis in the newborn.

　*o. prophylaxis* see Credé's prophylaxis.

*organogenesis* the segregation of tissues into various organs during embryonic development.

*os* (pl. ora) opening.

　*o. external* where cervical canal opens into the vagina.

　*o. internal* where cervical canal opens into the body of the uterus.

　*o. uteri* mouth of the uterus.

*ova* plural of ovum.

*ovary* female gonad in which the ova develop.

*oviduct* tube through which the ova are conveyed to the uterus. Synonyms: salpinx, fallopian tube.

*ovulation* rupture of the graafian follicle and discharge of the ovum.

*ovum* female reproductive element.

*oxytocic* agent that stimulates uterine contractions.

*oxytocin* oxytocic principle of the posterior lobe of the pituitary gland; may be prepared synthetically.

*palsy* synonym: paralysis.

　*Bell's p.* facial paralysis.

　*Erb-Duchenne p.* an upper arm paralysis.

　*Klumpke's p.* form of brachial palsy involving wrist and hand.

*Papanicolaou's stain* staining smears of exfoliated cells from the cervix for detection of malignant process.

*para* past pregnancies continued to period of viability; para refers to pregnancies, not to fetuses.

*parametritis* inflammation of the parametrium.

*parametrium* connective tissue around the uterus.

*parturient* pertaining to birth; giving birth.

*parturition* act of giving birth; process by which the baby is born.

*pelvimeter* instrument designed for estimating pelvic measurements.

*pelvimetry* measurements of pelvic dimensions.

*pelvis* structure formed by the innominate bones, sacrum and coccyx.

　*false p.* that portion above the linea terminalis (pelvic brim).

　*true p.* that portion of the pelvic cavity below the iliopectineal line.

*perinatal* period shortly before and after birth; generally considered from the twenty-ninth week of gestation until 1 to 4 weeks of the neonatal period have been completed.

　*p. mortality* the sum of deaths of fetuses with weight of 501 grams or more (20 weeks' gestation) and neonatal deaths.

*perineorrhaphy* suture of perineum for repair of lacerations.

*perineotomy* incision of the perineum.

*perineum* pelvic floor; the region between the fourchette and the anus.

*phenylalanine* an amino acid.

*phenylalanine hydroxylase* enzyme converting phenylalanine to tyrosine.

*phenylketonuria* metabolic hereditary disorder involving defective enzyme system resulting in faulty metabolism of phenylalanine and mental retardation.

*phenylpyruvic acid* metabolic derivative of phenylalanine.

*phimosis* tightness of the foreskin of the penis.

*phlebitis* inflammation of a vein.

*phlebothrombosis* clotting in a vein, not associated within inflammation of the vessel wall, if the clot detaches, it may result in pulmonary embolism.

*phlegmasia* fever or inflammation.

　*p. alba dolens* phlebitis of the femoral vein; if it occurs during the puerperium, it is then called "milk leg."

*phocomelia* improper development of the arms and legs.

*pinocytosis* ingestion of fluid material by phagocytic cells.

*Pitocin* proprietary name for an oxytocic fraction solution of the posterior pituitary gland.

*Pituitrin* proprietary name of a posterior pituitary injection.

*placenta* cakelike or flat mass; organ attached to the wall of the uterus through which the fetus derives its nourishment and oxygen.

　*p. abruptio* see abruptio placentae.

　*p. adherent* one that remains attached to the uterine wall longer than the usual time after birth of the infant.

　*p. battledore* one with the cord inserted along the margin instead of excentrally or centrally.

　*p. circumvallata* a placenta encircled with a white nodular ring.

　*p. previa* a placenta implanted in the lower uterine segment.

　*p. retained* the placenta separates but is retained within the uterus; muscular contractions fail to expel it spontaneously.

　*p. succenturiata* one with an accessory lobe attached to the main placenta by an artery and vein.

*platypelloid pelvis* flat pelvis, one contracted anteroposteriorly.

*polydactylia* extra digits on hands or feet.

*polygalactia* excessive secretion of milk.

*polyhydramnios* excess of amniotic fluid during pregnancy.

*polymastia* presence of more than two mammary glands.

*Porro's operation* removal of the uterus after a classical cesarean section.

*position* in obstetrics, the way the presenting part lies in relation to one of the four quadrants of the mother's pelvis.

*precipitate delivery* see under delivery.

*preeclampsia* state of severe toxemia preceding eclampsia.

*pregnancy* state of being pregnant.

    *pride of p.* characteristic stride the pregnant woman assumes to compensate for increased pressure of the enlarging uterus on the abdominal wall.

    *prolonged* one extending 2 or more weeks beyond calculated date of delivery.

    *psychogenic p.* see pseudocyesis.

*pregnanediol* excretion product of progesterone found in breast milk.

*premature infant* see under infant.

*premature labor* see under labor.

*prenatal* preceding the time of birth.

*prepuce* foreskin over the glans penis in the male.

*presentation* in obstetrics, that portion of the fetus presenting over the pelvic inlet—cephalic, breech, or scapula.

*primigravida* woman pregnant for the first time.

*primipara* a woman who had one pregnancy that was delivered after the period of viability.

*progesterone* steroid hormone obtained from the corpus luteum; also formed in the placenta.

*prolactin* hormone that stimulates lactation; lactogenic hormone, luteotropic hormone (LTH).

*promontory* projecting process.

    *p. of the sacrum* upper, projecting portion of the sacrum; that area between the last lumbar vertebra and the sacrum.

*proteinuria* protein in the urine.

*pruritus* severe itching.

    *p. vulvae* itching of the vulva; may be psychogenic or secondary to a dermatitis.

*pseudoanemia* a term used in obstetrics for a temporary anemia.

*pseudocyesis* condition in which a woman thinks she is pregnant but is not; false pregnancy.

*pseudomenstruation* slight vaginal spotting sometimes noted in the female infant due to sudden withdrawal of estrogen.

*ptyalism* excess in secretion of saliva.

*pudendum* external genitalia; the vulva.

*puerperal* pertaining to the puerperium.

*p. infection* wound infection of the birth canal.

*puerperium* period of 6 weeks after childbirth.

*pyrosis* burning sensation in the epigastric region associated with acid from the stomach. Synonym: heartburn.

*quickening* feeling of life experienced by the mother as the fetus makes its movements in utero.

*regurgitation* implies returning or spitting up of *small* amounts of a feeding.

*relaxin* ovarian hormone believed to contribute to the softening of the cervix and to have some influence on the water content of the uterus.

*restitution* spontaneous turning of the fetal head, to right or left, after it has extended through the vulva.

*retrolental fibroplasia* disease of premature infants, characterized by retinal detachment and fibrosis.

*Rh₀Gam* immune globulin; anti-D gamma globulin for Rh prophylaxis.

*Ritgen maneuver* performed by the obstetrician to ease delivery of the head over the perineum. Pressure is applied with the fingers one on each side of the anus while the other hand exerts downward pressure on the occiput.

*rugae of the vagina* transverse folds of stratified squamous epithelium along the walls of the vaginal canal.

*salpinx* the fallopian tube.

*Schultze mechanism* method of expression of the placenta; central portion of the placenta is forced into the vagina first.

*secundine* placenta and membranes expelled after birth of the infant. Synonym: afterbirth.

*semen* male urethral discharge that fertilizes the ovum.

*semination* introduction of semen into the vaginal canal.

*setting-sun sign* downward displacement of the eyes; said to be indicative of intracranial pressure.

*show* serosanguineous vaginal discharge usually tinged with blood resulting from changes occurring in the cervix before and during labor.

*Silverman-Andersen score* method for scoring the breathing performance of premature infants.

*Skene's glands* two small glands within the meatus of the female urethra; homologues of the prostate gland in the male.

*smegma* thickened, odoriferous secretions of sebaceous glands, found in the region of the labia minora and the clitoris.

*souffle* a soft sound; a murmur.

    *funic s.* sound produced by the blood as it courses through the umbilical arteries; synchronous with fetal heart sounds.

*placental s.* sound believed to be produced by blood flow in the placenta.

*uterine s.* sound produced by blood as it enters the dilated arteries of the gravid uterus; synchronous with maternal pulse.

*Spalding-Horner sign* overriding of the bones of the skull as seen in x-ray film; indicates fetal death.

*spectrophotometry* method used for analysis of amniotic fluid.

*spermatogenesis* development of male germ cells (gametes) into mature spermatozoa.

*spermatozoa* the male germ cell.

*spina* thornlike projection or process.

*s. bifida* defect in closure of the bony spinal canal.

*station* in obstetrics, the location of the presenting part of the fetus in relation to the ischial spines of the pelvis.

*stillborn* a fetus born dead.

*striae* (pl. of stria.)

*s. gravidarum* reddish, purple, irregular depressions that appear in the skin of the abdomen, thighs, and buttocks; caused by breaking of underlying connective tissue.

*subinvolution* in obstetrics, delay in normal involution of the uterus during the puerperium.

*succedaneum* see under caput.

*superfecundation* two ova liberated at one ovulation are fertilized by two separate acts of coitus.

*superfetation* impregnation of an ovum when there is a developing fetus in the uterus.

*surfactant* lipoprotein secreted by alveolar epithelium to decrease surface tension of the fluid and ease opening of the alveoli.

*symbiosis* mode of life; to live together; close union of two.

*symphysis pubis* thick mass of fibrocartilage formed at union of pubic bones.

*syncope* feeling of faintness.

*syncytium layer* outer layer of trophoblastic cells secretes estrogen and progesterone.

*syndactyly* webbing or fusion of the digits of the hand or foot.

*teratogen* agent causing a defect in developing embryo.

*teratology* study of monstrosities.

*testis* male gonad that produces the spermatozoa.

*tetany* syndrome manifested by muscle twitchings.

*thelitis* inflammation of the mammary papilla.

*thrombophlebitis* inflammatory process along the walls of the blood vessels.

*thrush* infection caused by *Candida albicans,* characterized by superficial white patches in the mouth; it may spread to other areas of the body.

*toxemia* toxic substances in the blood.

*t. of pregnancy* specific hypertensive disease of pregnancy or the early puerperium.

*tracheoesophageal fistula* congenital anomaly involving a fistula between the trachea and the esophagus.

*trophectoderm* outer layer of cells of the blastodermic vessicle; early trophoblasts.

*trophoblast* cells that form outer layer of the blastula.

*tympanites* distention of the abdomen with gas.

*tyrosine* amino acid produced in the metabolism of phenylalanine.

*umbilical cord* see funis.

*uteri inertia* see inertia, uteri.

*uterine atony* muscles of the myometrium fail to contract and retract normally.

*uterine milk* mucin and glycogen secreted by glands of the endormetrium as nourishment for the ovum.

*uterine souffle* see under souffle.

*uterus* hollow, muscular organ in which the fertilized ovum develops.

*vagina* tubular canal extending from the vulva to the cervix.

*varices* (pl. of varix) enlarged veins, arteries, or lymphatic vessels.

*vernix caseosa* greasy, white, sebaceous material distributed over areas of the newborn infant's body at birth.

*version* in obstetrics, manual turning of the fetus.

*Braxton Hicks's v.* combined external and internal maneuver to change position of the fetus.

*cephalic v.* turning the fetus to make the vertex the presenting part.

*podalic v.* turning the fetus to make the feet or buttocks the presenting part.

*vertex* anatomically, top or crown of the head.

*vestibule* space or cavity.

*v. of the vagina* area between anterior portion of labia minora and posterior fourchette.

*viable* in obstetrics, fetus capable of living outside of the uterus.

*von Fernwald's sign* softening and enlargement of the fundus at the site of implantation.

*vulva* external genitalia. Synonym: pudendum.

*Wharton's jelly* mucoid substance covering the umbilical vein and arteries.

*witch's milk* minute secretions from the papilla of the infant's breasts (resembling colostrum) due to transfer of maternal hormones.

*yolk sac* one of the embryonic membranes or outer cavity of the embryonic cell mass.

*zona pellucida* transparent, striated membrane surrounding an ovum.

*zygote* the fertilized ovum.

# Index

Labor—cont'd
  coaching, need for, during, 163, 164
  contractions during, 148, 149, 152, 153
    evaluating, 160, 161
    irregular, 186
    tetanic, 195
  crowning during, 152
  discomforts associated with, 148, 162
  drugs used during; *see* Analgesics; Anesthesia;
      specific drugs
  dry, 161
  duration of, 148, 149, 150, 153, 156
  dysfunctional, 183, 190, 191
  dystocia during, 185-191
  education in preparation for, 124-126; *see also*
      Cooperative childbirth
  effect of, on neonate, 166, 167, 241-243, 305
  elevated temperature during, 162
  enema during, 160
    contraindications for, during, 160
  engagement of presenting part during, 144, 145
  episiotomy during, 152, 200
  examination during, 160
  false, 59, 125, 148, 149
  fears associated with, 159, 160
  fetal adaptation to pelvis and birth canal during,
      151, 152
  fetal anoxia during, 162, 167
  fetal danger signals, 162, 163
  fetal distress during, 162
  fetal heart rate
    during, 160
    slowing of, during, 160, 167
  fetal hyperactivity during, 162, 163
  first stage of, 149, 150, 161, 162
    duration of, 150
    and nursing responsibilities, 159-164
    phases of, 161, 162
  fluids during, 161
  food during, 161
  fourth stage of, 156
    and nursing responsibilities, 166
  fundus, guarding, during, 166
  hemorrhage during, 154, 191, 193, 194
    and nursing responsibilities, 194
  high-risk
    part I, 183-196
    part II, 200-205
  hyperactivity of fetus during, 162, 163
  hyperventilation during, 132, 165, 166
  hypnosis during, 179, 180
  induction of, 200-202
    with hypertonic saline solution, 101, 170
  lacerations during, 191
    and degree of, 194
    and prevention by nurse, 165
  latent phase of, 149, 161
  leg cramps during, 164
  length of, 150, 162
  levator ani muscles, function of, during, 152,
      154
  maternal danger signals during, 162
  meconium, passage of, during, 162
  membranes, rupture of
    artificial; *see* Amniotomy
    during, 150

Labor—cont'd
  membranes, rupture of—cont'd
    premature and infection, 183, 187
      with breech, 187
    prolonged, 224
  multiple births, 192
  muscle cramps during, 164
  Nitrazine paper test during, 161
  nursing responsibilities during, 164-166
    in emergency situation, 165
  obstacles preventing normal progress, 189; *see
      also* Dystocias
  obstructed; *see* Dystocias
  onset of, 148
    teaching in preparation for, 124-126
  oxytocics during, 154, 156
    and precipitous delivery, 191
  pain, alleviation of, during, 175-180
  pain, attitude toward, during, 163, 176
  panting during, 132, 165
  perineum, bulging of, during, 152, 164
  phases and progress, 149
    and nursing responsibilities, 164, 165, 166
  position of patient
    during, 162
    for delivery, 165
  precipitate, and nursing responsibilities, 191
  premature, 183, 184
    definition of, 183
    drugs to halt, 184
    effect on neonate, 184
    incidence of, 184
    predisposing factors, 183
  preparation for onset of, 124, 125
  prolapse of cord during, 163, 189, 193
  prolonged, 184-185
    cause of hemorrhage, 193
    contributory factors, 185
    definition of, 185
    effect of, on fetus, 185
  protracted active phase, cause of dystocia, 190
    and nursing responsibilities, 191
  psychological support during, 132, 163, 164
  pulse during, 162
  rupture of membranes during, 150
    premature, 183, 187
  rupture of uterus during, 195, 196
  second stage of, 152
    with breech, 187
    duration of, 153
    and nursing responsibilities, 164
    signs of approaching, 152, 164
  stages of, 149-156
    most dangerous
      for fetus, 153
      for mother, 156
  stirrups, use of, during, 165
  teaching in preparation for onset of, 124-126
  temperature during, 162
  test of, 190
  third stage of, 154, 165, 166
    Brandt-Andrews maneuver during, 154
    duration of, 156
    hemorrhage during, 154
    nursing responsibilities during, 166
    oxytocics during, 155, 156
    phases of, 154

Prenatal clinics, 117-125
Prenatal examination, initial, 119
Prenatal period, teaching
  and counseling during, 121
  in preparation for onset of labor, 124, 125
Prepuce, 3
Presentations and positions, 140-143
  attitudes of, 144
  breech, 186
  brow, 186
  compound, 186
  duration of labor and, 149
  face, 186
  mentum; *see* Face
  sacrum; *see* Breech
  transverse, 186
  vertex, 141-143
Presenting part
  attitude of, 144
  dipping of, 145
  engagement of, 145
  fixation of, 145
  floating of, 145
  stations of, 145
Presumptive signs of pregnancy, 25
Pride of pregnancy, 59
Primigravida
  and complications, 190
  definition of, 26
Primipara, definition of, 26
Primordial follicles, 6
Probable signs of pregnancy, 25
Progesterone
  level and pregnancy tests, 22
  secretion of
    by ovaries, 7, 12, 13
    by placenta, 33
    by trophoblasts, 33
Prolactin, 12, 14, 64
  secretion of, inhibited during pregnancy, 63, 64
Prolapse of cord during labor, 163, 189, 193
Prolonged labor, 184, 185
Prolonged pregnancy, 35
Promazine hydrochloride; *see* Sparine
Proteins
  deficiency of, 84
  function and sources of, during pregnancy, 74
  inadequate retention of, 77
Proteinuria
  with preeclampsia, 94
  during puerperium, 217
Proteolytic enzymes, 30
Prothrombin level, 242
Pruritus during pregnancy, 86
Pseudoanemia during pregnancy, 60
Pseudocyesis, 66, 101
Pseudohermaphroditism, drugs as cause of, 48
Pseudomenstruation, 263
Psychogenic abortion, 101
Psychogenic pregnancy; *see* Pseudocyesis
Psychological adjustments to pregnancy, 64-66
Psychological aspects of puerperium, 211, 217
Psychological support during labor, 163, 164
Ptyalism, 86
Pudendal nerve block, 179
Pudendum, 3
Puerperal fever; *see* Puerperal infection

Puerperal hematomas, 226
Puerperal infection
  definition of, 223
  modes of, 223, 224
  predisposing factors, 224
  predominating organism as cause of, 224
Puerperal psychosis following eclampsia, 97
Puerperium
  abdominal wall during, 215
  after-pains during, 214, 215
  ambulation during, 216
  bathing during, 216
  bladder function during, 217
  bleeding during; *see* Lochia
  blood pressure during, 212
  blood vessels, injury to, during, 226
  bowel function during, 217
  breasts
    care of, during, 219
    engorgement of, during, 218
  cardiac patient during, 226, 227
  cervicitis during, 224
  cervix, physiology of, during, 213
  complications during; *see* Puerperal infections; specific complication
  cystitis during, 217
  diaphoresis during, 217
  diastasis of recti muscles during, 215
  discharge, preparation for, during, 234, 235
  diuresis during, 217
  drugs to contract uterus during, 155
  endometritis during, 224
  endometrium during, 123
  engorgement of breasts during, 218
  examination during, 234
  exercises during, 216
  fever during, 223
  Fowler's position during, 224
  fundus, height of, during, 213
  hematomas during, 226
  hemorrhage, delayed, during, 107, 108, 225, 226
  hemorrhoids during, 217
  high-risk, 223-227
  Homan's sign during, 225
  integrated mother-baby care during, 229-232
  involution of uterus during, 212
  lactose in urine during, 217
  leukocytosis during, 60, 224
  lochia during, 214
    and infections, 224
  lochiometra, 224
  mastitis during, 226
  menses, return of, during 235
  oliguria during, 108
  oxytocics for involution of uterus during, 155, 212
  parametritis during, 224
  pelvic cellulitis during, 224
  perineal care during, 214
  perineal discomfort during, 214
  perineum during, 214
  phlebothrombosis during, 225
  physiological, clinical, and nursing aspects of, 212-218
  postpartum blues during, 212
  preparation for discharge, 234-236
  proteinuria during, 217

Puerperium—cont'd
  psychological aspects of, 229-232
  pulse during, 212
  pyelitis during, 121
  pyelonephritis during, 217
  self-care at home during, 234, 235
  sitz bath during, 218
  striae during, 216
  subinvolution of uterus during, 226
  thrombophlebitis during, 225
  toxemia during, 97
  tub baths during, 216
  tympanites during, 217
  uterus during, 212
  vagina during, 213
  vital signs during, 212
  voiding during, 217
  weight loss during, 217
  white cell count during, 224
Pulse
  during labor, 162
  during puerperium, 212
Pyelitis during puerperium, 121
Pyelonephritis
  cause of, during pregnancy, 62, 108
  during puerperium, 217
Pyloric stenosis in neonate, 283
Pylorospasms in neonate, 283
Pyrosis; *see* Heartburn

**Q**
Quickening
  experience of, 37, 59, 124
  means of determining period of gestation, 124
  sign of pregnancy, 25

**R**
Recovery nursery; *see* Nursery
  responsibilities of nurse in, 241, 242
Rectal examination
  during labor, 160
  for palpation of presenting part, 145
Rectocele, 213
Recumbent position for delivery, 165
Reflex
  behavior development in neonate; *see* Neonate
  milk ejection, 274, 275
  stimuli of myometrium, 151
Regional anesthesia, 179
Rejections, maternal, toward neonate, 255
Relaxin hormone, 61, 62, 84
Renal agenesis, 32, 295
Renal glycosuria, 62, 121
Reproductive cycle, endocrine control of, 12
Respirations
  establishment of, in neonate, 166, 167
  intrauterine, 166, 167
  during labor, 162
  stabilization of, in neonate, 242
Respiratory
  disorders in neonate, 281, 282
  distress in neonate, signs and symptoms of, 242
  system, physiology of, during pregnancy, 62
Rest during pregnancy, 85, 121
Resuscitation of neonate, 169, 184

Retraction ring, of uterus
  Bandl's, 149, 195
  Braun's, 149
Retrolental fibroplasia, 308
Retroplacental bleeding, 106, 154
Rh factor, 49, 50
Rh isoimmunization, 49
Rh₀Gam, 52
Rhythm cycle, 22
Rickets, protecting fetus against, 72
Ritgen maneuver during labor, 152
Rubella,
  congenital, 45
  subclinical, 46
  transplacental transmission of, 45
Rugae, vaginal, 5
Rupture of uterus, 195, 196

**S**
Sacrum, 138
  presentation of; *see* Breech
  promontory of, 130
Saddle block anesthesia, 178
Salpinges; *see* Fallopian tube(s)
Scanzoni's maneuver, 186
Schultze method of placenta expulsion, 154
Scopolamine hydrobromide, 176
Sedation
  during labor and nursing responsibilities, 161, 176, 177
  over-, and dangers of, 190
Semmelweis, I. P., 223, 318
Sensory status of neonate, 258
Setting-sun sign, 249
Sex determination, 36
  from amniotic fluid, 35
Shirodkar technique, 102
Shoes, type to wear during pregnancy, 123
Show, bloody
  as premonitory sign of labor, 164, 194
  and tears, 194
Sign(s)
  Cullin, 103
  halo, 99
  Homan, 225
  of prgenancy, 25
  setting-sun, 249
  Spalding-Horner, 170
Silver nitrate, 249
Silverman-Andersen score, 307
Sim's position, 84, 85, 162, 163
Sitz bath
  to relieve pain from hemorrhoids, 85
  to relieve perineal discomfort, 214
Skene's ducts, 3
Skin changes
  of neonate, 246, 247
  during pregnancy, 61
Skull, fetal, 140
Sleep
  needs during pregnancy, 85, 121
  pattern of neonate, 255
Smallpox, transplacental transfer of, 46
Smegma on neonate, 249
Smellie-Veit (or Mauriceau) maneuver, 188